NEAL'S YARD REMEDIES

Natural Health & Body Care

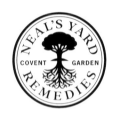

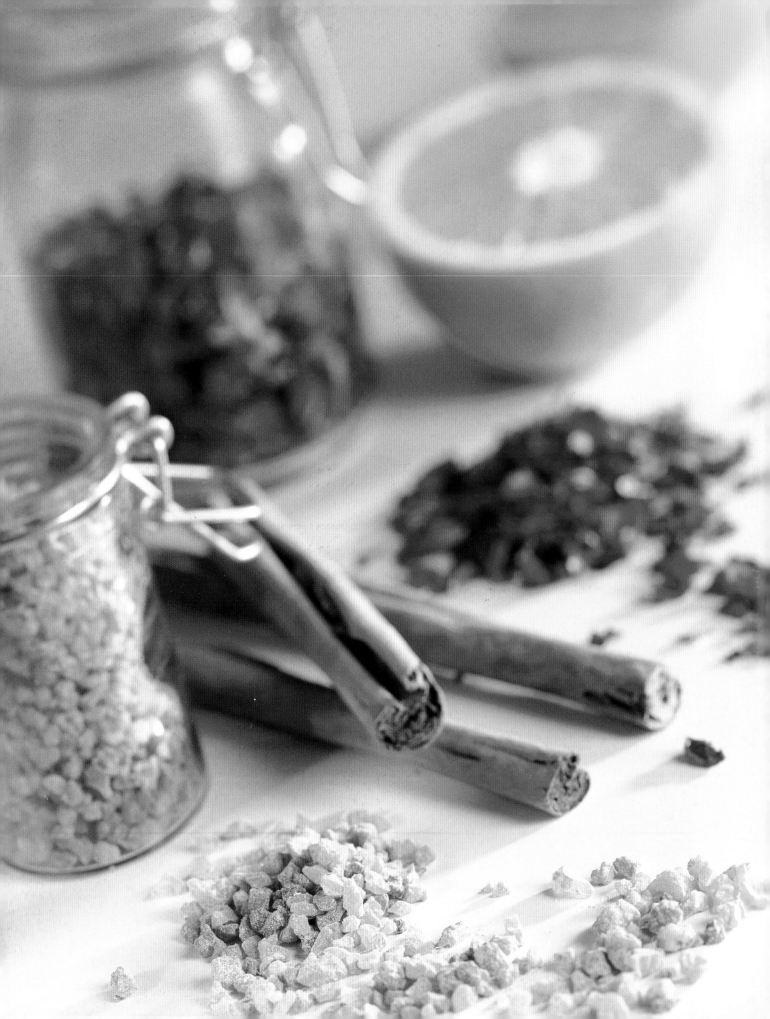

NEAL'S YARD REMEDIES

Natural Health & Body Care

A comprehensive and informative guide to natural remedies,
recipes and routines for the whole body

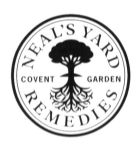

AURUM

First published in the UK in 2000 by

Aurum Press Ltd

25 Bedford Avenue

London WC1B 3AT

ISBN: 1-85410-705-4

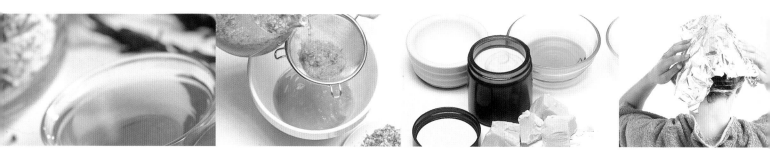

A HALDANE MASON BOOK

Conceived, designed and produced by Haldane Mason Ltd, London

Editorial Director: Sydney Francis

Art Director: Ron Samuel

Editor: Ben Keith

Design: Zoë Mellors

Picture Research: Ben Keith

Colour reproduction by CK Litho Ltd, UK

Printed in the United Arab Emirates by Emirates Printing Press

Acknowledgements

We would like to thank all the staff, past and present, at Neal's Yard Remedies for their help, including Louise Green, Stephen Frank, Wendy Lomas and all in the New Product Development team. In particular we would like to thank Alice Rhodes, Sandra Hill and Amendeep Sidhu for their contributions. Many thanks also to our patient editorial team at Haldane Mason, especially Ben Keith and Sydney Francis.

Picture acknowledgements

Cover photography by Andrew Sydenham and Amanda Heywood.
All photography by Andrew Sydenham with the exception of the following:
A–Z Botanical 64 (top right), 92 (top left), 169, 182, 204; **Chanel** 52 (top left, bottom left), 64 (bottom), 66 (left), 92 (top left), 97 (bottom), 116, 165; **Stephen Dew** 84; **Golgemma/Patrick Collin** 196; **Guerlain** 195; **Haldane Mason** 15 (all), **/Sue Ford** 8, 17 (all) 18 (both), 57 (both), 79, 96 (bottom), 103 (bottom), 109 (centre top), 113 (b. right), 114 (bottom), 138, 139 (left, right), 144 (right), 148 (top); **Amanda Heywood** 6 (centre left, centre right), 7 (centre right), 11 (centre right), 36, 37, 39 (all), 41 (all), 43 (all), 45 (all), 51 (top right, bottom), 55 (bottom), 63 (both), 64 (top left), 65 (all), 66 (centre, right), 67 (both), 68, 72 (left, right), 73 (left, centre right, right), 75 (top centre, bottom right), 81 (top left, top right, bottom right), 87 (all), 88, 89 (all), 90, 91 (all), 92 (centre top, centre top left), 93 (all), 97 (centre), 98, 101 (both), 103 (all), 105 (all), 106 (all), 107 (all), 108 (bottom right), 109 (top, centre bottom, bottom), 111 (both), 112 (right, bottom), 113 (top), 114 (top left, top right), 115 (top), 116, 117 (all), 119 (all), 120, 121 (right), 122 (right), 123, 124 (both), 125 (top), 126 (both), 127 (all), 131 (both), 132 (both), 133 (all), 137 (all), 140, 141 (all), 142 (all), 143 (top, centre), 144 (all), 145 (all), 146 (all), 147 (all), 148 (bottom), 149 (centre, bottom), 164, 166, 167, 170, 171, 172, 173, 174, 175, 176, 177, 179, 180, 181, 183, 184, 185, 186, 188, 189, 190, 191, 192, 193, 194, 197, 198, 199, 200, 201, 202, 205, 212, 213, 214, 215, 216 (both), 217, 218, 219, 221 (both), 222 (top), 223, 224; **Rowan McOnegal/McOnegal Botanical** 187; **Neal's Yard Remedies** 55 (top), 157 (top left, bottom right); **Christine Wilson** 178.

Every effort has been made to identify the correct photographers or copyright holders. We apologize in advance for any errors or omissions.

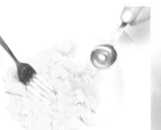 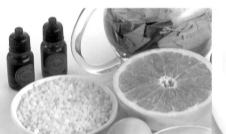 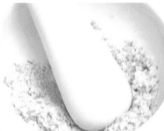 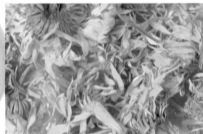

IMPORTANT

Contents

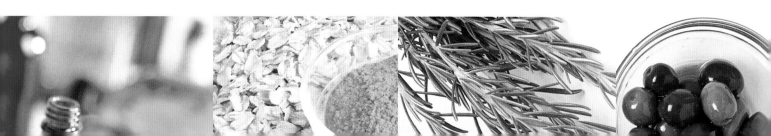

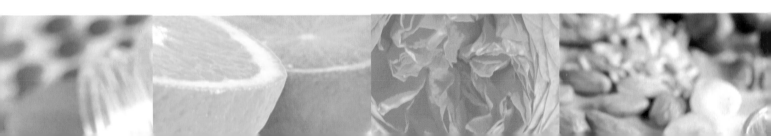

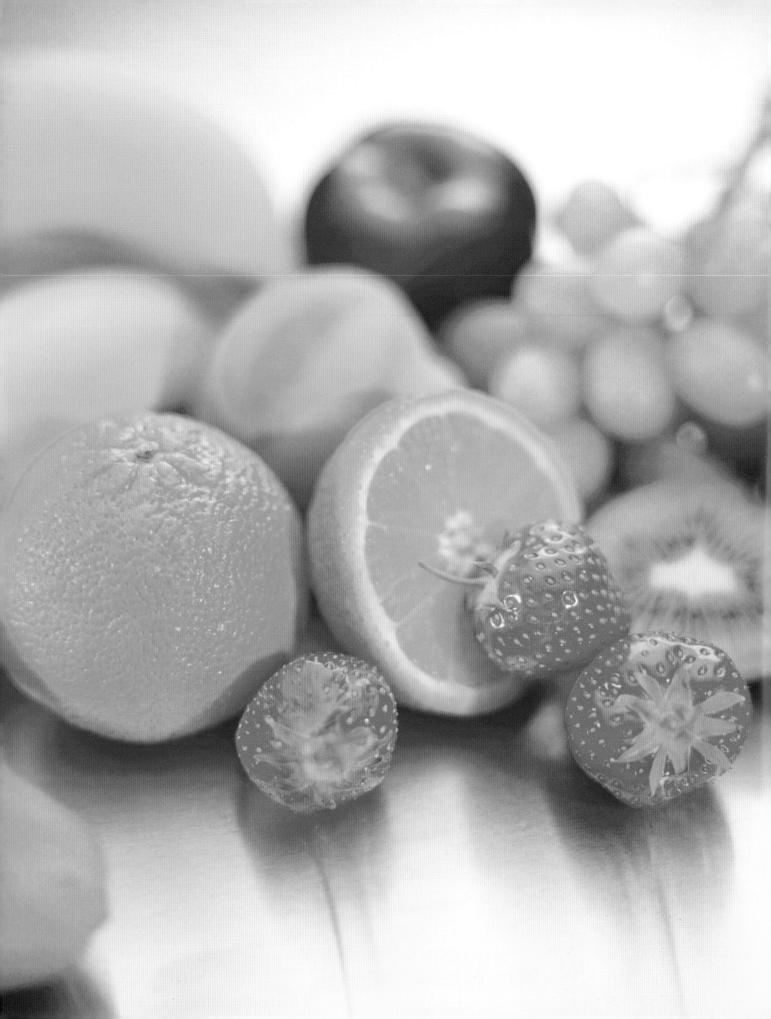

day-to-day body care the natural way

How we look and feel

depends on our health,

and this, in turn, is affected

by our lifestyle. Natural ways

to good health need to be

built into our daily routines,

and a balance must be struck

between psychological and

physical well-being.

body care the natural way

Natural health and body care is about developing energy and vitality as well as looking after your physical body. It also means caring for your body and feeling comfortable with it, whatever shape it is. Few people have the super-slim, boyish look currently promoted by the fashion industry and the media, but we can all take positive steps to improve our level of health and appearance. A healthy, smiling face has an inherent beauty, whether or not the individual features that make up that face conform to our preconceived ideas of attractiveness.

To enjoy good health and feel energetic we need to look after the spiritual, mental and emotional aspects of our lives, as well as our physical health. There is an intrinsic connection between these different aspects of ourselves, and this manifests itself in a flow of energy which, if positive, keeps us whole and healthy. After all, feeling good on the inside is vital to looking good on the outside.

In the external world, all the processes of Mother Nature are interconnected. In order for a meadow to produce sweet, healthy grass, for example, the soil must be uncontaminated and the meadow must be managed with an understanding of the natural cycles involved in creating good pasture. You cannot separate one part from the whole and expect it to remain healthy in isolation. In a similar way you cannot expect to have healthy, clear skin without taking your general level of health into account.

The underlying causes of skin problems can be difficult to unravel because they are generally a complex combination of diet, stress, hereditary factors, individual susceptibility and environment, not to mention general health. Coping with a skin problem without the use of strong, orthodox medication to suppress it is a real challenge for those people who would like to make the decision to switch to a more natural approach to leading a healthy lifestyle. A psychological approach to dealing with such physiological skin problems, however, could possibly include meditation, visualization, counselling or any of the other methods that are used to combat stress.

The link between the mind, the emotions and the skin is a complex one. If we have a skin problem it can be difficult not to feel self-conscious about it, and not to let it dent our self-confidence. On the other hand, many of us find that our skin condition is affected by the amount of stress we are experiencing, creating a vicious cycle. (For advice on psychological approaches and other complementary therapies that may help you to deal with stress and other such problems, please refer to the list of organizations, associations and societies on pages 243–8)

Daily stresses and life events tend to throw us into a state of imbalance. If we become stuck for too long in this imbalance our emotions may become toxic – which will almost inevitably affect our physical bodies, too, causing illness. Our ability to adapt and deal both practically and creatively with life's ups and downs will determine our capacity to expel any toxicity and re-establish good health. We all have an innate desire – the life force or vital force – to create the conditions for balance within ourselves and in our environment, and it is the aim of all of the various systems of natural healing to help us to achieve this.

Our potential for good health is based on the unique mixture of our parents' genes, the physical and emotional environment in which we were nurtured, and our individual ability to cope with these factors. We all need to strike a balance between accepting the basics of who we are – as man or woman, black or white, gay or straight, able-bodied or handicapped, and so on – and recognizing that there are also huge areas of choice about what we can do with our lives. One of the most debilitating states of mind, and frequently the cause of many people's depression and ultimately illness, is to feel that there are no options to choose from. It is vital to remember that there are always options, even if these are limited to a question of our attitude towards problems.

establishing good health

So, having established that all areas of our lives are interconnected, and that in order to be healthy physically we also need to be healthy spiritually, mentally and emotionally, how can we establish the conditions for good health in our life?

spiritual health

Most of us will recognize the experience of feeling in contact with something greater than ourselves at some time in our lives, and the aim of cultivating our spiritual life is to have greater access to this source of energy, to get it flowing through every aspect of our lives. Being in contact with your spiritual self is the same thing as being in contact with your sense of purpose, or your source of energy and inspiration.

There are many techniques that have evolved over the centuries to help us develop our spiritual selves. All of these require freeing ourselves to some degree from our habitual way of responding to things, and our unconscious behaviour patterns. They also enable us to reach beyond the rational part of our brain to the more abstract, intuitive mind, and then even beyond that. This is the aim of many self-development and meditation groups. If developing this side of your life appeals to you, but you are not sure how to start, you could contact one of the organizations on pages 243–8 which may give you a pointer in the right direction. If we are able to give and receive love, and feel positive about the way we are learning from our life, then nurturing our body will become a natural part of our daily life.

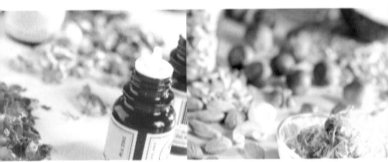
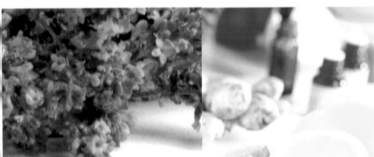

mental and emotional health

To be healthy mentally and emotionally we need to be able to accept the whole of our experiences. This is not so simple as it may sound. Most of us want to accept the nice things that happen to us, but not take responsibility for the unpleasant things. Similarly in our relationships, we want the good things that our partner has to offer, but may not want to recognize that there are also things about them that we do not like. Indeed, we may even develop an image of someone that is not based on who they really are, but on how we want to see them. Even closer to home, we have to be realistic about our own positive and negative attributes.

All our experiences and all our relationships enrich our lives and provide opportunities for us to get to know and understand ourselves better. It is by cultivating this attitude that we can become happier with who we are and also who we share our life with.

If being happy with who you are and with your relationships sounds to you like only a remote possibility, then it is probably because you have slipped into habitual thought processes and actions that no longer support your best interests. At times we all adopt behaviour strategies that may have been appropriate for a while in the past, but are inappropriate now. If, for example, you feel let down badly by your first relationship, leaving you in a distressed state, then feelings of suspicion and defensiveness are likely to feature in future

relationships. It is only by accepting and transforming these experiences into wisdom and not becoming embittered or ground down by them that we can be free to learn and move on.

Certain kinds of habitual behaviour, when they become deeply engraved into the lifestyle, will lead to addiction. There is often an emotional correlation to even the most seemingly physical addictions. Smoking, for example, helps us to feel less vulnerable, as well as providing a buzz from the nicotine. This is why addictions are so hard to give up – we have to deal with not only the physical withdrawal symptoms, but also the emotional need that the habit satisfied. Part of the key to giving up an addiction may be to become aware of the emotional need behind the prop. If we can satisfy that need in a more constructive way, then the possibility of giving up a damaging addiction becomes more real.

There are many ways of learning to become more aware of these unconscious patterns that we all develop and that hold us back. It is similar to the process outlined above, in that the first step is to become aware of how much of our behaviour is determined by habit and then begin to change some of the habits. It is much easier to change a habit for something more positive than it is to just stop it, because we will need to put the energy into something. So, the first step is to recognize the habit or underlying need behind the habit, and the next step

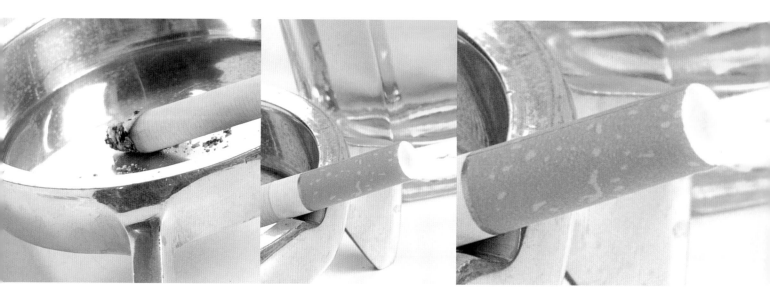

is to change the habit for a more positive, less damaging one. For example, it is only by changing our eating pattern to eat more healthy and fresh foods, and not by crash dieting, that we can make a lasting impact on our weight and well-being.

Counselling or psychotherapy can be of immense benefit if we are prepared to acknowledge that we need a helping hand to implement some changes in our emotional life. See the listings on pages 243–8 for some suggested organizations.

physical health

Staying healthy physically is an ongoing process. It involves living more or less in tune with the laws of nature. Life changes all the time and any organism must be able to adapt successfully to those changes – whether in circumstances or surroundings – in order to survive.

Living in tune with the laws of nature implies an attitude, but it also means that there are some basic requirements to be satisfied. Those are: living in a relatively non-toxic environment, eating nutritious food, drinking clean water and keeping the body exercised. It is the overall pattern that is most important here; we all have days when we eat badly or skip meals, or when we feel too lazy to exercise, but if our day-to-day habits are basically good, then our system should be able to cope with the odd lapse from a healthy lifestyle now and again.

If we are starting from a point of reasonably good health and vitality then building in good habits may be all that we need to keep us fit and healthy. Not everyone inherits good health, however, and most of us at some stage of our life will experience a period of illness. The experience of an illness may be the catalyst to get us to improve our diet or get more rest, or whatever it is that we feel needs adjusting to improve our well-being. If the symptoms of an illness persist or we simply do not feel quite right for more than a week or two, it may be time to consult a practitioner. A good practitioner should be able to help us re-establish good health and vitality, although we will have to give the process sufficient time to have an impact on our systems, especially if we have been unwell for a long period. Natural medicine will work with your own innate healing responses and will not brutally attempt to remove or suppress symptoms.

Choosing a particular therapy is not always easy. It is probably best to choose the one that you feel most drawn to, whether that be acupuncture, herbalism or whatever, and to seek advice from the professional bodies on your chosen therapy to ascertain if it is appropriate. The next step is to find a practitioner! Advice on therapies and practitioners is best sought from such organizations, associations or societies as those listed on pages 243–8 – qualified practitioners and therapists are most likely to be affiliated to such bodies.

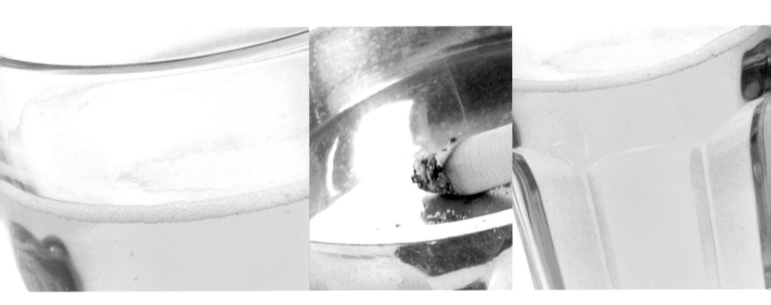

the environment

We all have mechanisms within us that have evolved to help us adapt to and cope with changing factors in our environment. One of the most important processes that we have for maintaining health is our ability continually to eliminate any toxins that may be taken into the system as a result of daily living. So long as we can keep on top of eliminating toxins, whether they are from our food, air, water, or emotions, then we have a good chance of keeping healthy. If the toxic load is too great, or if our channels of elimination become blocked, then disease will be the result.

The main organs of elimination are the bowels, kidneys and skin. The more toxic the external and internal environment, then the harder these organs have to work to get rid of the toxins.

It is easy to feel overwhelmed by the number of toxins to which we are exposed, but there are several steps that may be taken to minimize the impact that they may have. Identifying the more immediate hazards and choosing to do something about them can be a very empowering process. Some hazards that we do have the ability to avoid or change are habits like smoking, drinking alcohol, eating adulterated foods, taking drugs, wearing synthetic fibres and using chemical-laden toiletries and cosmetics. Other factors, such as environmental pollution and radiation, may seem beyond our control, but even here there are measures that each of us can take in order to cut down on exposure and minimize risks.

How to improve your environment

- Make sure any rooms you live or work in for lengthy periods of time are well ventilated.
- If you have air-conditioning units make sure that they are serviced regularly.
- If your living rooms have double-glazing and central heating the air can be very dry, so install a humidifier or buy plenty of plants.
- A build-up of positive ions can lead to feelings of lethargy and lowered vitality. Install an ionizer in any room containing a lot of electrical equipment such as televisions and computers.
- Use anti-glare screens on computers to reduce the positive ion effect.
- Make the most of natural daylight. Our nervous systems need full-spectrum light to maintain health, so if you are in artificial light for prolonged periods install full-spectrum lighting.

- Filter heavy metals and nitrates out of tap water for drinking and cooking.
- Green houseplants help to decrease carbon dioxide and benzene fumes.
- Choose natural furnishings such as wood, cotton and wool rather than synthetics.
- Use non-toxic paint when decorating and natural paper wall coverings rather than synthetic ones.
- Use natural flooring materials, such as ceramic tiles, cork or wood and natural fibres, such as wool, coir or cotton, rather than synthetic fibre carpets.
- Avoid using aerosols – as well as damaging the atmosphere they give off a fine mist of chemicals that are easily absorbed by the lungs and skin.
- Ask your dentist for porcelain or plastic fillings rather than amalgam ones, which contain toxic mercury.

the clothes we wear

We should not underestimate the potential impact that clothing may have on the general health of our bodies. The main function of clothes is to provide warmth and protection. However, little consideration is often given to the fabric that is used to make our clothes and what effect this may have on our health.

Adverse skin reactions may occur as a result of a detergent that is used to wash clothes, but we should also ask questions about the treatments used on the raw materials that go into making the fabrics that we wear. For example, what are the pesticides used in the cultivation of cotton and flax? What are the treatments used in the processing of wool and cashmere? And how does silk really get produced? Did you know that 18 per cent of the world's chemicals are used in the cotton industry? Lanolin, which is obtained from sheep's wool, will hardly ever cause allergic reactions, but the detergent used to clean the wool has been shown to cause problems. This is not to mention the fact that until recently sheep dips in the UK contained the notorious organo-phosphate compounds.

Make a positive decision concerning fabric, wherever possible, and ask questions – this way you will be acting in the interests of your body and the environment. Synthetic fabrics are frequently used to make garments and shoes, but some man-made materials do not allow the skin to breathe properly – a vital requirement for the clothes we wear every day. Particular care needs to be taken with underwear, socks and shoes; conditions such as thrush and athlete's foot can easily be avoided by ensuring that these are made from pure cotton – preferably unbleached and organically grown. Also, as we spend a considerable part of our lives asleep, it is worth investing in bedcovers and night garments that are non-synthetic and non-toxic, and are comfortable against the skin. For further information please refer to The Organic Cotton Site at *www.sustainablecotton.org*

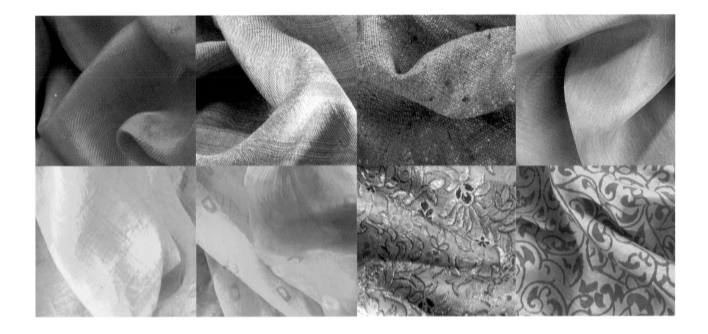

food

The phrase 'you are what you eat' has been understood by healers since ancient times, but in recent decades we seem to have lost sight of it. In Ancient Greece, Hippocrates (460–377 BC) outlined some illuminating truths about food, including: 'Let food be your medicine and let medicine be your food.' This illustrates very clearly how important our diet and eating habits are to our overall health.

If we eat nothing but refined, processed and polluted foods, we cannot expect to be healthy. In addition, since one of the primary functions of the skin is as an organ of elimination, if we eat foods laden with chemicals which the body then has to clear out, it is not surprising if unhealthy-looking skin is the result.

So what kind of food should we eat? Basically, the closer it is to its original state the more food retains its nutritional value. Food needs to be as fresh and as unprocessed and unrefined as possible. Ideally, we should eat as much of the whole product as possible, as with brown rice or wholemeal flour.

Refined foods are often low in vitamins, and to compensate for this, some foods actually have vitamins added. This seems rather a waste of resources. However, the fact that intensive agricultural methods have caused a decline in the natural vitamins and minerals in our food may mean that some of us will need to take food supplements. There is no substitute for good, fresh food, but if you feel that some supplement is necessary, choose an additive-free, well-balanced supplement or consult a nutritional advisor.

In the post-war period, factory farming in the UK was developed to help increase the self-sufficiency of the nation and to provide cheaper food. There have been some alarming incidents in recent years, however, which indicate that we need to reassess our attitude to producing food. For example, the battery farming of chickens has led to outbreaks of salmonella bacteria in eggs and poultry, feeding cows on an unnatural diet of meat products is implicated in the development of BSE, a disease for which our poor understanding of nature is responsible, and the overuse of nitrates in agriculture has led to the pollution of water supplies.

We are now having to accept irradiated food as an alternative to fresh food. Several supermarkets offer irradiated soft fruit because of its increased shelf life, and they do not have to indicate its status. In 1996, the first genetically modified soya beans arrived in Europe from the USA, and 60 per cent of the food we eat contains soya or its derivatives. This is despite the fact that the potential health implications such as increased food allergies have not been researched. Nevertheless, there are some steps we can take towards improving the quality of the food we eat and these are summarized on the opposite page.

If you are aware that you have not had a very good diet for some years, or that your diet is contributing to a particular disease, you could consider consulting a dietary therapist or a naturopath for specific advice. The naturopathic approach to health is that we need to be able to clear out impurities or toxins in our system, rather than allowing them to build up and contribute to disease. If we are reasonably healthy we should be able to eliminate a small amount of additives and toxins naturally through our bowels, bladder and skin. However, if the level of toxins in our diet is too high, or if our eliminative processes are blocked or under-functioning, symptoms of disease will result. A detoxifying or cleansing diet can be an effective way to clear out the system, and a good start to making improvements in your diet. The detoxifying diet shown on page 18 is effective and fairly gentle.

Alternatively, consult a naturopath or dietary therapist who will guide you through a cleansing regime to suit your particular needs – see pages 243–8 for naturopathic and dietary organizations. It is traditionally considered to be particularly beneficial to follow a cleansing diet in the spring and/or autumn.

If you have any particular health problem you should consult your health practitioner before going on a special diet.

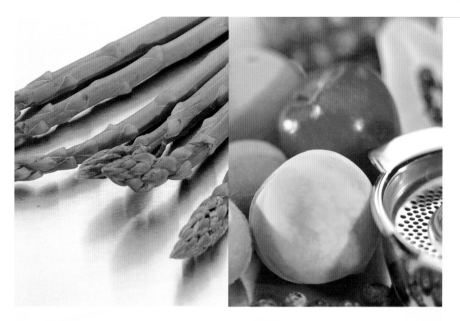

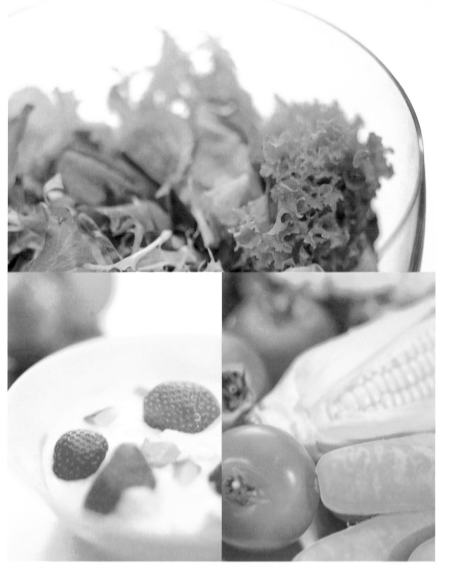

improving the quality of our diet

- Where possible, store food in glass or china containers, not in plastic or cling film (plastic wrap), which may leach toxic chemicals into your food.
- Avoid using aluminium foil wrappings on acidic food such as fruit or fruit cakes.
- Avoid using aluminium cooking utensils; choose instead glass, stainless steel or high-quality enamel (not chipped).
- Steam or stir-fry vegetables to retain the maximum amount of nutrients.
- Do not use microwaves for any food containing dairy products as the molecular structure of the proteins is altered and the effects of this are unknown. Also avoid heating food covered in plastic wraps which may allow the migration of toxic chemicals into your food.
- Avoid consuming large amounts of salt, refined sugar and animal fats.
- Avoid all food additives – i.e., foods containing E numbers – especially artificial colourings.
- Increase your intake of fresh vegetables, raw food and fruit.
- When possible, buy food that has been organically produced.

a detoxifying diet

Day 1

Fruit for breakfast, lunch and in the evening. Choose one type of fruit for each meal from the following: apples, pears or grapes. Eat as much fruit as you like at one sitting.

Day 2

Fruit for breakfast. Choose one type of fruit each day from: apples, pears, grapes, kiwi fruit, tomatoes and grapefruit. Eat raw vegetables for lunch. Make a mixture of at least five salad vegetables: mix roots (grated carrot and sliced beetroot and so on), sprouts and leafy vegetables. In the evening, eat cooked vegetables. Make a soup by boiling a mixture of at least five vegetables, preferably including onions. Do not add any salt or seasoning.

Days 3 – 6

See Day 2.

Day 7

Breakfast: as Day 2. Lunch: as Day 2, but in addition eat two pieces of dry crispbread or two rice cakes. Evening: as Day 2.

Days 8 – 9

See Day 7.

Day 10

Breakfast: as Day 2. Lunch: as Day 7. Evening: as Day 2, but in addition eat a baked potato with a small knob of butter.

notes

- Drink plenty of mineral water every day, and eat as much organically produced fruit and vegetables as possible.

- It is not unusual to get symptoms such as headaches, tiredness and skin eruptions during a cleansing diet. This is an indication that toxins are being released from the tissues and into the bloodstream before they are eliminated. If you drink enough water these symptoms usually disappear in a day or two.

- Important things to avoid completely throughout the diet are tea, coffee, cigarettes, salt, sugar, pepper, drugs, alcohol, antiperspirants and late nights.

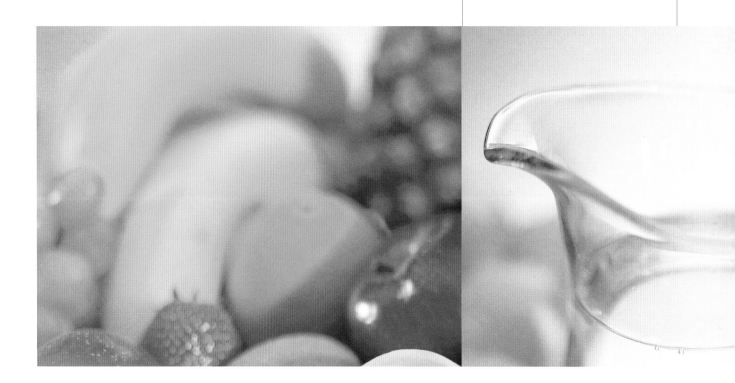

food supplements

A deficiency of vitamins or minerals can reduce our natural vitality and, over time, undermine our health. It used to be true that not everyone needed to take vitamin and mineral supplements, as a balanced diet of food grown in good soil should supply us with all the vitamins and minerals we need. Intensive agricultural practices, however, together with increasing levels of environmental pollutants, have reduced the quality of the foods we eat. Even a balanced diet based on organically grown food can leave our bodies deficient because so many minerals have been extracted from the soil. Stress and the consumption of stimulants such as alcohol, caffeine and smoking further leach minerals and vitamins from our bodies. And, if you live in a polluted city, are pre-menstrual, menopausal, pregnant or on the pill, exercise a lot, are fighting an infection or are over-stressed, your vitamin and mineral needs increase.

It is likely that most of us need a good multi-vitamin/mineral supplement on a daily basis; more specific supplements may also be needed as therapy when necessary. Not all supplements are the same, and it is advisable to buy them from a reputable company, such as a specialist health food store where the staff can help you choose those appropriate to your needs.

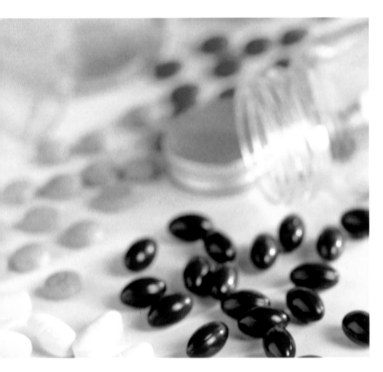

The ratios of the different vitamins and minerals can be important and some cheaper brands contain synthetic fillers and preservatives. Look for brands with descriptions such as 'contains no yeast, wheat, soy and dairy products and formulated without the use of preservatives, artificial flavours or colours'.

A multi-vitamin should contain at least the Recommended Daily Allowance (RDA) of the following vitamins: vitamin A, vitamin B1, vitamin B2, vitamin B3, vitamin B5, vitamin B6, vitamin B12, biotin, choline, vitamin C, vitamin D, folic acid and vitamin E.

A multi-mineral should contain at least the RDA of the following minerals: calcium, chromium, iron, magnesium, manganese, selenium and zinc.

free radicals and antioxidants

Free radicals are unstable molecules that are generated in the body. They contain extra oxygen and destroy unwanted invaders through oxidation. This is a beneficial and vital part of our immunity and we need a certain number of free radicals in our system for a normal, healthy metabolism. A number of factors can alter this healthy balance. Excess free radicals may be produced by stress, pollution and radiation (from TVs, microwaves, computers, mobile phones, sunlight and cosmic rays), or eaten with such things as overheated fats or oils found in fried foods. In excess, free radicals are thought to play a part in the development of many illnesses, as they attack normal body cells in an attempt to stabilize themselves. In particular, immune deficiency illnesses such as MS, ME and allergies, as well as some forms of cancer, are thought to be more prevalent today as a result of excess free radicals. This kind of cellular damage also accelerates the ageing process, causing such things as wrinkles and age spots.

Healthy cells with a good supply of oxygen are easily capable of warding off free radicals. Keep your cells healthy through exercise and eating foods that maximize oxygen in the body. Certain supplements, known as antioxidants or 'free radical scavengers', also prevent free radicals from stabilizing themselves. These are vitamins A, C and E, and the minerals selenium and zinc. Two substances with a renowned antioxidant action that may be easily incorporated into the diet on a daily basis are garlic and green tea.

vitamin and mineral chart

The following chart suggests good dietary sources of key vitamins and minerals. Vitamins tend to be specific to certain foods: a food may be an excellent source of one or more vitamins yet not contain other vitamins. This indicates the need for a varied and natural food diet. Processed foods are a very poor source of vitamins, hence the trend to add vitamins afterwards in synthetic form. Vitamins and minerals are essential to our health and vitality and we must ensure that we achieve the recommended daily allowance (RDA) either through the food we eat or the supplements we take.

Vitamin/ mineral	Average daily requirement	Deficiency symptoms	Dietary sources	Toxicity	Inhibiting factors
A	child: 800–1,000mcg adult: 800–2,000mcg	Mouth ulcers, poor night vision, acne, frequent colds or infections, dry flaky skin, dandruff, thrush or cystitis, diarrhoea.	Liver, carrots, watercress, cabbage, squash, sweet potatoes, melon, pumpkin, mangoes, tomatoes, broccoli, apricots, tangerines, asparagus.	Do not exceed: child: 4,000mcg adult: 8,000mcg	Heat, light, smoking, alcohol, coffee.
B1	child: 3.1–3.3mg adult: 3.5–9.2mg	Tender muscles, eye pains, irritability, poor concentration, 'restless legs', poor memory, stomach pains, constipation, tingling hands, rapid heartbeat.	Watercress, courgettes, lamb, asparagus, mushrooms, peas, lettuce, peppers, cauliflower, cabbage, tomatoes, brussel sprouts, beans.	Not a concern.	Alcohol, tea, coffee, birth control pills, tobacco, stress, refined foods and drinks.
B2	child: 1.8–2mg adult: 25–100mg	Burning or gritty eyes, light sensitivity, sore tongue, cataracts, dull or oily hair, eczema or dermatitis, split nails, cracked lips.	Almonds, wild rice, mushrooms, mackerel, cabbage, parsley, cashew nuts, broccoli, sesame seeds, sunflower seeds, lentils, mung beans, avocado.	Loss or excess may result in bright yellow-green urine.	Alcohol, tea, coffee, refined foods and drinks.
B3	child: 25mg adult: 25–30mg	Lack of energy, diarrhoea, insomnia, headaches, migraines, poor memory, anxiety or tension, depression, irritability, bleeding or tender gums, acne, eczema or dermatitis.	Mushrooms, tuna, chicken, peanuts, wild rice, sesame seeds, kelp, sunflower seeds, rice, wheat, wheatgerm, barley, almonds, dates.		Alcohol, tea, coffee, birth control pills.
B5	child: 10mg adult: 25mg	Muscle tremors or cramps, apathy, poor concentration, burning feet or tender heels, nausea, vomiting, lack of energy, exhaustion even after light exercise, anxiety, tension, teeth grinding.	Mushrooms, watercress, broccoli, alfalfa sprouts, peas, lentils, tomatoes, cabbage, celery, strawberries, eggs, avocados, wholewheat.		Stress, alcohol, tea, coffee, food processing and cooking.
B6	child: 2–5mg adult: 10–25mg	Irritability, depression, emotional instability, insomnia, migraines, nausea and vomiting, constipation, poor or dry condition of skin, hair and nails, joint or body aches, lack of energy, cold hands or feet, bad menstrual cramps or PMT, unhealthy cardiovascular system.	Wheatgerm, walnuts, fish, sunflower seeds, soya beans, brewer's yeast, wholegrain cereals, rice, avocado, bananas, egg yolk, liver, chicken, pork, molasses, green leafy vegetables, potatoes, dried beans.	Very large doses can result in neuritis.	Alcohol, smoking, birth control pills, high protein intake, processed foods.
B12	child: 2mcg adult: 2–3mcg	Poor hair condition, eczema, dermatitis, over-sensitive mouth to temperatures, irritability, anxiety or tension, lack of energy, constipation, tender or sore muscles, pale skin.	Oysters, sardines, tuna, lamb, eggs, shrimps, cottage cheese, milk, turkey, chicken, cheese.		Alcohol, smoking.
folic acid	child: 300mcg adult: 400–1,000mcg	Fatigue, depression and pallor. Deficiency can result from a poor diet, alcoholism, or from impaired absorption. Elderly people in particular can fall into this category. Deficiency can also occur during any serious illness.	Green leafy vegetables, sprouts, mushrooms, avocados, micro-algae and all chlorophyll-rich foods. Also found in wheatgerm, wheat bran, nuts, liver, kidneys, eggs and fish. The richest source remains brewers' yeast. Also found in mothers' milk.	Folic acid supplements may block the absorption of zinc.	Folic acid is very heat sensitive, so is easily lost in cooking. To obtain sufficient quantities, foods containing folic acid should be eaten raw or lightly steamed.

Vitamin/ mineral	Average daily requirement	Deficiency symptoms	Dietary sources	Toxicity	Inhibiting factors
C	child: 150mg adult: 400–1,000mg	Recurrent colds, flu or other infections, slow wound healing, loss of skin elasticity, weak and brittle fingernails, soft and bleeding gums, tooth decay, nosebleeds, tender joints, premature ageing, emotional instability, nervousness, irritability, depression, cold hands or feet, menopausal discomfort.	Broccoli, peppers, kiwi fruit, lemons, parsley, watercress, cauliflower, strawberries, cabbages, fresh fruits and vegetables, currants, rosehips, cherries, tomatoes, potatoes.	Very large quantities over a long time would need to be taken to produce symptoms of toxicity. The first symptom is usually diarrhoea.	Considerable amounts of vitamin C are lost during the processing or storage of food.
D	child: 10–20mcg adult: 10–20mcg	Joint pain or stiffness, backache, tooth decay, muscle cramps, hair loss.	Herrings, mackerel, salmon, oysters, cottage cheese. eggs.		Lack of sunlight, fried foods.
E	child: 70mg adult: 100–1,000mg	Destruction of red blood cells, coronary problems, cardiovascular disease, stroke, cramps at night, 'restless legs' or extremities that tend to fall asleep, osteoarthritis, high cholesterol, below par sexual behaviour, bad menstrual cramps or PMT, menopausal hot flushes, infertility.	Cold pressed vegetable oils (especially wheatgerm oil), nuts, seeds, soya, lettuce and green leafy vegetables, meat, egg yolk, rice. Dietary shortages rarely occur.	Very little.	High temperature cooking, especially frying. Air pollution, birth control pills, excess intake of highly processed fats and oils.
calcium	child: 350mg teens: 1,000mg adult: 800mg	Muscle cramps, brittle bones, tooth decay and retarded growth, excessive bleeding, insomnia, nervousness, irritability, anxiety, depression, palpitations.	Green leafy vegetables, cauliflower, brewers' yeast, parsley, beans, yoghurt, milk, cheese, cream, molasses, rhubarb, egg yolk, sesame seeds, almonds, walnuts, millet, hard water.	Large doses taken over a long period can lead to calcium deposits, e.g. kidney stones. There may be loss of appetite, constipation, nausea, abdominal pains, and poor muscle tone.	Alcohol, tea and coffee, lack of exercise.
iron	child: 7–10mg adult: 15mg	Anaemia, paleness, lowered vitality and libido, lowered resistance to infection, abnormal fatigue, headache, shortness of breath during exercise. The most common cause of iron deficiency is heavy periods.	Meat, liver, kidneys, raw clams and oysters, pumpkin seeds, parsley, almonds, asparagus, apricots, dried fruits, wholegrain cereals, dried pulses, sunflower and sesame seeds, walnuts, brewers' yeast, bananas, molasses, beans, spinach, alfalfa, egg yolk, red wine and seafoods.	Excess iron can cause nausea, vomiting, intestinal upsets, constipation, black stools, exhaustion and rapid breathing. Young children should not be given iron supplements; it could damage their kidneys.	Vitamin C in the diet may help absorption of non-meat iron sources. Tea and coffee at mealtimes inhibits absorption. Iron bonded with carbon (chelated iron) is absorbed more easily.
magnesium	child: 85–350mg adult: 85–350mg	Muscle cramps, numbness and tingling, tremors, confusion/disorientation, memory impairment, insomnia, depression, vertigo, apathy, weakness, loss of appetite, swallowing difficulties, hypoglycaemia, PMT, menopausal problems, premature wrinkles, kidney damage, heart attack and epileptic seizure.	Wholegrains, fruits, green leafy vegetables, soya beans, alfalfa and all sprouted seeds, nuts, seafood, milk and bananas. Because magnesium is widely distributed in foods, deficiency rarely occurs.	Excess magnesium may cause nausea, vomiting, diarrhoea, dizziness and muscle weakness.	High levels of calcium from milk products, proteins, fats.
potassium	child: 1,600mg adult: 2,000mg	Muscle weakness, lack of energy, listlessness, irritability, nausea, vomiting, diarrhoea, swollen abdomen, cellulite.	Watercress, cabbage, mushrooms, parsley, cauliflower, courgettes, celery, molasses, peanuts and wild rice.		Excess salt in diet, alcohol, sugar, stress.
selenium	child: 50mcg adult: 100mcg	Fatigue, frequent infections, loss of tissue elasticity, muscle degeneration, premature ageing, male infertility or overactivity, cataracts, heart disease, high blood pressure, multiple sclerosis, rheumatoid arthritis, cancer, cystic fibrosis, menopausal discomfort.	Shellfish, herrings, kelp, molasses, raw wheatgerm, garlic, onions, nuts and seeds, (selenium fed brewer's yeast), mother's milk, fish, cereals, grains, organ meats, garlic, mushrooms, eggs and dairy products.	Over 750mg per day can produce hair and nail dysfunction and nervous system disorders. A garlic like smell may occur on the breath.	Crops often lack selenium due to deficiency in the soil. Selenium is lost when food is refined.
zinc	child: 7mg adult: 15–20mg	Lowered resistance to infection, skin problems, slow healing of wounds, dandruff and hair loss, white spots on finger nails, lethargy, depression, low male sexual energy, bad menstrual cramps or PMT, impairment of taste and loss of appetite, night blindness, joint or body aches and pains, 'restless legs'.	Fresh oysters, ginger root, pecan nuts, split peas, pumpkin seeds, meat, shellfish, herrings, nuts, bananas, wholemeal bread.	Take supplements 1 hour away from meals to prevent interaction with other dietary nutrients (may inhibit copper and iron absorption). Excess may cause pains, nausea, vomiting, fever, headaches, fatigue, poor muscle co-ordination.	Zinc bonded with carbon (chelated zinc) is more easily absorbed into the body.

exercise

When it comes to maintaining a good level of physical health, environmental and dietary considerations are important, but keeping fit is fundamental. This becomes more true the older we get. Keeping fit does not necessarily mean lifting weights every day or jogging for 30 minutes before breakfast, but it does require a commitment to regular, moderate exercise. The type of exercise that is most likely to be sustained is that which you can build into your lifestyle, such as walking the children to school, doing 20 minutes of yoga before lunch and cycling to work. Getting some exercise every day will help you to feel more energetic.

Remember, there is no need to develop huge muscles or be super-thin to feel good about your body, but regular exercise will help you to feel trimmer, better about your body and better about yourself.

movement and relaxation

To allow the body to function well, we need a good balance of movement and relaxation. Both movement and relaxation are essential to keep our blood circulating, allowing nutrients and oxygen to reach each cell. This is how we make our energy. The main causes of ill-health, or simply feeling out of balance, are stagnation and blockage of this natural flow of life. Many of these blockages are caused by tension, which may be of physical or emotional origin, and learning to relax is one of the most important things that we will ever do. Bringing relaxation into movement is the key to restoring health and balance with exercise.

It is often the simplest exercises which are the most effective. The human body has developed in a specific way in order to perform particular physical movements, and one of these basic movements is walking. Learning to walk consciously, with the back straight and the arms and shoulders relaxed is the best all-round form of exercise and is easily done by everyone.

conscious walking

Walking can become a dynamic exercise by paying attention to your posture and your breath – consciously let your shoulders drop, breathe deeply and regularly, at times allow the arms to swing loosely from the sides. If you are walking to work, invest in a good rucksack which will enable you to maintain a straight spine and dropped shoulders. Carrying a bag on one shoulder will create an imbalance in the posture, and eventually the musculo-skeletal system. If you have to carry a bag, change it to the opposite shoulder now and again.

Try to be aware of how you hold yourself when you walk; extend your spine to give space to your internal organs, which are gently massaged by the natural rhythm of walking. The body loves natural rhythms; walking regularly every day will aid your digestion and ability to eliminate waste, and help to regularize the menstrual flow. Creating a good rhythm of breathing will strengthen the lungs and the heart. Strenuous aerobic exercise can help to develop strength and muscle, but it is also easy to create stress in the body and any benefit tends to be short-term. The heart and lungs prefer regular, rhythmic movement, and will react more healthily to slow, steady strengthening.

Include the occasional uphill walk to increase the activity of both heart and lungs. Remember to breathe deeply and evenly, as you would when walking on the flat, and keep the shoulders open and relaxed. The lungs need space to expand and contract to their full capacity, especially with the increased exertion, so try to keep the diaphragm relaxed. This can be helped by gently swinging the arms as you walk.

Both movement and relaxation can be achieved by walking. The body is naturally toned, the breath deepened and regularized. It is our most accessible way of exercising, so simple that we tend to underestimate its benefits.

warming-up exercises

In all traditions of exercise some kind of warming-up process is used to ease the body into movement. In the east, a very similar form of warming-up is often used in both the yoga and martial arts traditions, the aim being to aid the flow of blood and energy through the body by moving each of the main joints in sequence. Oriental medicine claims that much imbalance in health is due to a stagnation of blood and energy, and this stagnation is most likely to occur at the joints. The exercise sequence aims to move each joint in flexion, extension and rotation, as appropriate.

Standing with the feet parallel to each other and at hip-width apart, take a few deep breaths. Feel that the feet are firmly in contact with the ground. Imagine for a few seconds that you are growing roots through the balls of your feet deep into the ground. These roots are your stability.

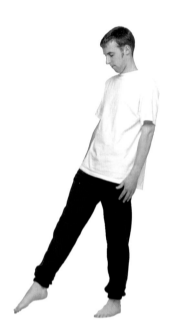

1 Feet and ankles: Lift up the right foot and slowly extend, pointing the toes, then pull up the toes towards the shin bone. Keep the left foot rooted into the ground. Repeat slowly 5 times, breathing in with the flexion, out with the extension. Then repeat with the left foot. As you move, bring your awareness into the foot and ankle. Feel whether the stretch is even on the inside and the outside of the foot. Try to correct any feeling of imbalance, but if this is difficult, just bring awareness to the area. Then move each foot in a circle, bringing a small movement of rotation to the ankle joint. Move the feet in both a clockwise and anticlockwise direction. Again pay attention to any areas of pain and tension.

2 Knees: Bring your feet together, regain your balance and feel rooted in the ground. Place the hands on the knees for support, bend the knees as you squat down, then extend the knees as you bend forward. Keep the hands on the knees, and rotate the knees in a circle. You will feel a rotation in both the knees and ankles.

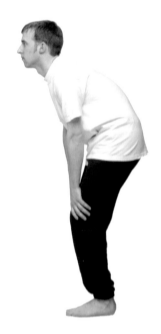

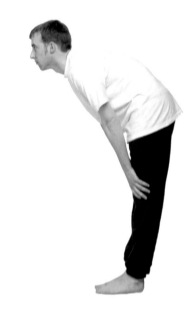

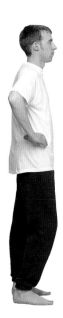

Hips: With the feet slightly wider apart, and hands over the hip joints, bend the right knee as you take the weight on to the right foot. Make sure that the bent knee is directly over the foot, and that the spine is straight. You should feel a slight stretch in the left hip joint. Move the weight to the left and repeat to the left. Repeat the whole exercise five times. This is a very subtle movement but brings stretch to a part of the body which is rarely moved, so go carefully. Aim to exhale as you stretch, and inhale as you move back to the centre position. If you feel no stretch, move the legs a little bit wider. Move the feet slightly closer together and bring the hands to the top of the hip bones. Rotate the hips in a clockwise and then in an anticlockwise direction.

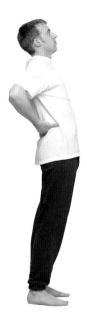

Lower back: Place the hands at the back of the waist over the kidneys. Take a deep breath in and as you breathe out bend backwards, supported by your hands. Stretch your spine upwards out of the lower back, try to relax your neck and expand your chest. Inhale as you return to the upright position. Exhale as you allow the body to relax forwards, hands moving towards the ground. Inhale as you slowly return to the upright position. Repeat three times.

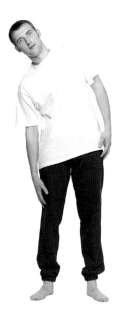

Waist and sides: Stand straight with the arms by the sides. Bend the body to the right, allowing the right hand to move down the side of the right leg. Repeat to the left. To increase the stretch, repeat the movement with the right hand stretching down the leg and the left arm stretched over the head close to the ear. Breathe out as you stretch to the side.

Remain in the position for a few breaths, breathing naturally. Return to the centre as you inhale and repeat to the left. Keep the body in alignment, not bending forward or back. Consciously relax the side that is stretching, particularly the side ribs and the neck. Complete five stretches to each side.

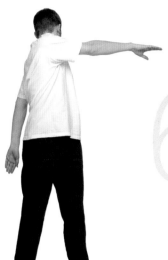

6 Keep breathing evenly and keep your attention focused on the part of the body which you are stretching. Breathing out with any stretch or exertion will help you to relax and release any tension that you are holding.

Move the feet wider apart, and with the hands by the sides twist to the right. Look over your shoulder towards the left foot as you point with the right hand at the heel of the left foot. Repeat to the left.

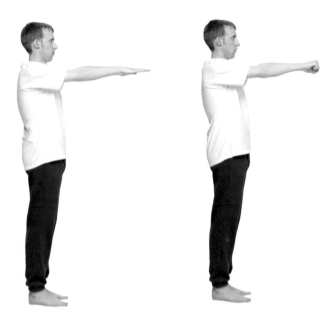

7 With the arms outstretched in front of you, breathe in as you consciously draw in the fingers to make a fist. Breathe out as you stretch the fingers, imagining that you are projecting energy through the finger tips. Repeat five times.

With the arms still outstretched, bend the hands backwards and forwards. Use your concentration to keep the movement evenly distributed through the wrist, trying to move the little finger side of the hand as much as the thumb. Repeat.

Rotate the hands in clockwise and then anticlockwise circles, five times each.

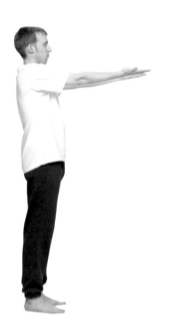

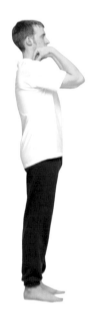

Stretch and flex the elbows by stretching out the arms in front of you with palms raised, and then bringing the hands to touch the shoulders. Repeat five times.

9 Keeping the hands on the shoulders, make large circles with the elbows, bringing them together to meet at the centre of the chest and then circling upwards and outwards. Repeat five times and then change the direction of the rotation. Shake the arms and shoulders well, releasing any tension.

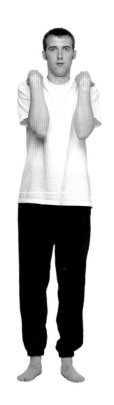
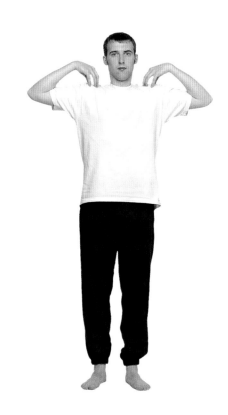

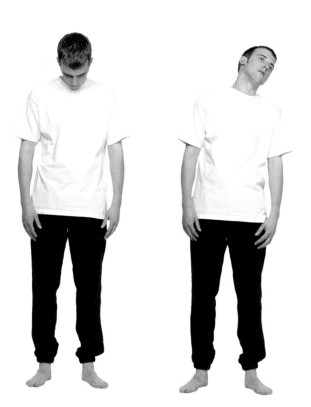

10 Neck stretches: Breathe in deeply and, as you exhale, bring the chin down towards the chest. Breathe in as you return to the centre. Breathe out again as you move the head back. Repeat five times. Never force the neck; always allow the weight of the head to create a natural stretch. Work with the breath to keep the movements slow and controlled.

From the upright position, stretch to the side, allowing the ear to move towards the shoulder. Again, work slowly as you exhale and allow the weight of the head to create the stretch. Breathe in as you return to centre. Repeat the movement to the other side. Repeat five times to each side.

Keeping the head on a straight vertical axis, take a deep breath in, as you breathe out move the head around, looking with the eyes over the shoulder as far as you can. This exercises the eyes as well as the neck. Repeat five times to each side.

Rub your hands together until the palms are hot and place them over the eyes. Repeat five times.

11 Place the hands over the eyes and then with a long sweeping movement bring the hands over the top of the head, down the back of the neck, over the front of the chest, to the back of the waist. Finally, sweep down the back of the legs to the ground. Repeat this movement five times.

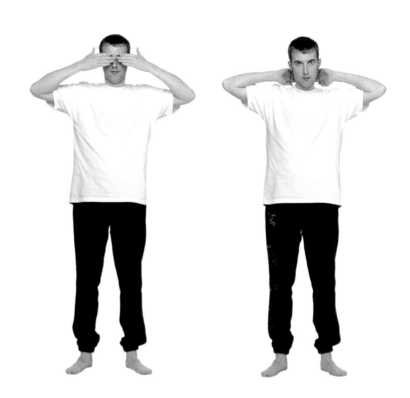

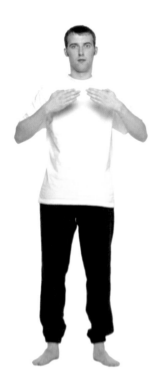

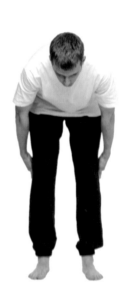

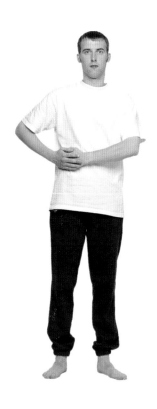

abdominal massage

Place the left hand to the right side of the navel and place the right hand on top of the left. Guiding with the right hand, move in clockwise circles around the navel. This simple massage may be performed over the clothes, or on the skin using a suitable massage oil. The movement should be in a clockwise direction to follow the natural direction of the intestines. It is an effective massage for constipation, period pains, and abdominal bloating. For constipation use a stimulating massage oil, and for a nervous knotted stomach use a calming blend. At least 50 rounds should be counted each time.

breathing

The heart and lungs respond well to the calm of meditation and the controlled rhythm of the breath. Repetition of simple breathing exercises will calm the mind and the heart. Breathing deeply and rhythmically aids the uptake of oxygen and releases tension throughout the whole system.

---

breathing exercises

- Sit with the spine straight in any position which feels comfortable to you. If you are sitting on a chair, make sure that your feet are flat on the floor. Allow your hands to relax in your lap, or on your knees. Take in a deep breath and then exhale deeply, expelling all the stale air from the lungs. Repeat a few times and then allow the breath to return to normal. Breathe in a deep and relaxed way, counting to ten on each breath. Be aware of the feeling of the air in the nose. Breathe very gently as if you do not want to disturb the nose or make any sound. When you reach to the count of ten, begin again. If your mind wanders and you lose count, just begin again. Continue for ten minutes.

- If you suffer from stress, you may find that your breathing has become very shallow, utilizing only the upper part of the lungs. Feel the lungs expanding to their full, the diaphragm relaxing and releasing downwards with the inhalation. If you have problems sleeping, try this exercise before you go to bed.

To be effective these exercises need to be repeated frequently: a little exercise every day is the best way to create new patterns of health and well-being.

qi gong: balancing heaven and earth

The ancient Chinese practices of tai ji quan and qi gong create a balance between the body and mind by working with the subtle energy channels. In qi gong the movements are simple, but by using the breath and focusing the attention they provide the most effective tool for combating stress and allowing the body to return to its own natural rhythms. According to the ancient Chinese, life exists on earth due to a balance of the energies of heaven and earth. Heaven brings warmth, movement, inspiration and energy, and is known as yang; earth brings moisture, nutrition, stability and form, and is known as yin. As a plant draws food from the soil and energy from the sun, inner transformations allow it to flourish and grow. It is much the same with us. Yin and yang combine to create life in a constant process of change and interchange, balance and counterbalance. The interaction of yin and yang and heaven and earth is made possible by the dynamic life force known to the Chinese as qi.

Qi gong literally means 'working with qi'. Qi flows in our bodies through a system of channels known as the meridian system. Complex in its details, this system is actually based on the simple assumption that yin energy flows up from the earth, yang energy flows downwards from heaven. The yin channels flow from the earth, through the feet and the inner legs into the abdomen, from where they spread into the chest. From the chest they pass through the inner arm, ending in the finger tips. The yang channels flow downwards, beginning in the finger tips, flowing into the head, down the back of the body and to the toes.

Qi gong is very simple and very subtle. We are working with energy, helping the balance and interchange of yin and yang and tuning in with the natural rhythms of heaven and earth. As tension is released from the body, the movements begin to take on a natural flow, until you feel as if the qi is moving you. There is no effort, no strain and no stress.

basic stance

Standing with the feet parallel and shoulder width apart, slightly bend the knees. The feet should feel in contact with the ground, so spend a few moments checking that the balance is equal between the heels and the toes, the outer and inner edges of the feet. In the centre of the sole of the foot, the yin meridians contact the ground, giving rooting and stability to the body. Begin to imagine these roots growing through the feet down towards the centre of the earth.

Consciously tilt the pelvis forward, stretching the lower part of the spine and slightly contracting the lower abdomen. This is a feeling or sensation more than a real muscular contraction, but do not worry if you cannot quite feel it, it will come. Gently swing the arms as you rotate the waist, allowing tension to fall from the shoulders.

Close your eyes and concentrate on your weight and gravity. The whole area below the waist should feel heavy and solid. Imagine your weight sinking down, through the waist, and the hips, down through the legs into the feet and through the soles of the feet deep into the earth. Feel rooted like a tree feels rooted.

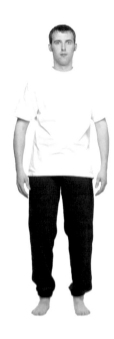

1 Let the hands rest gently on the lower abdomen wherever they feel comfortable. Bring your attention to your breath, breathing naturally and regularly.

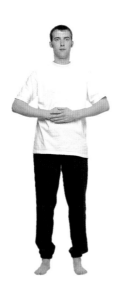

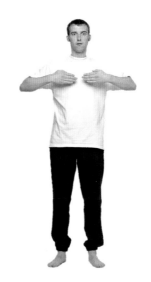

2 When the body feels completely relaxed, take a breath in, drawing the hands slowly apart, and at a distance of 5–7.5 cm (2–3 inches) from the body follow the line of the central energy channels from the lower abdomen to the chest.

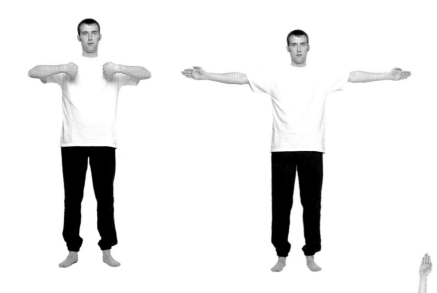

3 With the hands in front of the chest and the elbows raised begin to exhale, move the hands across the chest fingers pointing inwards towards the arm pits, and gradually, with the exhalation, stretch the arms to a fully extended horizontal position, following the yin meridians flowing from the chest, along the internal face of the arm into the finger tips.

4 Take a few deep breaths and with another inhalation stretch the arms and hands out and move them upwards as if embracing the heavens. Breathe out with the hands stretched above the head.

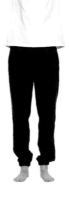

5 After a few breaths, slowly bring the hands down to just above the top of the head. Then move them down over the back of the head and neck to the shoulders, tracing the surface of the body but keeping the hands about 5 cm (2 inches) away.

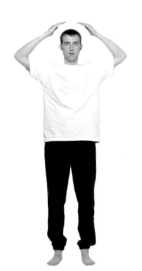 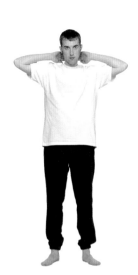

6 The hands follow the centre front and around the lower rib cage, while the concentration remains on the spine. The hands finally come to rest on the back at waist level, over the kidneys. Take a few breaths.

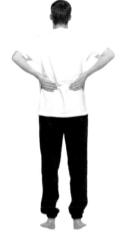

7 On an exhalation, bend forward, follow the yang meridians on the back of the legs with the hands, until the hands reach the floor. Bend the knees as much as is necessary. Remain for a few moments contacting the yin and the earth.

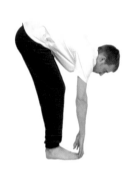

8 With the hands facing the inside, yin part of the legs, draw the yin energy up through the legs into the groin and come to rest on the lower abdomen.

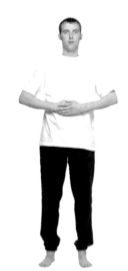

This sequence of movements forms one cycle and should be repeated many times until it becomes fluid.

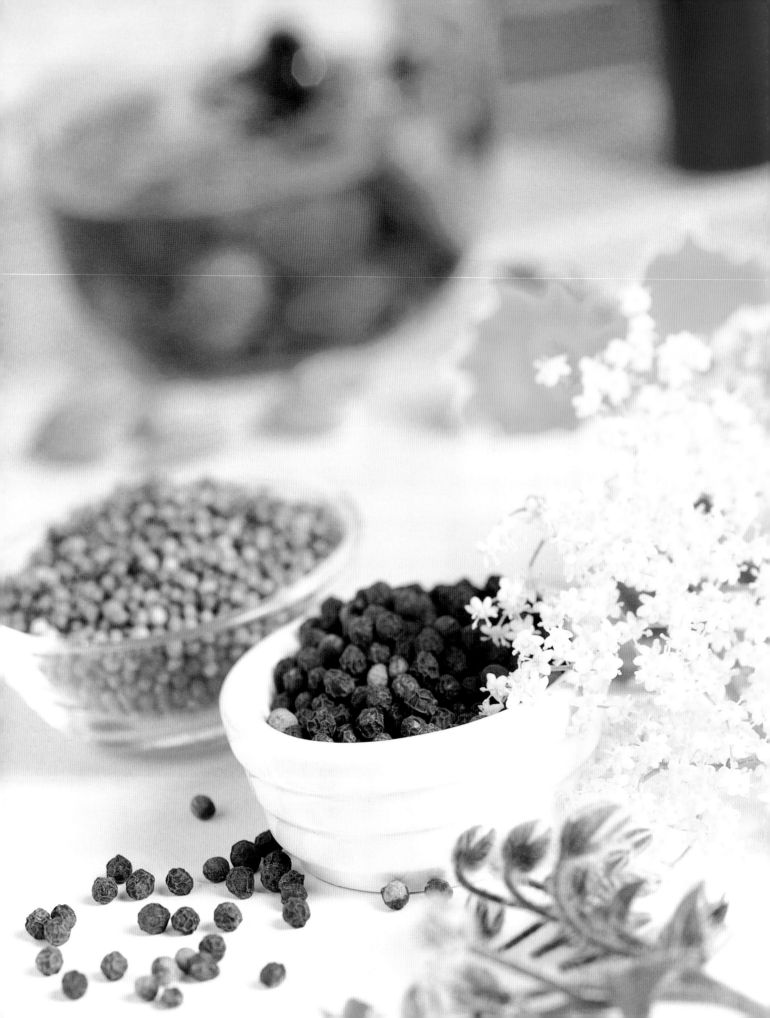

making the best of natural ingredients

When adopting natural methods for improving your health it is fundamental to use fresh, good quality ingredients, not only as part of your diet but also when making your own cosmetics. The fresher the ingredients, the more effective will be the end product.

choosing what to make

Being clear about what you want to make is the first step to making successful health and beauty products. This is not as obvious as it sounds! Ask yourself who the product is for; you can then choose the appropriate ingredients to suit their needs. Products for elderly skin require different ingredients to those for a young one. Asian skin will have different demands from black skin types, and white skin will be different again. Below are some guidelines to consider when you are deciding what to make, but keep in mind individual preferences and types within each group.

babies

We all started our lives with skin that was soft and very delicate, but from the time we are born our skin is subjected to the harsh rays of the sun. With the thinning of the ozone layer, it is becoming more and more important to protect skin from the damage of UV rays. Babies' skin is particularly susceptible not only to the sun but also to any pollutants found in the air, water, food or toiletries. Great care must be given to the quality of oils and other ingredients used. Try to resist the temptation to make your baby product smell fragrant. Instead, use herbs infused in either water or a base oil (see pages 59–60). Babies do not generally need anything more complicated than a plain olive oil soap to wash with and simple almond oil (organic) to moisturize or rehydrate dry skin. By adding some chamomile, lavender or marigold tea to the bath, these simple infusions can help alleviate most skin problems. (See also pages 148–9 for other baby products.)

teenagers

During the difficult time of hormonal changes, young adults have particular beauty requirements. Use cleansing herbs and oils for the ingredients. This is a time when teenagers are very sensitive about their appearance, so help and advice will be appreciated. Try to involve them in the making of their own skin preparations, which will hopefully encourage them to develop a positive attitude towards themselves. The lure of advertised commercial products and peer pressure will demand that any product you make is effective and pleasant to use. Blends of herbs are good for facial cleansing, and the recipes for relaxing bath oils on page 107 may give you some ideas.

pregnancy

During pregnancy, women go through many changes that may affect both the physical body and the emotions, so take extra care to find out what the person needs and would like. In the main, the body provides for itself, but it may be that the hair could do with extra nourishment, or the skin could be dry. The best products are those which aid relaxation and a sense of well-being.

Remember that everything will have an effect on the growing foetus in one way or another. Do not use anything strong and, as with baby products, be extra vigilant with the quality of the ingredients you use. Always check the list on pages 56–7 for oils and herbs that must not be used during pregnancy.

ageing skin

As chemical medicine, surgery, and genetic modification make it more possible for us to live longer, we try to put off the signs of ageing. Many of us seek to maintain a fresh, young look throughout our lives. This attitude exists even among school children. We are all obsessed with the desire for eternal youth! The best attitude to have is to strive for good health. A healthy, radiant person is attractive whatever age they are and keeping the skin cleansed free of pollutants and well nourished with natural moisturizers will go a long way towards keeping a youthful appearance.

There are many recipes to use in this book, for men, women and children of all ages. They can be fun to make for your own beauty needs or for the special requirements of others. Take time to work out the appropriate product, bearing in mind the skin type and the general health of the person.

the elderly

There are many products that you can make to enhance the quality of life of the elderly. As it ages, the skin gets thinner, drier and more brittle. You can focus on making products that are rich in oils and vitamins but which are also easy to apply. Older people need gentle cleansers for the skin, hair and bath. Sometimes the olfactory sense becomes less acute with age, so it might be necessary to increase the percentage of aromatic oils where a fragrance is desired, but be careful, as elderly skin can become very sensitive. If you are making a product for someone else, find out if an invigorating or relaxing product is required; many elderly people lead active lives.

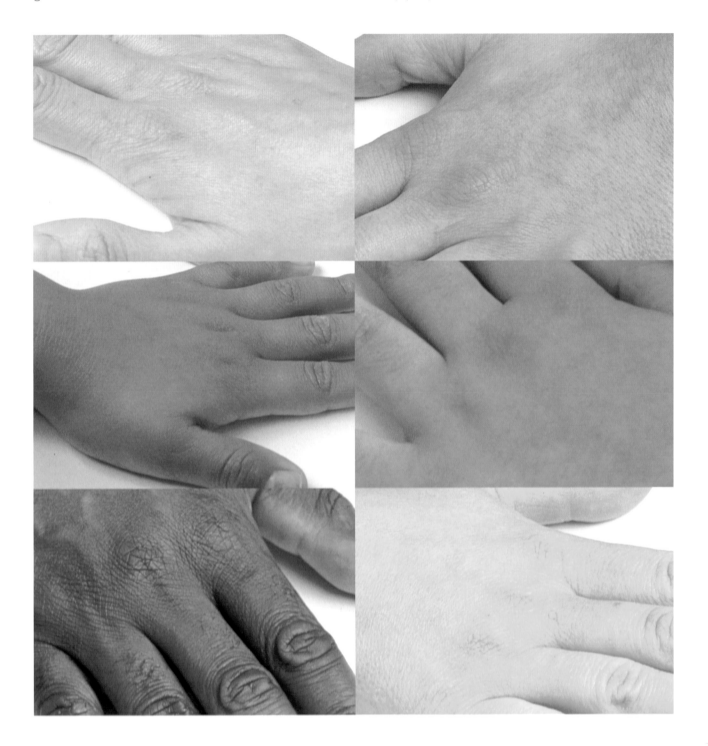

equipment and utensils

Very little specialized equipment is required to make the recipes in this book, and most of the utensils needed will be found in the average kitchen. Before you begin to make any of the products, read quickly through the recipe to check that you have everything you will need. The list below summarizes the items used, but you can, of course, improvise with your own kitchen utensils.

A bain-marie is used to soften ingredients gently, through indirect heat. Most kitchen stores will sell customized bain-maries, but if you do not have one, simply place the ingredients to be heated in a heatproof bowl that will sit on the rim of a saucepan one-quarter to one-third filled with water. As the water in the base pan is heated, the bowl becomes warm and the heat permeates to the ingredients and softens them.

Jars sold for homemade preserves are ideal for storing many of the recipes, and good cookware stores supply a range of sizes. The smaller ones are especially useful. Preserving jars are usually made of clear glass, with glass lids that are held in place by metal wires, which are flipped over to seal the jar shut. Some types also have rubber rings around the lids, which provide a completely airtight seal. Creams and balms are best stored in wide-necked, dark-coloured glass jars and bottles.

Before you begin, sterilize your equipment, including the jars and bottles (and their lids) that will hold the finished product, by immersing them in boiling water for 20 minutes. Remember, too, to wash your hands thoroughly.

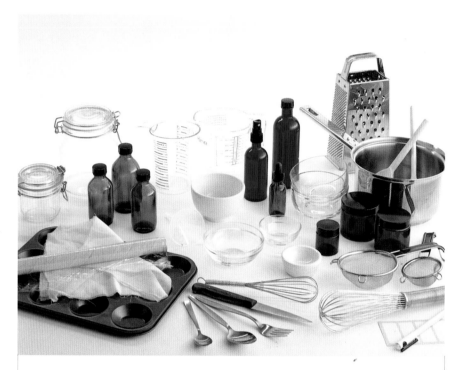

basic kit

- Atomizer spray
- Bain-marie or double saucepan, or saucepan with heatproof bowl
- Bun tin (cookie pan)
- Clingfilm (plastic kitchen film)
- Coffee filter (unbleached)
- Fork
- Funnel
- Glass bowls (at least two sizes)
- Clear and dark glass bottles (various sizes)
- Sealable screw-top or preserving jars (various sizes)
- Grater

- Hand whisk
- Kettle
- Knife
- Labels and pen
- Measuring jug
- Muslin (cheesecloth)
- Pestle and mortar
- Saucepan
- Wooden spoons
- Metal spoons
- Strainer or sieve
- Tea pot
- Teaspoon and tablespoon or measuring spoons

knowing the right ingredients

Throughout this book you are encouraged to use natural remedies and to learn ways of keeping healthy that work in harmony with the environment. As we have become more aware of the world in which we live, so we have developed our knowledge of plants and how to use them. It can become a life-long interest, and the more you can experience through growing, collecting, and cooking plants, the more they will become familiar and effective in your products. Use all your senses: taste the herbs, smell the oils, feel the texture of the clays. Use the book to discover the basic guidelines, and in time you will develop your preferences so that you can experiment with your own creations.

Follow the guidelines on pages 38–47 on making the different plant extracts. This will help you to use your chosen ingredients in the best ways for the product. Just as it is important to source quality plant materials, so you also need to find the purest, least adulterated ingredients for the clays, lanolin or beeswax. Smaller producers are often able to supply products that are fresher and less processed than those supplied by more commercial companies. Large companies usually need to provide a consistent quality in what they sell, and cannot afford the time or money to allow for seasonal variations, manual collection or sorting, and so on. As a result, the product may have less inherent vitality due to heat or to other forms of processing.

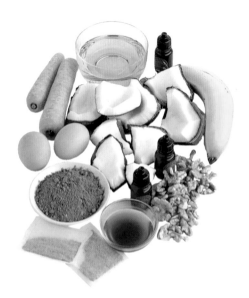

Be adventurous! Flower remedies and vitamins and minerals are effective when used internally, so it may be worth including some of these natural remedies in beauty care. Read the glossaries on pages 212–39 – propolis, benzoin and vanilla tincture, for example, can all help preserve your preparations and prolong their shelf life, and bee pollen and honey are excellent to use for their enriching and nourishing properties.

The colour of your created product will depend on the natural colour of the ingredients. If you want to add a more definite shade then consider adding some of the following: spirulina will turn your products green (and add a strong fragance) and can easily be added to bath products. Beetroot, blackberry and mulberry will all add a red to purple tone. Artichoke, nettles and comfrey all give a green to brown colour. When adding extracts for colour remember to consider the overall therapeutic effects that the additions will make.

creating the best combinations

Herbs and oils work well in blends. When they are blended, they work in synergy; learning what goes with what is simply a matter of practice. It is the same when you are developing a mixture of herbs for internal use; they need to be blended for their taste as well as for their function.

Once you have decided which product to make, write a list of the raw materials you intend to use and then think about how best to combine them. Very different products may be created simply by varying the method of extraction. Use an infusion of herbs for the water part of what you are making, or make an oil extraction of herbs if the product needs a richer and a more moisturizing function. Guidance on this is given in the basic recipes on the following pages.

basic recipes

The recipes in this section – for infusions, decoctions, tinctures, macerated oils, cream base and balm base – form the basis for the other recipes in this book. Use them in conjunction with the more detailed information on quantities and ingredients to complete the individual recipes with your own choice of herbs and essential oils.

Infusions and decoctions are best prepared on the day they are to be used, so that they are absolutely fresh. Tinctures, macerated oils, creams and balms will all keep for a little longer – the exact length of time is given with each basic recipe.

infusions

An infusion is the appropriate way to harness the properties of the softer, green or flowering parts of a plant. Infusions are made like a tea, so are very easy to make. They may be used instead of water in any of the recipes in this book and are a simple way of including a specific herb for a particular skin type or condition.

herb or mixture of herbs	Chop the herb or mixture of herbs. Transfer to a cup or teapot. Pour on boiling water. Leave to steep for 10 minutes, preferably covered to avoid the loss of volatile oils in the steam. Strain before use. Make up as required.
boiling water	
cup or teapot	
sieve or tea strainer	

decoctions

This is the appropriate way to use the woodier parts of a plant – its roots, bark, berries and seeds. When making decoctions, use a steel or enamelled cast iron saucepan in preference to an aluminium one, as the aluminium can react with anything cooked in it, and so taint the decoction.

herb or mixture of herbs	Place the herb or mixture of herbs in a saucepan. Pour on water, cover and bring to the boil. Simmer for 10 minutes. Strain before use. Make up as required.
cold water	
saucepan (with lid)	
sieve	

herbs used in infusions include:

- borage
- chamomile
- cleavers
- comfrey leaf
- elderflower
- lavender
- lemon balm
- marigold
- marsh mallow leaf
- rose petals

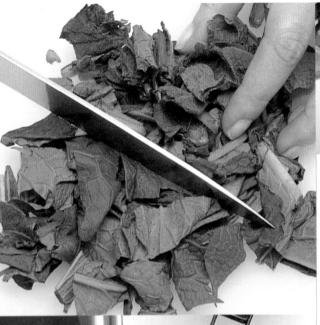

1 chopping herbs for the infusion

2 straining the infusion

quantities

The quantity of herb varies according to the herb used, the strength of the infusion or decoction required and its desired purpose. Unless otherwise stated, the standard measurement is 1 heaped teaspoon of dried herb to 1 cup of boiling water. Wherever possible use fresh herbs and double the quantity.

1 boiling the decoction

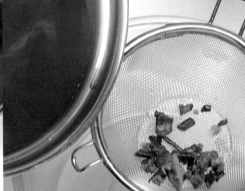

2 straining the decoction

herbs used in decoctions include:

- burdock root
- echinacea
- fennel
- ginseng
- marsh mallow root
- quassia

macerated oils

The volatile oils contained in aromatic plants can be released by soaking them in vegetable oil. This is called an infused or macerated oil. Macerated oils can be used as carrier oils or they can be incorporated into cosmetic recipes. There are two methods of preparation.

the sun method

This method can also be used with cider vinegar or witch hazel instead of vegetable oil. The oil will keep for up to 12 months.

finely chopped fresh herbs
vegetable oil (e.g., virgin
   olive oil, sweet almond oil
   or sunflower oil)
sealable jar
sieve
dark glass bottle

Pack a sealable jar tightly with finely chopped fresh herbs. Cover the herbs with a good-quality vegetable oil. Virgin olive oil and sweet almond oil are best, although sunflower oil is a good alternative. It is very important that the plant material is completely covered by the oil both for full extraction and to exclude contamination. Seal the jar and leave in direct sunlight for 2 weeks, shaking daily. Strain and repeat with fresh plant material. Leave for another 2 weeks, shaking daily. Strain, pour into a dark glass bottle and label with the name and date.

the heat method

This method is faster and possibly more practical, especially if the oil is needed for immediate use. If the oil is not needed immediately, it will keep for up to 12 months. It is not necessary to use a cold-pressed oil for this method, as the oil is heated, which ruins the benefits of cold pressing.

finely chopped fresh herbs
vegetable oil
boiling water
heat proof bowl
saucepan
sieve
dark glass bottle

Place the finely chopped herbs in a bowl. Cover with vegetable oil. Place the bowl containing the mixture over a pan of boiling water, cover and heat for 1 hour. Remove from the heat, strain and repeat with fresh herbs. Strain, pour into a dark glass bottle and label with the name and date.

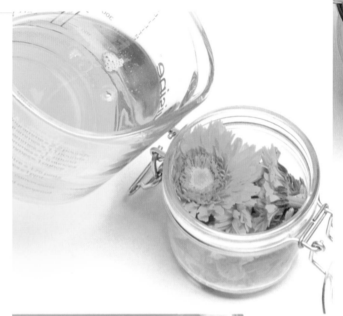

1 the sun method: filling the jar

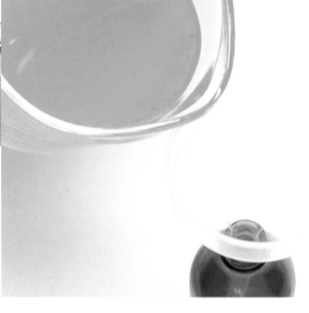

herbs used in macerates include:

- calendula
- carrot
- comfrey
- garlic
- mullein
- St John's wort

2 the sun method: straining the oil

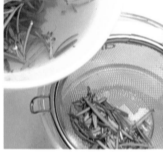

1 the heat method: straining the oil

2 the heat method: pouring into a dark glass bottle

cream base

This is a simple cream base that can be used to carry essential oils and herbal tinctures for external application. It will keep well in the refrigerator for up to 2 months. The ingredients given here are sufficient to make about 100 g (3½ oz).

8 g/2 tsp beeswax (granules
   or grated)
10 g/2½ tsp cocoa butter
30 ml/2 tbsp almond oil
15 ml/1 tbsp wheatgerm oil
45 ml/3 tbsp spring water
5 g/1¼ tsp emulsifying wax
2 saucepans
dark glass jar

Heat the beeswax, cocoa butter and base oils together in a bowl over a saucepan of water until the ingredients have melted. Warm the spring water in another saucepan and dissolve the emulsifying wax into it. Take the oily mixture off the heat. Slowly add the spring water mixture to the oily mixture and stir until cool. Add the essential oils or herbal tincture. Store in a dark glass jar in the refrigerator.

balm base

This is a simple base that does not require an emulsifier. It works well, but does not have the creamy texture of the previous recipe. It can set quite hard, depending on the ratio of beeswax to oils, and will last for 6 months if it is stored in an airtight jar. The ingredients given here are sufficient to make about 100 g (3½ oz).

8 g/2 tsp beeswax (granules
   or grated)
45 ml/3 tbsp almond oil
15 ml/1 tbsp wheatgerm oil
10 ml/2 tsp herb tincture
5 drops essential oil
saucepan
dark glass jar

Heat the beeswax and almond oil in a bowl over a saucepan of boiling water until the beeswax has melted. Add the wheatgerm oil and tincture and gently stir together. Remove from the heat and allow to cool slightly. Add the essential oils and mix thoroughly. Pour into a dark glass jar and allow to set.

**1 heating the
cream base**

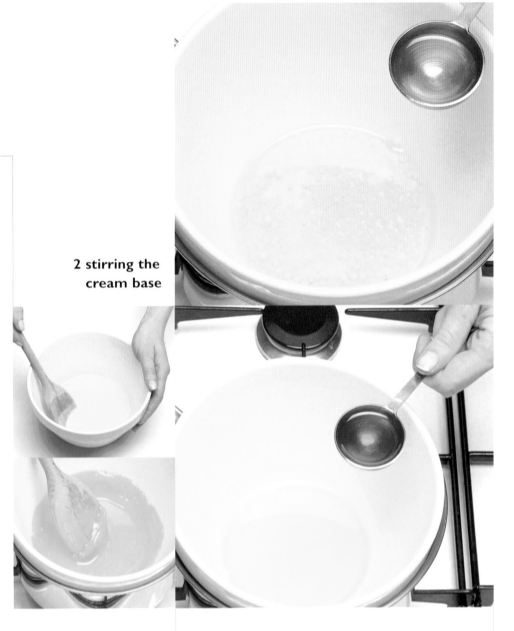

variations

You can replace the
spring water with an
infusion, which will
allow you to include
herbs that suit your
own skin type and
skin requirements. You
could also substitute
other oils of your
choice for the almond
or wheatgerm oils.

**2 stirring the
cream base**

**1 heating the
balm base**

**2 adding oils to
the balm base**

variations

As with the Cream Base,
you can use oils of your
choice instead of the
almond and wheatgerm
oils. It is an ideal recipe
to use for making up

first-aid remedies. If
you learn the properties
of the herbs you will
discover that there is
an endless range of
opportunities available.

tinctures

The medicinal properties of herbs can be extracted using a mixture of water and alcohol. The resulting preparation is known as a tincture. The ratio of water to alcohol varies from herb to herb in accordance with the constituents required, (see pages 46–7 for more details). It is standard practice to use one herb per tincture, although it is possible to combine tinctures.

The final volume is based on 100 per cent proof alcohol (available from duty-free shops); we therefore recommend using high-proof vodka when making tinctures. The alcohol acts as a preservative, making this an excellent way to store herbs out of season. A tincture will keep for up to 12 months.

Volume for volume, tinctures are a lot stronger than either infusions, decoctions or macerates, so they only need to be used in small quantities. This is just as well when making cosmetics as most tinctures have quite distinctive smells which, in large quantities, would be hard to mask.

finely chopped (fresh) herbs

high-proof vodka

water

sealable jar

muslin (cheesecloth)

sieve

unbleached coffee filter

dark glass bottle

Pack a sealable jar tightly with finely chopped herbs – ideally fresh herbs should be used where possible, but if necessary dried or even powdered plant material can act as substitutes. Immerse the herb totally in vodka and water. Seal the jar and store for 2 weeks away from direct sunlight, shaking occasionally. Strain the mixture through muslin (cheesecloth) and then filter through an unbleached coffee filter. Pour into a dark glass bottle. Label clearly with the name and date, and store in a cool place away from sunlight. Make up as required.

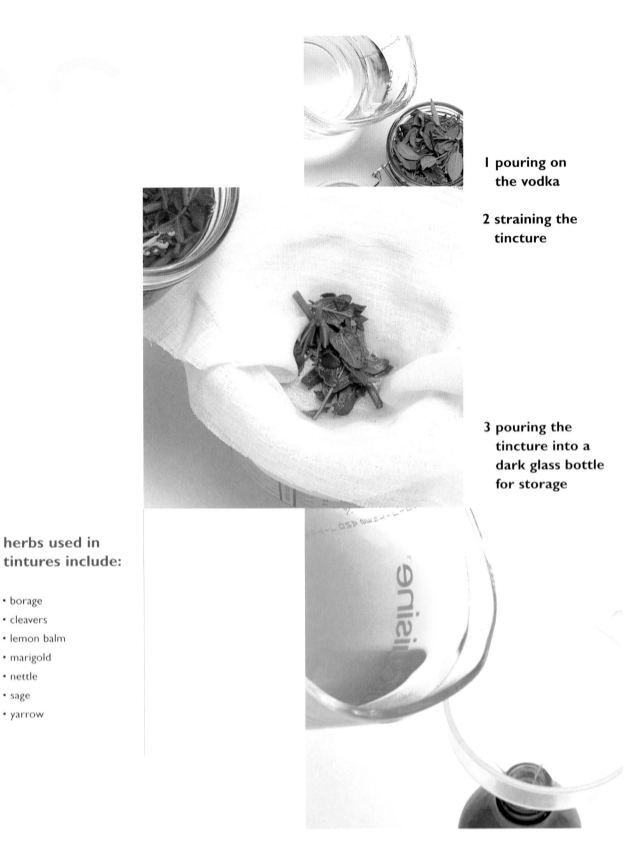

1 pouring on
   the vodka

2 straining the
   tincture

3 pouring the
   tincture into a
   dark glass bottle
   for storage

**herbs used in
tintures include:**

- borage
- cleavers
- lemon balm
- marigold
- nettle
- sage
- yarrow

tinctures

To make tinctures (see page 44), follow the ratios between the plant material and the water/100% alcohol mixture shown in the wt/vol column. The proportion of alcohol to water required is given in the % alc column.

Latin name	Common name	wt/vol	% alc
Achillea millefolium	yarrow	1:5	25
Acorus calamus	sweet flag	1:5	60
Aesculus hippocastanum	horse chestnut	1:5	25
Alchemilla xanthochlora	lady's mantle	1:5	25
Aletris farinosa	unicorn root	1:5	25
Aloe ferox	cape aloe	1:40	45
Alpinia officinarum	galangal	1:5	25
Althaea officinalis	marsh mallow	1:5	25
Ammi visnaga	khella	1:5	25
Angelica archangelica	angelica	1:5	45
Aphanes arvensis	parsley piert, breakstone parsley	1:5	25
Apium graveolens	celery	1:4	60
Arctium lappa	burdock	1:5	25
Arctostaphylos uva-ursi	bearberry	1:5	25
Armoracia rusticana	horseradish	1:10	45
Arnica montana	arnica	1:10	45
Artemisia abrotanum	southernwood	1:10	45
Artemisia absinthium	wormwood	1:10	45
Artemisia vulgaris	mugwort	1:10	45
Asclepias tuberosa	pleurisy root	1:10	25
Avena sativa	oats	1:5	25
Baptisia tinctoria	wild indigo	1:10	60
Berberis vulgaris	barberry	1:5	25
Betula pendula	birch	1:5	25
Borago officinalis	borage	1:5	25
Calendula officinalis	marigold	1:5	25
Capsella bursa-pastoris	shepherd's purse	1:5	25
Capsicum frutescens	cayenne pepper	1:20	60
Carum carvi	caraway seed	1:5	45
Centaurium erythraea	centaury	1:5	25
Cephaelis ipecacuanha BP 1983	ipecacuanha	1:10	90
Chamaelirium luteum	false unicorn root	1:10	90
Chamaemelum nobile	Roman chamomile	1:5	45

Latin name	Common name	wt/vol	% alc
Chondrus crispus	Irish moss, carrageen	1:5	25
Cinnamomum zeylanicum	cinnamon	1:5	45
Cola nitida	cola	1:5	25
Collinsonia canadensis	stone root	1:5	25
Commiphora myrrha	myrrh, oleo gum	1:5	90
Cytisus scoparius	broom	1:5	25
Drimia maritima	squill	1:10	60
Echinacea angustifolia	coneflower	1:5	45
Eleutherococcus senticosus	Siberian ginseng	1:5	25
Equisetum arvense	horsetail	1:5	25
Eschscholzia californica	Californian poppy	1:5	45
Eucalyptus globulus	eucalyptus	1:5	45
Euphorbia hirta	euphorbia, spurge	1:5	60
Euphrasia officinalis	eyebright	1:5	25
Foeniculum vulgare	fennel	1:5	45
Fucus vesiculosus	bladderwrack	1:2	25
Fumaria officinalis	fumitory	1:5	25
Galega officinalis	goat's rue	1:5	25
Galium aparine	cleavers, goosegrass	1:5	25
Gentiana lutea	gentian	1:5	45
Geranium maculatum radix	cranesbill root	1:5	25
Geum urbanum	avens	1:5	25
Ginkgo biloba	maidenhair tree	1:5	25
Glechoma hederacea	ground ivy	1:5	25
Grindelia camporum	grindelia	1:10	25
Guaiacum officinale	lignum vitae	1:5	90
Hamamelis virginiana	witch hazel	1:5	25
Harpagophytum procumbens	devil's claw	1:5	25
Humulus lupulus	hops	1:5	60
Hydrangea arborescens	hydrangea	1:5	25
Hydrastis canadensis	golden seal	1:10	60
Hypericum perforatum	St John's wort	1:5	45

Latin name	Common name	wt/vol	% alc	Latin name	Common name	wt/vol	% alc
Hyssopus officinalis	hyssop	1:5	45	Rubus idaeus	raspberry	1:5	25
Jateorhiza palmata	calumba	1:10	60	Rumex crispus	yellow dock	1:5	25
Juglans cinerea	butternut	1:5	25	Ruta graveolens	rue	1:5	25
Juniperus communis	juniper	1:5	45	Salvia officinalis	common sage	1:5	45
Lactuca virosa	wild lettuce	1:5	25	Sambucus nigra	elder	1:5	25
Lamium album	white deadnettle	1:5	25	Sanguinaria canadensis	bloodroot	1:5	60
Larrea divaricata	chaparall	1:5	25	Senna alexandrina	senna	1:5	45
Lavandula angustifolia	lavender	1:5	45	Serenoa repens	saw palmetto	1:5	90
Lycopus virginicus	bugleweed	1:5	25	Smilax regelii	sarsaparilla root	1:5	25
Mahonia aquifolium	oregon grape	1:5	25	Solidago virgaurea	golden rod	1:5	25
Marsdenia cundurango	condurango	1:5	45	Stachys officinalis	wood betony	1:5	25
Matricaria recutita	German chamomile	1:5	45	Stellaria media	chickweed	1:5	25
Medicago sativa	alfalfa, lucerne	1:5	25	Stillingia sylvatica	queen's delight	1:5	45
Melilotus officinalis	melilot	1:5	25	Symphytum officinale	comfrey	1:10	25
Melissa officinalis	lemon balm	1:5	45	Tabebuia impetiginosa	lapacho	1:5	45
Mentha x piperita	peppermint	1:5	45	Tanacetum vulgare	tansy	1:5	45
Ononis spinosa	restharrow	1:5	45	Tanacetum parthenium	feverfew	2:5	25
Panax ginseng	Korean ginseng	1:5	25	Taraxacum officinale	dandelion	1:5	25
Parietaria judaica	pellitory-of-the-wall	1:5	25	Teucrium chamaedrys	germander	1:5	25
				Teucrium scorodonia	wood sage	1:5	25
Passiflora incarnata	passion flower	1:8	25	Thuja occidentalis	thuja	1:10	60
Persicaria bistorta	bistort	1:5	25	Thymus vulgaris	thyme	1:5	45
Peumus boldus	boldo	1:10	60	Tilia x europaea	lime	1:5	25
Phytolacca americana	pokeroot	1:5	45	Toona sinensis	toona	1:5	25
Pilosella officinarum	mouse-ear hawkweed	1:5	25	Trifolium pratense	red clover	1:10	25
				Trillium erectum	birthroot	1:5	45
Pimpinella anisum	aniseed	1:5	45	Turnera diffusa	damiana	1:5	60
Piper methysticum	kava kava	1:5	25	Tussilago farfara	coltsfoot	1:5	25
Piscidia piscipula	Jamaican dogwood	1:5	30	Ulmus rubra	slippery elm	1:5	25
Plantago lanceolata	ribwort	1:5	25	Urtica dioica	stinging nettle	1:5	25
Populus tremula	white poplar	1:5	25	Verbascum thapsus	mullein	1:5	25
Potentilla erecta	tormentil	1:5	25	Veronicastrum virginicum	blackroot	1:5	70
Prunus serotina	wild cherry	1:5	25				
Pulmonaria officinalis	lungwort	1:5	25	Viburnum opulus	crampbark	1:5	25
Pulsatilla vulgaris	pasque flower	1:10	25	Viburnum prunifolium	black haw	1:5	25
Quercus robur	oak	1:5	25	Vinca major	greater periwinkle	1:5	25
Ranunculus ficaria	pilewort	1:5	25	Viola odorata	sweet violet	1:5	25
Rhamnus purshianus	cascara sagrada	1:5	25	Viola tricolor	heartsease	1:5	25
Rheum officinale	rhubarb	1:5	25	Vitex agnus-castus	chaste tree	1:5	25
Rhus aromatica	sweet sumac	1:5	25	Zea mays	corn	1:5	25
Rosmarinus officinalis	rosemary	1:5	45	Zingiber officinale	ginger	1:2	90

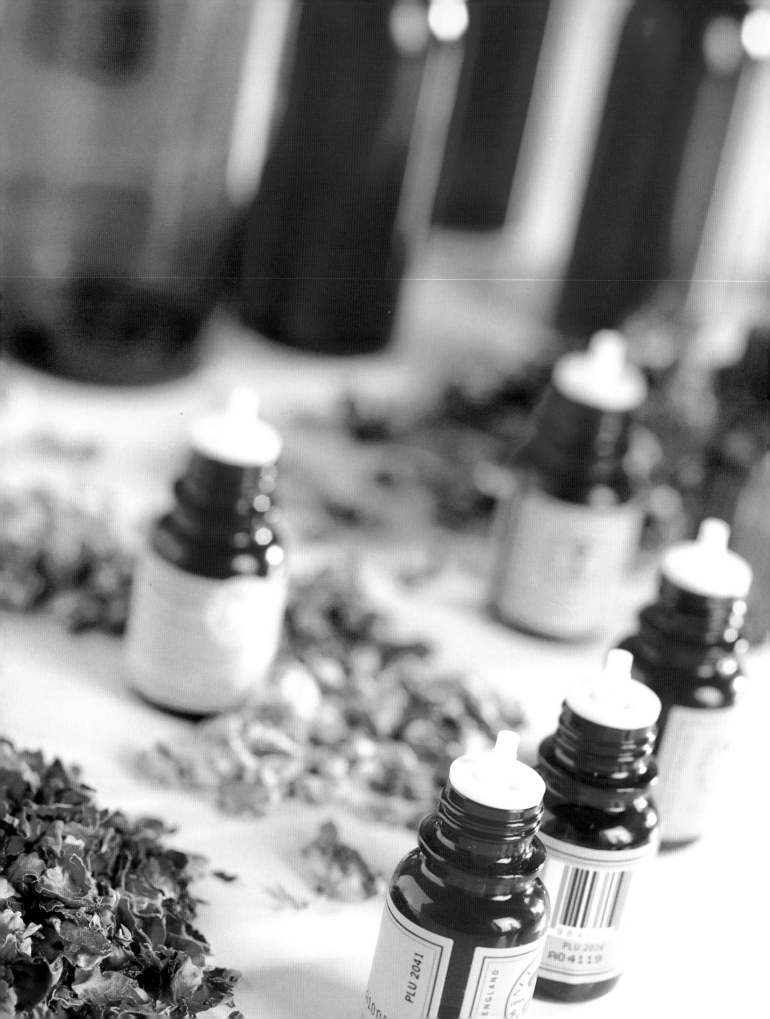

using essential oils

Essential oils have been used for cosmetic, perfumery and therapeutic purposes for thousands of years. They are an invaluable part of today's food and flavouring industry and in more recent years have also been incorporated into a wide range of commercial household and pharmaceutical products. Peppermint oil, for example, is used in confectionery, drinks, washing-up liquid, air fresheners, toothpaste, shaving foam and indigestion tablets, to name but a few. Many of the recipes in this book use essential oils both for fragrancing and for their therapeutic properties. These pages show how to choose, use and store the oils, and how they work.

Aromatherapy as we know it today has been developed during this century, originally by a small number of researchers investigating the antiseptic properties of essential oils. These became particularly important during the First World War, when certain oils were widely used to treat trench foot and infected wounds. One of these researchers was the Frenchman René-Maurice Gattefossé, who, in the 1920s, became the first person to use the word 'aromatherapie'.

In the 1960s aromatherapy was introduced to Britain by a remarkable woman called Marguerite Maury. In France, Maury developed a system of aromatherapy that utilized both the medicinal properties of essential oils and their ability to rejuvenate the skin and maintain a youthful appearance. She then set up a clinic in England and began to teach her system to beauty therapists, who became the first generation of holistic aromatherapists in Europe.

One of the areas that aromatherapists have researched is the method of absorption of essential oils into the body. Gattefossé discovered that it takes between 30 minutes and 12 hours for an essential oil to be absorbed into the various systems of the body after it has been massaged on to the skin. Since then, tests have shown that essential oil molecules can be detected in urine only an hour after the oil has been rubbed on to the back of the hand. A simple test that you can do yourself is to rub a sliced garlic clove on to the soles of a friend's foot; after about 30 minutes you will be able to smell the essential oil from the garlic on his or her breath.

Most essential oils should be diluted before being applied to the skin, although there are a few exceptions. These include lavender, jasmine, neroli, sandalwood and rose, which can generally be used neat as a perfume. Furthermore, some wonderful blends can be made using these particular oils. Lavender and tea tree can be applied neat as a remedy for insect bites and minor burns, and also to disinfect wounds.

how do essential oils work?

The use of essential oils is one of the fastest-growing forms of natural medicine and is indeed an excellent example of a holistic approach to health – first because essential oils can be used to treat the whole person, body, mind and spirit, and second because, unlike conventional medicine, which targets drugs to eradicate a particular disease process, the oils may have a specific action on a disease process but will also support and strengthen the person to throw off the disease. Tea tree oil, for example, will have a direct anti-viral effect on the common cold virus and will also act as an immuno-stimulant, encouraging the body itself to fight the infection.

When choosing an essential oil, either for yourself or for someone else, it is important to consider the specific physical properties of the oil, along with its more profound characteristics. Look closely at the oils' physiological, psychological and spiritual properties, bearing in mind that each of these areas are active simultaneously in all individuals.

Choose an oil that seems to offer the greatest benefits on all levels. Pine oil, for example, is an excellent respiratory antiseptic and decongestant, useful for the treatment of bronchitis. In addition, it is stimulating and refreshing – particularly useful for general feelings of fatigue. The psychological profile of pine oil is suited to those who are emotionally closed and suffer feelings of guilt. Using pine oil will help to revive and refresh the body, dispersing rigidity and guilt, and allow sensitivity and openness to be better expressed.

mind and body

An essential oil is composed of individual chemical constituents that, in combination, provide its physiological properties. Rosemary oil, for example, is known to have among its properties those of being antiseptic, antispasmodic, carminative and stimulant. This indicates that it will be useful for treating infections, period pains, flatulence and tiredness.

During the early part of this century, scientists believed that if the chemical constituents thought to be primarily responsible for certain properties were isolated they could be concentrated and rendered even more effective. The constituent could then be synthesized, thus becoming much cheaper to produce than an essential oil. Thymol, for example, a constituent

of thyme oil, was used for many years as a disinfectant in hospitals and surgical wards.

It is now becoming more generally appreciated that an essential oil is a very complex combination of hundreds of different constituents and that many of these individual constituents work synergistically together. This means that the combination of constituents as found in an essential oil is more effective and more appropriate in use than an isolated constituent. For example, it has now been discovered that thyme oil is effective against a much wider variety of pathogens than thymol (its main constituent) and, when used at normal aromatherapy dilutions, is much less likely to be an irritant when applied to the skin. Indeed, most essential oils are better tolerated than their isolated components, which tend to be very much more aggressive in action than a complete essential oil.

This is not to say that essential oils are not toxic – several that are safe to use externally are toxic when taken internally, for example, eucalyptus. Others are safe to use at normal dilutions but are likely to irritate the skin if not diluted before use. There are even some oils that are so toxic they are not available, such as wintergreen. This means that a user of essential oils needs to learn about them in order to employ them with confidence.

An interest in the chemistry of essential oils can be a very useful basis for understanding both the likely properties of an essential oil and any potential toxicity it may have. In France, a system of using essential oils known as clinical aromatherapy has been developed. This is practised by doctors who have acquired a

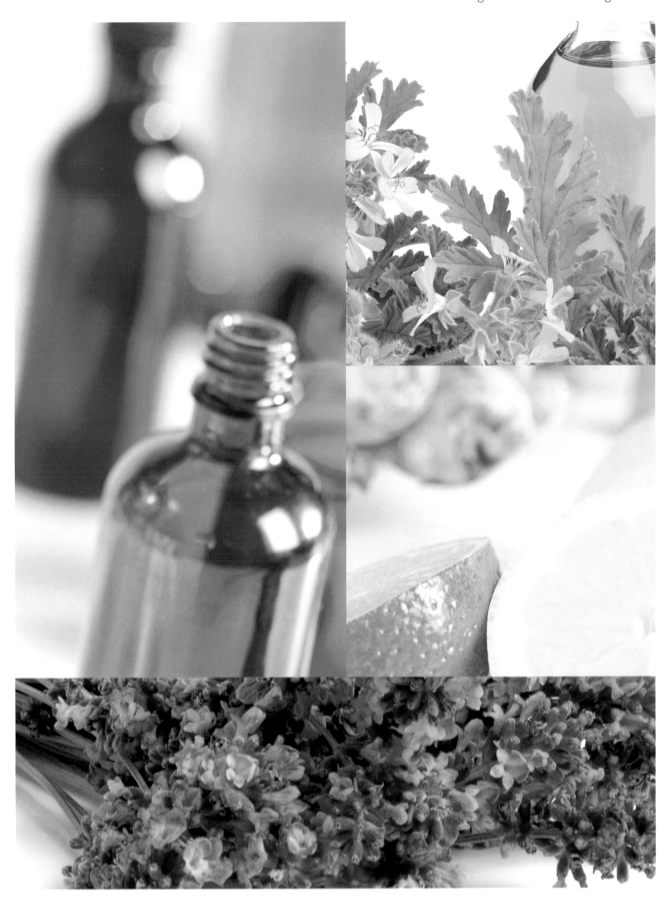

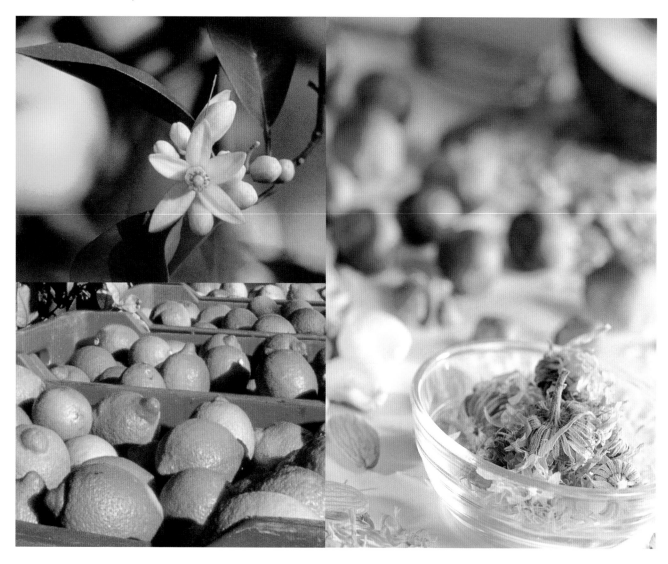

thorough understanding of the physiological properties of essential oils, and who are thus able to prescribe them internally for specific physical ailments.

While the physiological properties are very varied, there are several main areas of action for which essential oils have established their deserved reputation. The first of these is their antiseptic action: all essential oils are antibacterial, although each oil is effective against different pathogens. There have been hundreds of laboratory tests which have shown just how effective these oils can be against bacterial, viral, fungal and parasitic infection. Tea tree oil, for example, is effective against streptococcus, gonococcus, pneumococcus, candida albicans, trichomonas vaginalis, herpes simplex, wart virus and scabies, among others. Some clinics, particularly in France, will culture bacteria

taken from a site of infection and expose them to different essential oils to see which oil is most effective against the particular pathogens involved. This process is known as creating an aromatogram. A study in 1971 showed that lemongrass oil was more effective against *Staphyloccocus aureus* (associated with many skin infections) than penicillin and streptomycin.

Essential oils are known to stimulate the immune response and thereby aid the body in fighting infection. All essential oils stimulate phagocytosis, or the ability of white blood cells to dispose of invading bacteria. For example, thyme oil and tea tree oil have been used to benefit people suffering with HIV-related diseases, as they are both strongly antiseptic and excellent immuno-stimulants, as well as being powerful germicides. Many essential oils have a blood purifying action that works by stimulating the various processes of elimination. This cleansing action means that toxins and metabolic residues which may otherwise lead to a variety of diseases are removed from the system, an effect that is very beneficial in many chronic diseases such as arthritis, as well as helping to reduce cellulite and clear skin problems. Good examples of detoxifying oils include juniper and rosemary.

A further physiological action of essential oils is upon the endocrine system. This is a group of glands that produce hormones and regulate reproduction, growth, metabolism, our response to stress and the levels of various vital nutrients in the bloodstream. Some essential oils contain phytohormones or 'plant hormones', which act within the body in a similar manner to our own hormones. Phytohormones can reinforce or replace the effects of the corresponding human hormones. Fennel oil, for example, contains a plant oestrogen which stimulates the production of breast milk and can be beneficial in treating symptoms of premenstrual tension.

Other essential oils influence the hormone secretion of certain endocrine glands. For example, rosemary oil has a stimulating action on the adrenal cortex, and will help to increase vitality; rose oil has an effect on many of the hormones involved in reproduction and is an excellent treatment for many menstrual and menopausal disorders; while geranium oil tends to have a balancing effect on the endocrine system in general and can help to redress an excess or deficit of various hormones.

The endocrine system is a two-way link between our body and our emotions: our hormone secretions affect our moods (such as in premenstrual tension), and our moods affect our hormone secretions (for example, when a sudden shock or fright triggers the secretion of adrenaline). This is why essential oils, by having a therapeutic action on our endocrine system, can have a beneficial effect on both our body and our emotions.

Essential oils also have a beneficial effect on our well-being by virtue of their action on the nervous system. Much research has been done to illustrate the sedating or calming properties of certain essential oils such as lavender and neroli, and the stimulating properties of oils such as rosemary. These essential oils have been shown to have a measurable effect on brain activity. Here lies part of the reason why aromatherapy has such wonderful results in the treatment of people who are suffering from stress. Another important factor here is the many benefits that will be obtained through receiving a therapeutic massage from an aromatherapist; it is true of many conditions, and stress-related ones especially, that much may be gained from the healing touch of the experienced masseur.

body energy

Another interesting way in which essential oils bring their healing properties to the individual is through their action on what is often called the 'qi' or energy system of the body. The 'qi' as it is known to the Chinese, or 'prana' to the Indians, or 'vital force' in the language of homoeopaths, is becoming understood more generally as the electromagnetic field that radiates from the body and gives dynamism and integrity to a living being; when someone dies, their electromagnetic field disintegrates.

In a healthy person, the picture of their electromagnetic field, as shown by Kirlian photography, extends well beyond their physical form and looks vibrant and colourful. In a tired or sick person, however, the electromagnetic field is weak and dull. Essential oils have been shown by the Italian researcher Professor Rovesti and others to have an influence on cellular magnetic fields, and thus their use actually has a direct effect on the dynamic energy system that integrates life itself.

Having considered some of the measurable effects of essential oils, it should be realized that one of the great things about aromatherapy is that it is about pleasure as well as healing. When choosing an essential oil for a treatment, it is important to make sure its odour is pleasing to the recipient. Part of the benefit of using an essential oil will come from enjoying it, and that is also one of the ways that essential oils can enhance our feeling of well-being. Some essential oils, such as jasmine, are appreciated by most people, whereas others (patchouli being a prime example) provoke a more extreme reaction, being loved by some but heartily disliked by others.

how oils enter the body

The quickest way of drawing an essential oil into the system is by inhalation through the nose. When an odorous vapour is inhaled (for example, by wafting a tissue with a few drops of eucalyptus oil on it under the nose) the vapour is warmed and mixed with water vapour from the mucous membrane in the nasal cavity. The vapour molecules are then diffused over hundreds of microscopic hairs called cilia which are located in the olfactory organ at the root of the nose. Particular cilia are stimulated by different odours and a nervous impulse is sent to the adjacent olfactory bulb and then straight to the hypothalamus and limbic portions of the brain. (This part of the brain is the seat of the emotions, which explains why certain smells affect our moods and stir our memories so profoundly.) Neurochemicals are then released which are passed on, via the nervous system, to the rest of the body.

Inhaled essential oils will also pass into the lungs via the trachea and the bronchi, and from there into the bronchioles and eventually to the microscopic alveoli, where gaseous exchange with the blood takes place. The circulatory system will then transport them around the rest of the body.

There are a number of ways in which you can apply essential oils to the skin. Essential oil molecules are minute and penetrate the skin by diffusing through the hair follicles and sweat glands. They also permeate between the skin cells by combining with the skin's lipids (fats) and thereby enter the dermis (the layer of skin beneath the epidermis). Once in the dermis they can enter the blood capillaries and lymph vessels, which then transport them around the rest of the body by the circulatory systems.

absorbing oils through the skin

Exactly how much of an essential oil applied to the skin is absorbed into the body is variable, and depends on the particular oil being used, on the type of carrier – whether oil or water – on the temperature of the surrounding air and of the oil itself, as warmth increases absorption.

One of the main functions of the skin is as an organ of protection for the body, and this makes it particularly suitable as a route for the intake of essential oils, because the skin contains enzymes that can break down or inactivate several of the more potentially toxic constituents of the oils.

(There is no such protective system when the oils are taken internally – see below.) The layers of the skin also act as a kind of reservoir for essential oils, which are then 'time-released' into the circulatory system. This means that essential oils are released into the body more slowly via the skin than if they are taken internally.

taking oils internally

Taking essential oils internally can be extremely effective in the treatment of certain ailments and diseases. However, they should only be used in this way if they are specifically prescribed by a qualified medical practitioner who is specially trained in the oral administration of essential oils. The same is true for rectal administration and vaginal douches: the mucous membranes of these areas are so delicate that these methods of application should be supervised by experienced practitioners. (See also information on safety on pages 56–7, and the safety notes on individual oils.)

When taken internally, essential oils are absorbed through the gastrointestinal tract straight into the bloodstream and then on to the liver, in some cases causing liver failure. Oral administration of essential oils means that the entire dose is released into the system at once. One result of this is that any toxicity is most hazardous if the oil is taken internally; there is also the risk of irritation and damage to the lining of the gastrointestinal tract.

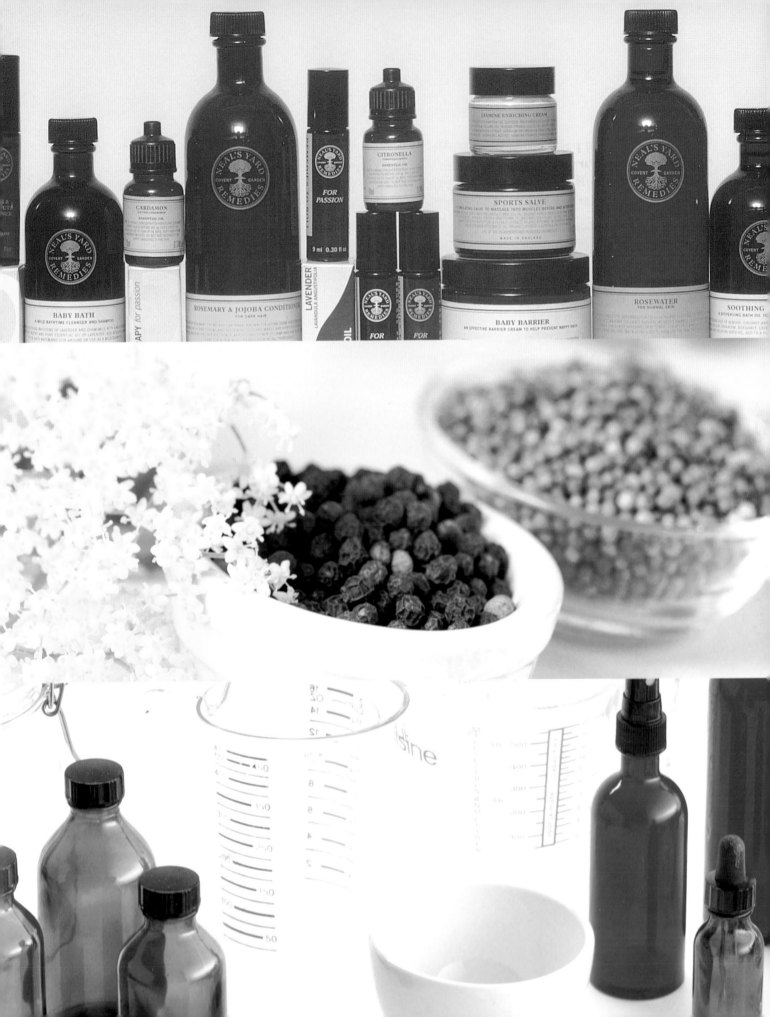

safety

When properly diluted and used with common sense, essential oils are safe, pleasurable and therapeutic and can greatly enhance a healthy lifestyle. They are, however, extremely concentrated plant essences and need to be treated with respect. Never apply any oils except those you know to be totally non-toxic and non-irritant directly to the skin without diluting first as detailed in this book. Do not take essential oils internally without supervision from an experienced and qualified practitioner. Do learn about the individual oils and use them cautiously at first and then with more confidence as your experience and knowledge grow.

Always do a patch test before using a new oil, particularly if you have sensitive skin. Apply the diluted oil to a small patch of skin on the inner wrist or elbow and wait for an hour to check that no irritation or redness develops before using the oil more widely. If any adverse reaction at all develops after using a particular essential oil, discontinue its use immediately. It is possible to develop a sensitivity to any substance, including an essential oil, even after you have used it many times before.

The following guidelines will help you to use the oils discussed in this book safely, however, if you have a professional interest in aromatherapy, we would recommend that you read *Essential Oil Safety* by Robert Tisserand and Tony Balacs, a useful and detailed book (see list of further reading on pages 249–50).

accidents with essential oils

If you accidentally spill a neat essential oil on your skin, or develop an allergic reaction to an oil, splash plenty of cold water over the area and continue applying cold water for at least 20 minutes. If any irritation remains, consult your health practitioner. If any essential oil gets into the eyes, splash copiously with cold water and get urgent medical help if any redness or irritation persists. Several essential oils that are safe to use externally are toxic if taken internally, for example, tea tree or clove. If poisoning from an essential oil is suspected, telephone a general practitioner or go to the hospital accident and emergency department. If there are any serious signs of poisoning, such as seizures or unconsciousness, or a young child has ingested some essential oil, call the emergency services.

essential oils to avoid

The following essential oils should not be used by anyone. Many are not available as they are already on government 'Poisons Lists' and are not allowed to be sold: armoise, bitter almond, boldo, buchu, cade, calamus, camphor (brown and yellow), cassia, cinnamon bark, costus, elecampane, exotic basil (high estragole), fig leaf, ho leaf (camphor and saffrol chemotypes), horseradish, hyssop, mustard, pennyroyal, sage (Dalmatian), sassafras, tansy, tarragon, thuja, verbena, wintergreen, wormseed, wormwood.

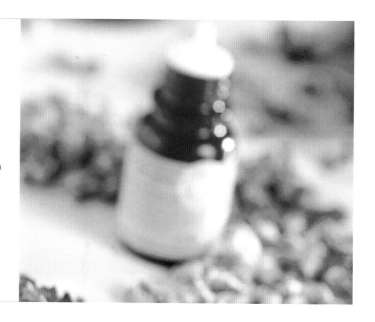

high blood pressure

Certain aromatherapists have suggested that some of the more stimulating essential oils, such as rosemary, should be avoided by people with high blood pressure. There is in fact no evidence to support this view. The only exception is for people who suffer from cardiac fibrillation, who should avoid peppermint oil.

pregnancy

Some people believe that all essential oils should be avoided during pregnancy, but most are perfectly safe to use externally at normal aromatherapy dilutions, and oils such as juniper, marjoram, rose and rosemary can be very helpful in dealing with any problems or discomforts that arise during this time. Mandarin and neroli are the most commonly recommended essential oils to use during pregnancy; they have been included in the massage blend on page 67, which will help to nourish the skin and prevent stretch marks.

babies and children

0–6 months:

The only oils that should be used at this stage are lavender and Roman chamomile. Add 1 drop of essential oil to 10 ml (2 tsp) of sweet almond oil or jojoba oil for a massage, or use in a room fragrancer.

6–12 months:

Use only chamomile and Roman chamomile, lavender, mandarin, neroli and rose.

1–6 years:

Use only chamomile and Roman chamomile, coriander, lavender, mandarin, neroli, orange, palmarosa, rose, rosewood and tea tree.

7–12 years:

Use essential oils as indicated in this book, but avoid basil. Quarter the dosage given for adults of all the oils.

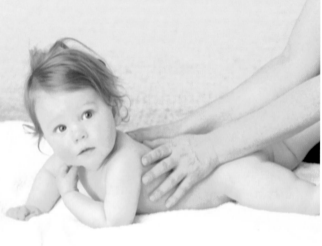

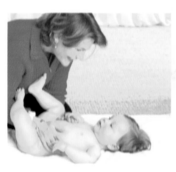

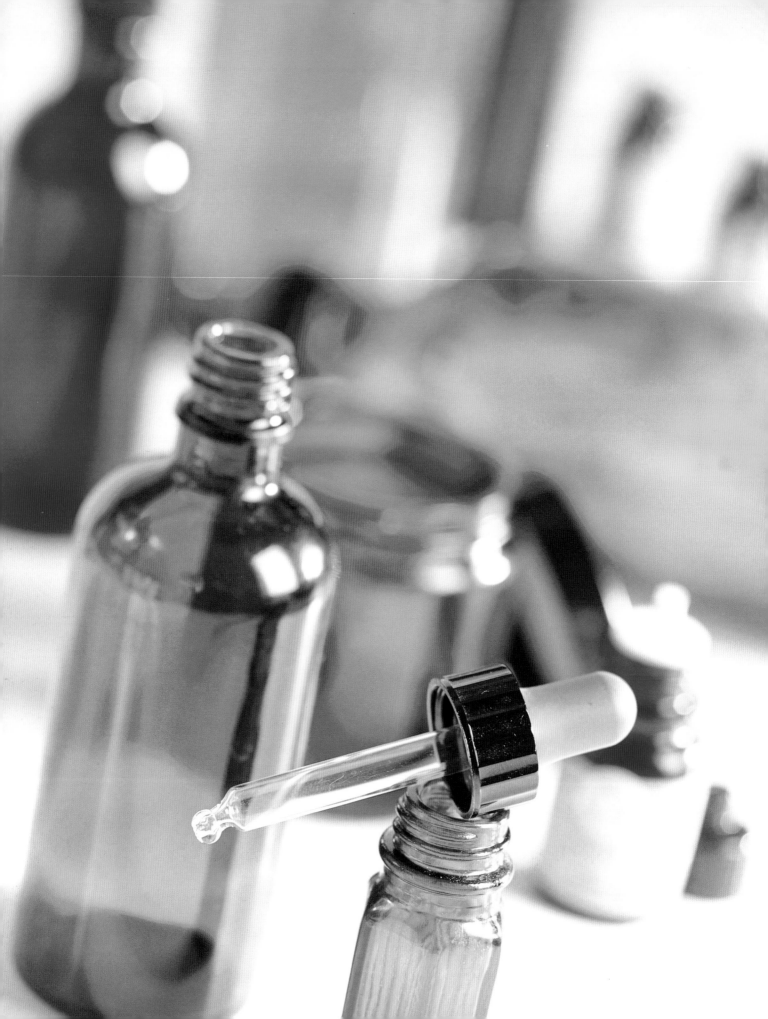

blending essential oils

All essential oils can be blended to create new combinations. Recommendations of oils that combine well are given in the oil profiles on pages 164–205, and recipes of favourite blends are contained on pages 63–7 – use the ideas as a starting point and experiment to create your own blends. Most essential oils need to be diluted in a base oil before being applied to the skin; following are details of the best base oils to use. Remember, blending is an art, requiring a combination of technique and creative flair.

base oils

Base oils, or carrier oils, are used as a medium in which to dilute the essential oils before applying them to the skin. There are a number of base oils that are suitable, all with slightly different properties. Use only vegetable, nut or seed oils as mineral oil tends to block the pores and is not as readily absorbed. Wherever possible buy machine-expressed or cold-pressed oils in preference to heat- or solvent-extracted oils as the former will retain more of the plant nutrients. Some organically produced oils are also available, and these are free of biocide and synthetic fertilizer residues.

Macerated oils can also make an excellent base for the addition of essential oils. These are plant oils, such as sunflower or olive, that have had a herb steeped in them so that the properties of the herb are infused into the oil. See pages 40–1 on making macerated oils.

All base oils should be as fresh as possible. Any oil that smells rancid or is more than two years old should not be used.

almond oil (sweet)

One of the most popular of all the base oils, almond is a nearly odourless, fairly light oil that is readily absorbed by the skin. It has a soothing effect and is well tolerated by most skin types, although sensitization is possible. It makes a good general-purpose massage base. Almond oil is usually available cold-pressed, when it contains vitamins A, B1, B2, B6 and a small amount of vitamin E.

apricot kernel oil

Apricot kernel oil is a light and odourless oil similar in properties to almond. Being light, it is suitable for applying to the face and other areas of delicate skin. It contains vitamin A and some B group vitamins.

arnica oil

This is a macerated oil made with the herb *Arnica montana*, which is renowned for its therapeutic properties. It is excellent for treating bruises, bumps, aches and pains, over-exertion, backache, injuries, strains and sprains. However, do not use arnica oil on broken skin.

avocado oil

Avocado is a thick green oil when cold-pressed, more viscous and pale yellow when heat-extracted. Cold-pressed avocado oil is rich in nutrients (vitamins A, B and D and lecithin) and keeps fairly well. It is excellent for dry and ageing skin. Because of its viscosity it should be used as part of a massage base blend, for example 10–25 per cent in a lighter base oil such as almond.

calendula oil

This is a macerated oil containing the herb marigold (*Calendula officinalis*), which has excellent healing and anti-inflammatory properties. Calendula oil is suitable for any damaged skin, especially wounds, ulcers, bed sores, eczema, scars, and chapped and cracked skin. It will also help to prevent stretch marks during pregnancy and may be massaged on to sore nipples. It may be used on its own or blended with other base oils.

carrot oil

Carrot oil is a nourishing orange-coloured oil made by blending carrot extract with a vegetable oil. It is rich in beta-carotene and vitamins B, C, D and E. This oil is excellent for prematurely ageing, inflamed, damaged or scarred skin. When buying it, check that it is in fact made from carrots as commercial carrot oil is often produced from *Tagetes* flowers instead. The orange colour of carrot oil can stain the skin and clothing, so allow plenty of time for the oil to be absorbed before getting dressed, or use in a partial dilution with other base oils.

coconut oil

Coconut oil is solid at room temperature but liquefies at body heat, so before use melt it by warming it in your hand or on a radiator. It is traditionally used for dry skin and especially for hair and scalp treatments. You can melt the coconut oil, add the essential oils and stir before allowing the oil to set again so that you can use a little of the prepared oil as required.

comfrey oil

This is a macerated oil using the herb comfrey (*Symphytum officinale*), renowned for its healing properties. Comfrey oil is excellent for treating scars, rheumatism and arthritis, aches and pains, broken bones, bruises, wounds and burns.

evening primrose oil

Evening primrose oil is rich in linoleic acid and also contains gamma linoleic acid (GLA) and other vitamins and minerals. It is excellent in the treatment of eczema, psoriasis and dry and ageing skin but is rather expensive. Use as 10 per cent or more of a base oil blend.

grapeseed oil

Grapeseed is a light and odourless oil that is particularly suitable for the massage of oily skin. It contains linoleic acid and a small amount of vitamin E. It can be blended or used as a 100 per cent base oil.

hazelnut oil

A rich and nourishing oil that has a pleasant nutty smell. It contains oleic acid, linoleic acid, vitamins and minerals. Hazelnut oil is particularly useful for treating acne and scarred or ageing skin. It may be used as part of a blend or as a 100 per cent base oil.

jojoba oil

This is not actually an oil but a liquid wax. It is stable and keeps well, but is rather expensive. Jojoba oil combines readily with sebum and is highly penetrative. It is a balancing oil, good for treating acne and oily skin as well as dry and dehydrated skin. It is also anti-inflammatory and may be used for the treatment of eczema and psoriasis.

olive oil

As well as being a culinary oil, olive oil has been used for centuries for cosmetic and therapeutic purposes. It is particularly beneficial for treating rheumatism, aches and pains and dry or inflamed skin. Cold-pressed olive oil is rich in a number of vitamins and minerals. Because it is rather thick and green, it is more pleasant to use if diluted 10–50 per cent with other base oils.

St John's wort oil

A macerated oil made with St John's wort herb (*Hypericum perforatum*), which has antiseptic, healing and pain-relieving properties. It has the ability to soothe nerve pain and is excellent for treating sciatica, backache, neuralgia, lumbago and shingles; it may also be used for damaged skin, burns, wounds and ulcers. Good-quality St John's wort oil is traditionally made using olive oil and should be a beautiful deep red colour.

sunflower oil

This is a pleasant, light oil that is available organically produced and cold-pressed. It is often used as the base for good-quality macerated oils. Cold-pressed sunflower oil contains vitamins A, B, D and E. It makes an excellent massage oil base.

wheatgerm oil

Wheatgerm is a thick, amber-coloured oil that if unrefined is naturally rich in vitamin E. It is suitable for dry, damaged, ageing or scarred skin and will help to prevent stretch marks during pregnancy. Wheatgerm oil is rather viscous so should be blended with other lighter base oils at a dilution of 10–20 per cent. Despite the anti-oxidant properties of vitamin E, wheatgerm oil tends to deteriorate quickly so should be used within 12 months of purchase.

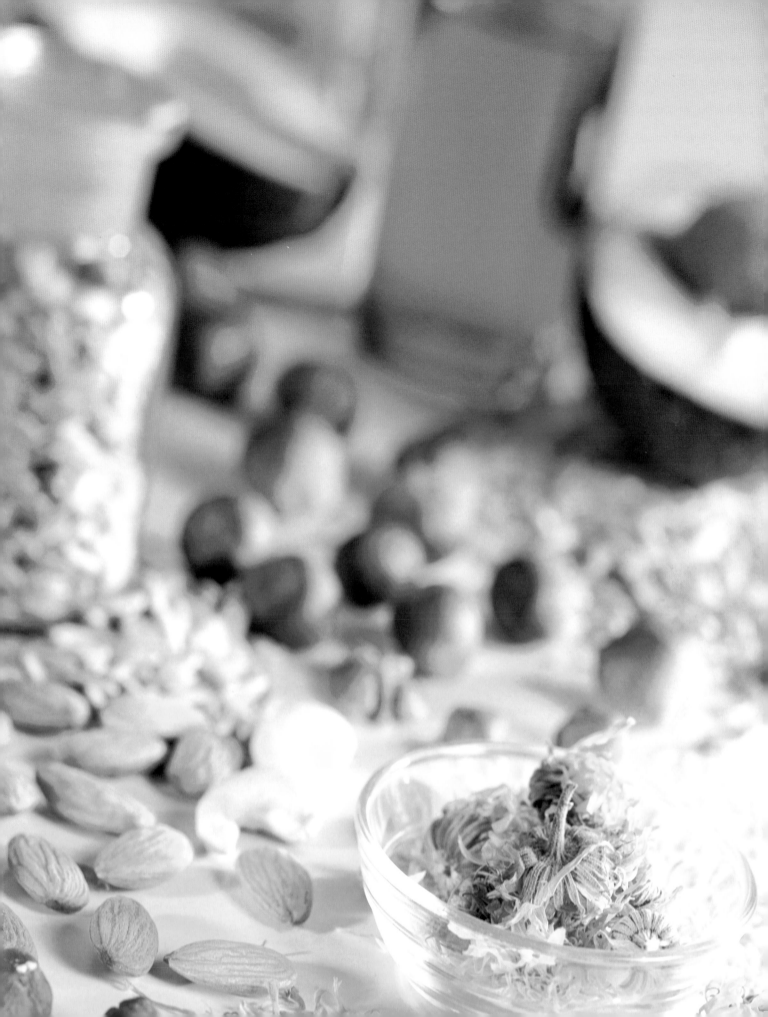

essential oil blends

Some favourite recipes are given here for you to follow, but once you are a little more confident you should begin to experiment – it will help you to learn about the oils as well as giving you the opportunity to make a unique oil combination of your own.

blending

When blending oils yourself, bear in mind the following guidelines:

- Blending is an art, and like all arts it is a combination of technique and creative flair.
- The most pleasing blend is likely to have a balance of what perfumers call 'base', 'middle' and 'top' notes. Base notes have a deep, rich smell, for example sandalwood, vetiver and ylang-ylang. Middle notes include most of the floral smells such as geranium and lavender. Top notes have a light, refreshing smell, such as is found in the citrus oils.
- Do not use too many essential oils in any one blend – between four and seven is usually about right.
- If you spoil a blend by a poor combination it is unlikely that you will be able to correct your mistake; it is better to start again.

- Make a record of your blends as you go along; smell, evaluate and write a comment after each addition of an oil.
- Less is more; just two drops of an essential oil can transform a blend.
- If you like a blend you are more likely to use it; be good to yourself.
- Most people find blending easier if it is done into an odourless base oil such as almond. Try using 30 ml/1 fl oz/2 tbsp of base oil. Assuming that 20 drops of essential oil is 1 ml, making a 2 per cent massage blend will require 12 drops of combined essential oil (blends should be 1–3 per cent).
- Make your blend in a small beaker, a tea cup or a wide-necked bottle.
- Once complete, store your blend in a glass bottle and label with the details of the mixture (or a name) and the date that you made it.

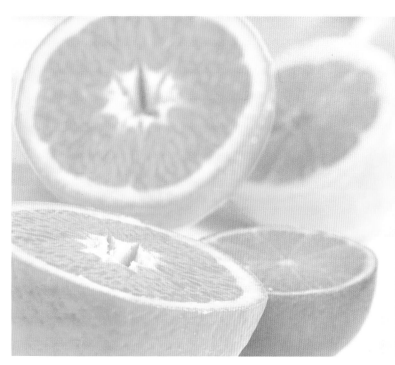
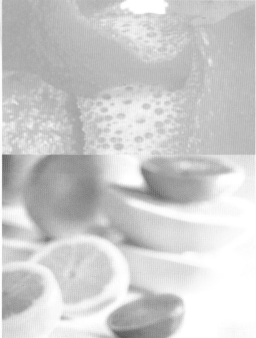

sensual massage oil – feminine

A relaxing and fragrant blend of oils, this is an ideal massage oil.

2 drops bergamot essential oil
4 drops geranium essential oil
6 drops lavender essential oil
4 drops marjoram essential oil

Add these oils to 30 ml (2 tbsp) almond oil for an excellent general massage oil. For a bath oil, double the amounts of the essential oils and mix with 30 ml (2 tbsp) almond oil, using 10 ml (2 tsp) for each bath. Or, mix the essential oils into an empty 10 ml (2 tsp) bottle, adding a few drops at a time to an essential oil burner to fragrance the room.

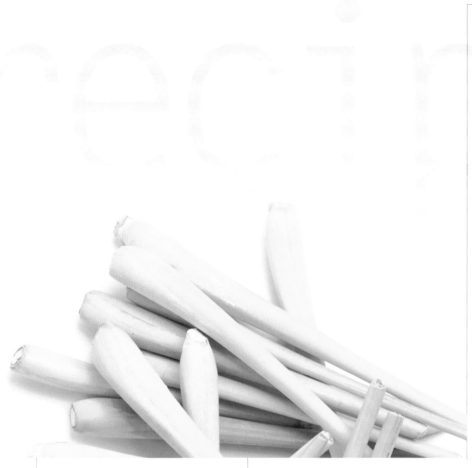

stimulating sports oil

An excellent rubbing oil to help with the warm-up process or to relieve over-exertion after sport. Rub into areas of muscle, paying particular attention to any painful areas, before and after activity.

1 drop ginger essential oil
4 drops lavender essential oil
3 drops lemongrass essential oil
4 drops rosemary essential oil
3 drops vetiver essential oil

Add to a base of 10 ml (2 tsp) arnica oil and 25 ml (5 tsp) almond oil.

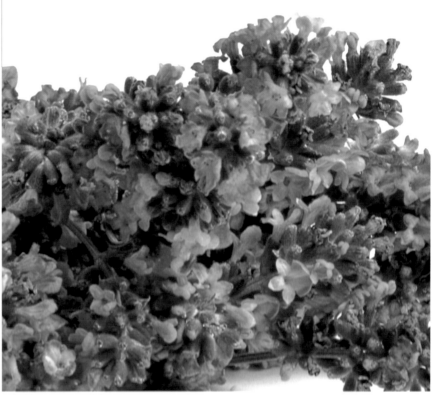

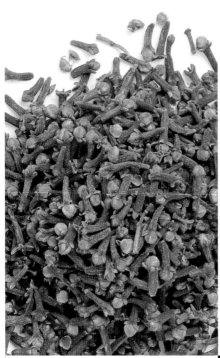

sensual massage oil – masculine

A fragrant, aphrodisiac blend of oils excellent for a sensual massage.

4 drops cedarwood essential oil
2 drops frankincense essential oil
2 drops orange essential oil
8 drops sandalwood essential oil
2 drops vetiver essential oil
2 drops ylang-ylang essential oil

Add to a base of 30 ml (2 tbsp) almond or grapeseed oil.

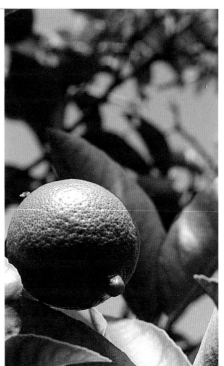

focus the mind

An excellent aid to concentration and memory. Use when studying for exams, for example, or during meditation.

4 drops cedarwood essential oil
1 drop clove essential oil
6 drops frankincense essential oil
2 drops lemon essential oil
2 drops orange essential oil
2 drops rosemary essential oil

Add to 30 ml (2 tbsp) almond oil and use as a massage oil. Alternatively, mix the essential oils into an empty 10 ml (2 tsp) bottle and add a few drops at a time to an essential oil burner.

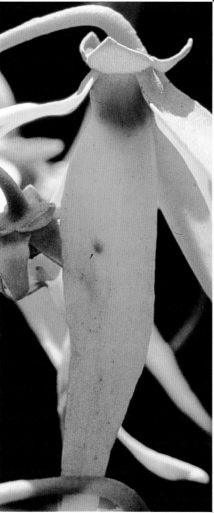

relaxing blend

A relaxing and fragrant blend of oils, this is ideal to use for general massage.

2 drops bergamot essential oil
4 drops geranium essential oil
6 drops lavender essential oil
4 drops marjoram essential oil

Add these oils to 30 ml (2 tbsp) almond oil for an excellent general massage oil. For a bath oil, double the amounts of the essential oils and mix with 30 ml (2 tbsp) almond oil; add 10 ml (2 tsp) to each bath. Mix the essential oils into an empty 10 ml (2 tsp) bottle and add a few drops at a time to an essential oil burner to fragrance the room.

nerve soother

A soothing blend of oils that will help relieve nerve tissue damage or sensitivity caused by sciatica or shingles.

    4 drops lavender essential oil
    1 drop melissa essential oil
    2 drops sandalwood
        essential oil
    2 drops Roman chamomile
        essential oil

Add the mixture to 15 ml (3 tsp) St John's wort oil, 5 ml (1 tsp) calendula oil and 10 ml (2 tsp) almond oil. Dab on to sensitive areas or mix with warm water to apply as a compress.

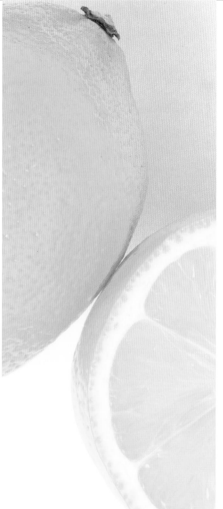

rheumatism blend

A warming blend of oils to relieve stiffness and pain in inflamed muscles and joints. Also use for sprains, strains and backache.

    2 drops cypress essential oil
    3 drops ginger essential oil
    4 drops juniper essential oil
    4 drops lavender essential oil
    2 drops pine essential oil

Add to a mixture of 10 ml (2 tsp) comfrey oil and 25 ml (5 tsp) almond oil and massage into painful areas. To make a bath oil, double the quantity of essential oils and add to the same mixture of base oils; add 10 ml (2 tsp) to each bath. For a compress, mix the oils in an empty bottle and add 4–6 drops to a bowl of warm water.

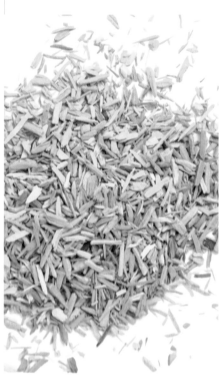

lung decongestant

    3 drops pine essential oil
    3 drops cedarwood essential oil
    2 drops lemon essential oil
    2 drops cypress essential oil
    3 drops ravensara essential oil

Add the mixture to 30 ml (6 tsp) seje oil and massage into the chest area, or put 8–10 drops in hot water and use to inhale the vapours. The mixture can also be used in a diffuser to fragrance the air.

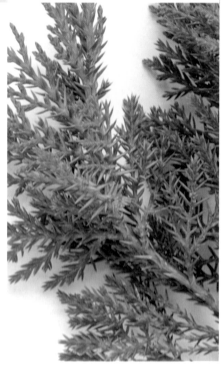

stress-reliever

A soothing and uplifting blend of essential oils guaranteed to relieve feelings of stress.

2 drops basil essential oil
4 drops clary sage essential oil
4 drops lavender essential oil
4 drops neroli essential oil
2 drops palmarosa essential oil

Add to 30 ml (2 tbsp) almond oil as a massage oil. For a bath oil, double the quantities of essential oils and add to 30 ml (2 tbsp) almond oil; add 10 ml (2 tsp) to each bath. Mix the essential oils into an empty 10 ml (2 tsp) bottle and add a few drops at a time to an essential oil burner to fragrance the room.

detox blend

A detoxifying oil blend that will help stimulate the lymphatic system and break down cellulite.

2 drops black pepper
    essential oil
2 drops cypress essential oil
2 drops frankincense
    essential oil
6 drops geranium essential oil
2 drops grapefruit essential oil
4 drops juniper essential oil
2 drops sandalwood essential oil

Add to 30 ml (2 tbsp) almond oil and massage into areas of cellulite on a daily basis.

immuno-stimulant blend

A blend to stimulate the immune system and help fight off any infection, especially colds, flu or coughs.

4 drops lavender essential oil
2 drops lemon essential oil
4 drops pine essential oil
6 drops tea tree essential oil
1 drop thyme essential oil

Add to 30 ml (2 tbsp) almond oil and use as a massage oil for over the kidney area or as a chest rub. Alternatively, put the blend in a 10 ml (2 tsp) bottle and add 4–6 drops to a footbath or use as a steam inhalation.

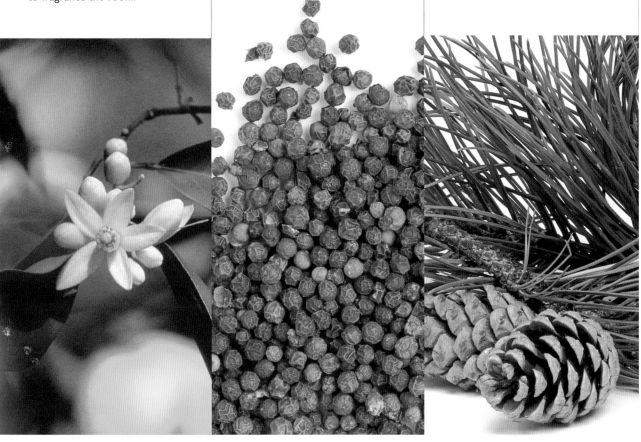

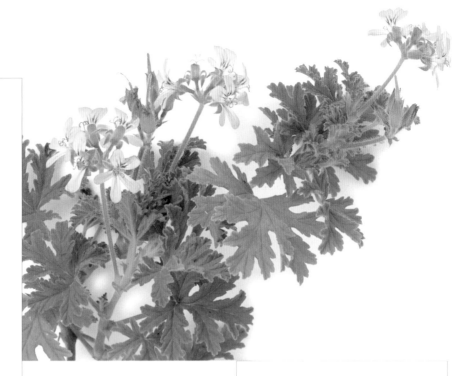

constipation blend

A blend to stimulate the gut and relieve occasional constipation.

2 drops black pepper
    essential oil
2 drops fennel essential oil
2 drops geranium essential oil
3 drops grapefruit essential oil
3 drops orange essential oil

Add to 30 ml (2 tbsp) olive oil (which itself has a laxative action) or almond oil. Massage into the abdomen with the flat of the hand using clockwise circular movements for 2–3 minutes.

pregnancy blend

A simple and non-toxic blend of oils that will nourish and promote suppleness of the skin, and help to prevent stretch marks.

5 drops mandarin essential oil
5 drops neroli essential oil

Add to a mixture of 10 ml (2 tsp) wheatgerm oil and 30 ml (2 tbsp) almond oil, or to 30 ml (2 tbsp) calendula macerated oil; massage over thighs, abdomen and breasts.

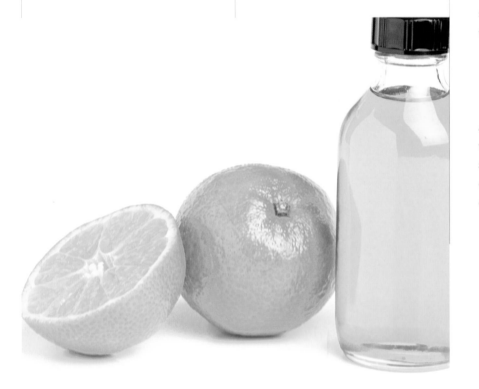

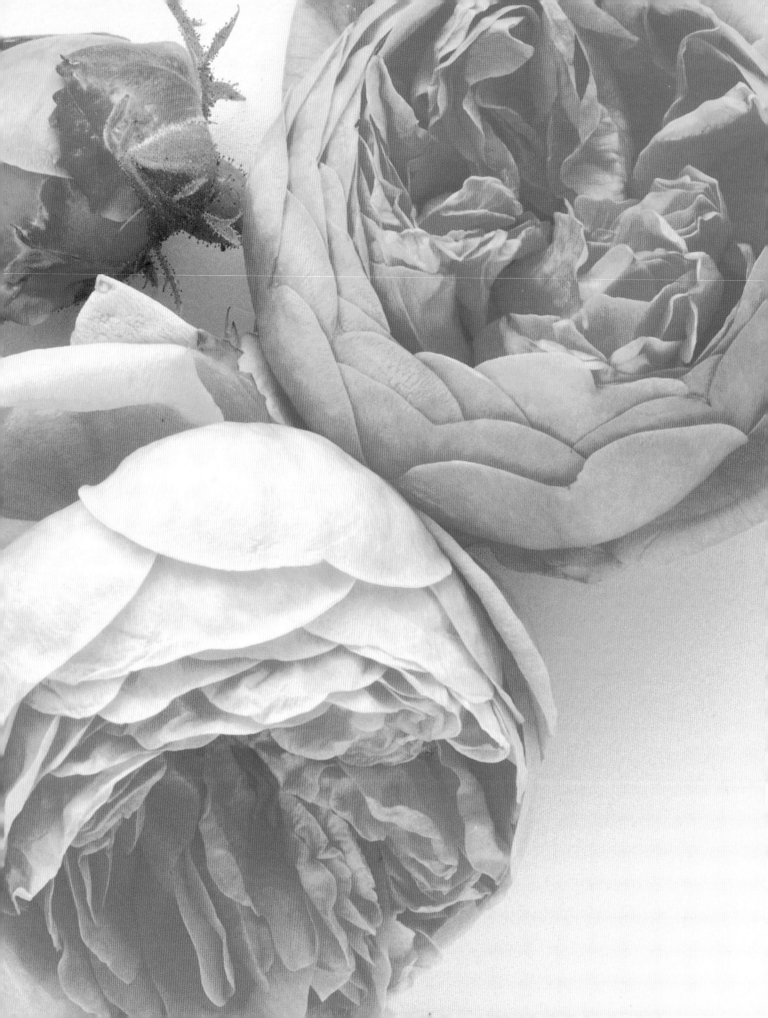

perfumery and fragrancing

Commercial perfume producers may choose from 3,000 individual elements to create a single perfume, but such complexity is not necessary. Using just a few essential oils and learning how to combine the individual fragrances into a subtle, balanced whole is not difficult, with a little practice. Simply refer to the guidelines on the pages that follow, and be prepared to experiment.

We are so accustomed to interpreting the world we live in by what we see and hear that it is easy to underestimate the part played by our sense of smell. We would be surprised to realize how greatly the way we feel about the people we meet and the places we visit is affected by our sense of smell. Our memory stores up associations of fragrances, and the art of fragrancing is to evoke these connections.

As we breathe in air through our noses, fragrant molecules are drawn up past the smell receptor cells, which react to each new odour. This reaction triggers an electrical signal to the part of the brain that is associated with feelings and emotions, so it is not surprising that what we smell connects us to the feelings we associate with it. Research has shown that the aromas of certain essential oils will bring about specific mood changes. We are beginning to see the potential in essential oils for affecting how we feel – the floral oils, for example, have been shown to be mood-enhancing.

We rely more on our olfactory sense than we may first think. As babies, we learn to recognize our mother by her smell. Imagine a warm sunny walk through a meadow and not being able to smell the fresh, green fragrance. Try walking into a coffee shop without the aroma of coffee brewing and freshly cooked pastries! If we were unable to smell, our days would seem drab and dull, and we would feel strangely lost without this sense of connection to our past.

We know that the human ability to distinguish smells is far inferior to that of other animals. For example, the male Emperor moth can detect a female moth over 10 kilometres (6 miles) away; an Alsatian dog has 220 million sense cells in its nose compared to a human with a mere 10 million!

It is interesting that we are largely unaware of our sense of smell and the part that it plays in our lives. We have hardly developed a language to describe what we smell. When it comes to our other senses we have a whole vocabulary to describe what things look like or how they sound, and it is possible that as humans have evolved, the olfactory sense has become less significant. It is known that humans are sexually attracted to each other through the pheromones or body smells that we all possess, but throughout history we have striven to mask these smells and replace them with expensive perfumes, many of which now contain synthetic sexual attractants.

using essential oils in perfumery

The use of oils in perfumery goes back a long way in history. Simple equipment used for making essential oils dating from around 3000 BC has been found in the Indian subcontinent. Oils such as jatamansi and cedarwood were used to excite the senses; eucalyptus was used for its therapeutic properties; olibanum, myrrh and cinnamon were used to raise the level of the soul of the individual and to exalt the spirit. Fragrant oils, waxes and unguents have long been used to enhance the body and add allure. It is said that Cleopatra painted her ship's sails with fragrant oils to attract Mark Antony as he sailed towards her across the Mediterranean. Different religious traditions around the world still burn oils and incense in places of worship.

Towards the end of ancient times, condiments and spices began to be used more and more widely, and trade in these commodities developed around the world. Oils such as ylang-ylang, vetiver and patchouli came to be produced, marking the first stages in perfumery as we know it.

The fragrance of a plant is present in minute glands. If you pick a leaf of peppermint and rub it gently between your finger and thumb the familiar mint smell is released when the cell walls containing volatile oils are broken down. Volatile oils are present in plants for different purposes: for example, eucalyptus has insecticidal properties to protect the plants from being eaten by insects, while roses contain fragrant oils to attract insects so that pollination can occur, and the frankincense tree produces resin to heal wounds or damage to the tree itself.

The volatile oils are found in different parts of the plant – in the flowers of mimosa, rose and ylang-ylang; in the flowers and leaves of peppermint, lavender, rosemary and violet; in the leaves and stems of geranium, thyme and petitgrain; in the bark of cinnamon; in the roots of vetiver and ginger; in the fruits of lemon, lime and bergamot; in the resins of frankincense, myrrh and benzoin; in the seeds of dill, fennel and aniseed; and in the wood of cedar, pine and sandalwood.

Most oils are produced by steam distillation. Water is heated and the rising steam passes into a receptacle containing the plant material. The heat causes the fragile oil sacs to break, and the volatile oil passes into the steam. When the steam cools, reverting to a liquid, the water and oil separate and the oil is drawn off. The water can be used as a flower water or 'hydrolat'. Steam distillation is a very similar process, but the water does not actually touch the plant. This is preferable because the plant is less likely to be damaged.

In the case of citrus fruit, the volatile oil is found in the peel and is extracted by expression after the peel has been removed from the fruit. New types of extraction processes involving carbon dioxide and nitrogen are now being used, and these cause even less damage to the plant and are less energy-consuming. They may be among the extraction processes of the future.

As the art of distilling oils developed, so did the art of fragrancing as we now know it. Grasse, in the south of France, became recognized as the centre of a perfume industry, and oils were produced from locally grown crops such as jasmine, lavender and narcissus. Today, perfume crops are grown and distilled all over the world.

Oils of any one type can vary enormously depending on the variety of the plant, the climate in which it is grown and the way the oil is extracted. The yields can range from plant to plant. Lavender produces around 1 kg (2.2 lb) of oil to 100 kg (220 lb) of flowers and leaves, whereas violets may produce as little as 3 g (less than 1/8 oz) of oil to 100 kg (220 lb) of flowers!

Oils are produced for different purposes, and different qualities are required for the various industries that use them. In the flavouring industry, for example, oils are added to confectionery and other foods. One of the largest crop of oils is peppermint – for example, in the late 1990s over 5,500 tonnes (5,400 tons) of the species *Mentha arvensis* and *Mentha* x *piperita* were produced each year in the USA alone. Incidentally, peppermint oil is also widely used in the pharmaceutical industry.

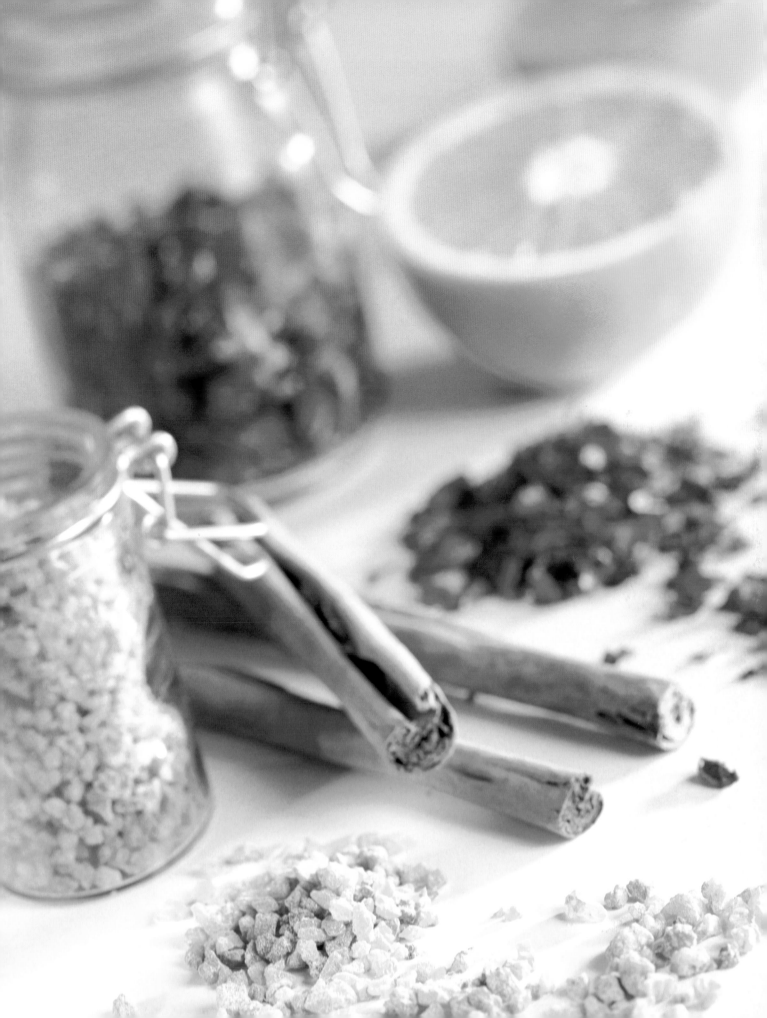

the ingredients you use

Whatever you are making, the ingredients you use will give your product its basic look and fragrance. This is why it is always worth making certain you use good quality ingredients. If, for example, you use cheap malt vinegar in a hair rinse, it is likely to smell like something from a chip shop! Similarly, using over-ripe fruit in a face mask will make the mask less effective, and it will smell less fresh.

It is worthwhile experimenting with your products by varying the ingredients and thus changing the colour, texture and fragrance. Make sure that you have thought through the reason for including each ingredient. It is best to be guided by the properties of the plant, which may appear to be a simple approach, but it seems to be the best policy, and it is certainly what we try to adhere to at Neal's Yard Remedies. In this way, the formulation has a clear function and the fragrance always seems to be appropriate. If the fragrance doesn't seem right, it could quite easily be because one or other of the ingredients is not the best one to use.

base oils

The fragrance of the base oils will vary. Wheatgerm oil has a strong, earthy smell; hazelnut oil gives off a delicious, nutty odour, which can significantly enhance the depth of a fragrance; olive and sesame oils are also distinctive; and oils such as grapeseed, almond and sunflower are lighter. When you are creating your own mixtures, it is probably best, in the first instance, to be guided by the purpose of your creation. Thus, if you want an enriching face cream with a high nutritive base, use oils such as avocado and almond, which will create a base cream that smells rather buttery.

tinctures

The main aroma of tinctures is generally that of alcohol, which will evaporate away, leaving behind the herbal odour. This is not generally very strong and will not tend to dominate a mixture, although tinctures will colour the product.

macerated oils

Generally, these oils have quite a mild fragrance of the particular herb used – unless you are macerating something like garlic! They can be added to a mixture and, in the case of St John's wort or carrot macerates, are more likely to alter the colour than the fragrance.

infusions

An infusion is a water extract of plants, which is similar to a tincture but which will add a mild, herby fragrance to your mixture. Depending on the strength of the infusion and the colour of the plant, the look of the resulting cream or shampoo will vary significantly, much less than the smell, unless you use something like seaweed, which is a wonderful ingredient, rich in minerals, but nevertheless strong smelling!

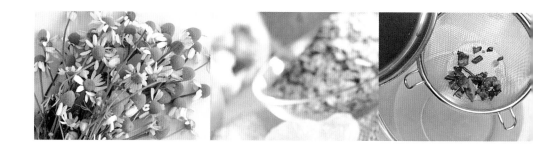

finding the appropriate fragrance

It is worth remembering that we do, in general, have an idea of how things should smell. The science behind fragrancing is to recognize what we expect different products to smell like, and to design a fragrance that is appropriate. Often a fragrance is used to mask unpleasant odours, but this will rarely be the case when you are making simple recipes for your skin and hair, which will, if no essential oils are added, smell of the ingredients, rather than oily or buttery.

Getting to know essential oils by actually using them is the best way to gain the basic memory building blocks. Start by learning about their properties and what contribution they can make to the function of your products.

When you make a product to stimulate and nourish the hair, you would probably expect it to smell rather 'herby'. Rosemary is an excellent essential oil to use for a hair product, but if you had decided to use, say, orange, you might not believe that it was quite as effective, simply from the fragrance, and in this instance, your instinct would be quite correct. Orange, however, blends very well with other oils, notably spicy or sweet oils, to lighten or lift the fragrance. Be guided by its function as a good toning and detoxifying essential oil, which will help you to recognize when to include it. Similarly, when you smell tea tree or eucalyptus in a product, you automatically associate it with an antiseptic function.

the classification of oils

Unlike other senses, the sense of smell does not have many descriptive words connected with it – smells are never big, red or loud! Adjectives like these belong to the vocabulary of the other senses. We tend to describe smells by referring to a past memory or by connecting a smell to something that we feel is similar.

Perfumers have created a language specifically to describe fragrances. They use an analogy with musical notation, referring to levels and types of fragrance as notes. Top notes are seen as being sharp (in Chinese terms 'yin') – for example, bergamot and lemon. In a blend, the smell of these oils will be the first to be perceived and the first to disappear, leaving the next level, or middle notes. This group has a more even, balanced odour. It is the heart of a fragrance, or its deep note, and gives the body of fragrant blend – as with geranium, cinnamon and marjoram, for example. Oils described as having a base note, such as vanilla, vetiver or patchouli, can be used as fixatives. They hold a fragrance together, giving it depth and endurance.

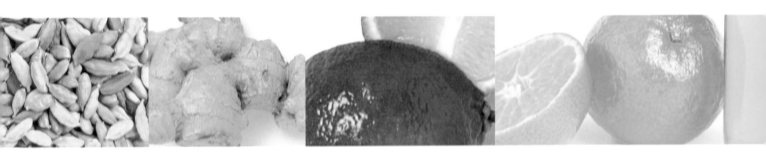

creating a perfume

Creating a balanced perfume requires a blend from each group of oils. A single perfume may be made up of as many as fifty ingredients, which have been selected from the 3,000 that are available, not all of which are natural. Since it was discovered how to create different fragrances using synthetics and extracts from other oils, it is increasingly common to find perfumes with only a small percentage of natural essential oil. In some instances this is a positive development, because in the past, animal extracts were used. Animals such as the civet cat, the musk deer and the beaver suffered in the pursuit of the very expensive ingredients the animals produced.

Perfumes are classified into odour groups. Perfumers will use terms like citrus, woody, green, floral, spicy, amber and leathery to describe a raw material. It is useful to have a basic awareness of these different fragrance classifications so that you can create a balanced fragrance. More important, however, is always to use good quality, reliable ingredients. As you spend more time working with essential oils, you will acquire a memory of them, and then making a fragrance will simply become a work of the imagination – visualization.

It is worth reiterating that being clear about what you want to achieve is most important. At Neal's Yard Remedies we ask ourselves what we would like to achieve from a product before asking how we would like it to be. This isn't the only way, but it is important to clarify what the product is for and how you would like it to smell. Once this is established, make a preliminary selection of oils. Again, when it comes to developing our own ideas, choices will be made according to the function we envisage for the finished product. For example, one project was to create a foaming bath, which we wanted to be as effective as possible. It was intended to soothe aching muscles, to help with tiredness and to leave the user feeling rejuvenated. Choosing the ingredients was not that difficult – pine, lemon and juniper essential oils, arnica tincture and infusions of seaweed, juniper berries and comfrey. Balancing the fragrance of the product was

more difficult, however, and we would proceed in a similar way to that outlined below.

Once the purpose of the product has been established, prepare some smelling strips. These can be made by cutting blotting paper into thin strips. It will be useful to number the strips. Arrange the oils around you for easy reference and place a drop of each oil that you think you would like to include on a smelling strip. This will give you a very broad idea of how well the oils work together. The next step is to record the combination of oils used. Make a note of the number of the strip you have used and then write down what you have just done.

If you like your newly created fragrance, try mixing it in a small beaker and adjust the quantities until it seems more balanced and no particular oil overpowers another. Creating a blend by using a top note oil, a middle note and a base note will give you a fragrance in which each individual oil is enhanced by the others. Each oil remains distinct yet is a part of the whole. Often a mix that seems so promising when you begin becomes confused and messy, so don't be afraid to start again!

To help you choose the oils to add to the product you are making you need to consider two main factors – what purpose the oil will have and what mood do you want to create? The answers to these two questions are not necessarily different, but it is worth defining your expectations at the outset so that you make the correct choices.

dilutions

Following are rough guides to the proportions in which the fragrance you have just made should be added into the mixture. If you wish to keep your mixture as a perfume, the base can be either alcohol or jojoba.

alcohol

As with making tinctures (see pages 44–5), it is probably better to use vodka or buy some ethyl alcohol from the chemist. This is especially appropriate when creating a perfume. The blend of essential oils should be added to form between 3 and 8 per cent of the whole.

flower waters

These products already contain essential oils, but will allow an extra 1 per cent of oil blend to be added. These are excellent for room sprays, insect repellents and so on when a predominant water base is required.

A blended fragrance of essential oils will be therapeutically effective above 2 per cent. It is best to keep below this level unless a specific effect is required. Do not forget that oils are readily absorbed through the skin.

cream base

Making your own cream is described on pages 42–3. The base will smell of the ingredients, so you will need to consider this when you come to add a fragrance. A creamy, honey base will be enhanced by a sweet, floral blend of oils, and this would be appropriate for a rich night cream. A soothing aftersun cream with aloe vera and chamomile in the base may well benefit from something lighter and a more cooling fragrance. Add your fragrance at a percentage of between 1 and 3 per cent of the total.

making your own fragrances

Use the table on pages 208–9 to help you select essential oils to blend together to make your own fragrance. Select an oil from each of the three groups – to provide top, middle and base notes of the fragrance – using the suggestions in the second column to create a well-balanced mixture that you can use in other recipes.

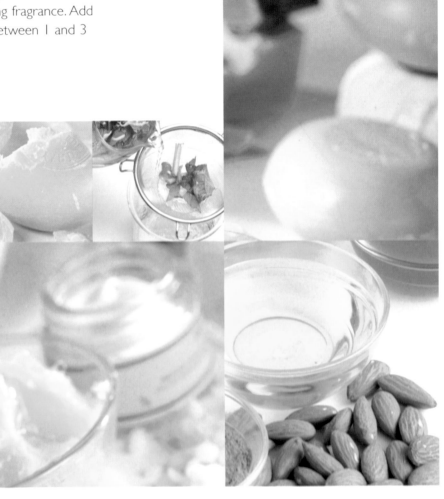

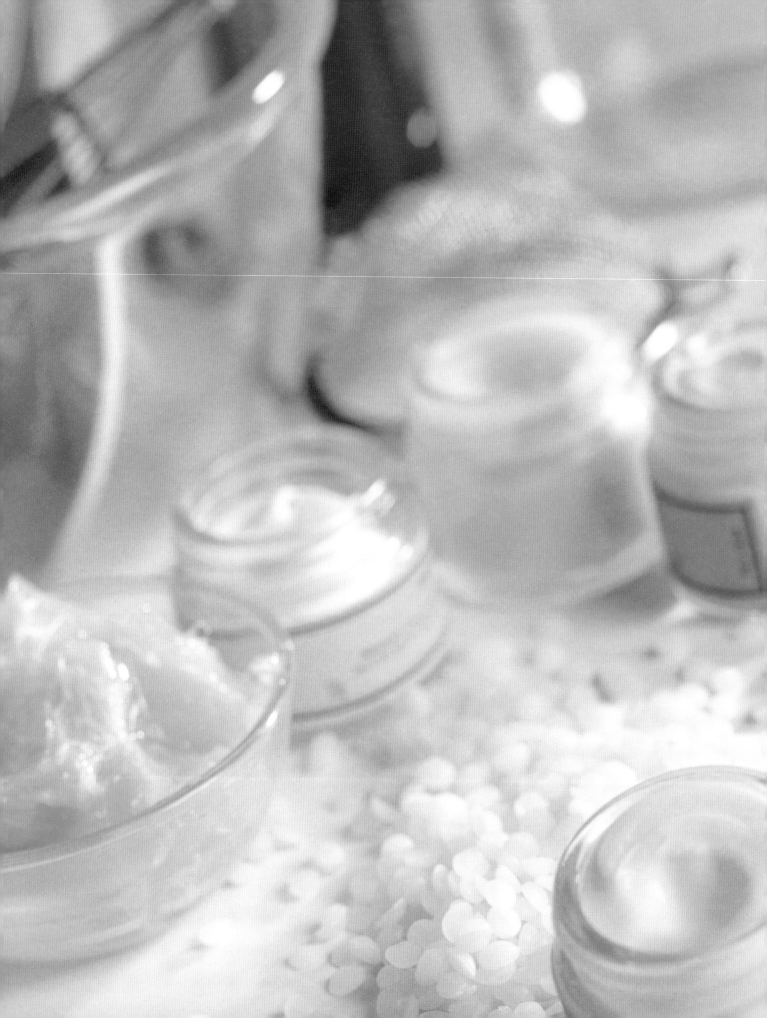

recipes & routines

3

Too often we step quickly from under the shower with barely a thought to the drying effects of soaps and water on our skin. Use the recipes that follow to exfoliate and smooth your skin. Massage your skin with fragrant lotions to soften and refresh it, and protect it from the harmful rays of the sun with some easily prepared oils.

introduction to the recipes

Not many of us have been taught how to make our own skin care preparations. Only a few generations ago many people would have known how to make up a cream for rough hands, a conditioner for the hair or a paste to redden the cheeks. Although the making of these beauty products was probably no more complicated than cooking food, it was vital to know what resources were available locally. It was also important to know which ingredients were nutritious to eat and which could be used in cosmetics or to treat illness.

There are many historical accounts which give details of traditional methods of doing everyday things, such as washing your hair. Many of the products were made in the home from natural ingredients found locally or grown in the garden. Wood ash, for example, could be collected and put in a bucket with a few bay leaves and water poured on. It was then left overnight and, in the morning, used to cleanse the hair. In addition, olive oil has long been used to improve the condition of hair. These are examples where knowledge of the environment and nature can be put to use in simple and effective ways. There are thousands of these creative beauty care traditions throughout the world that make use of local plants and other natural materials.

The aim of this section is not only to provide useful recipes but also to set up a framework and inspire confidence for you to make your own products using the plants and other materials available around you. If some of the materials cannot be found locally it is often possible to order them through mail catalogues.

These days most of us are too busy to embark on making beauty products – it is not until something goes wrong with our skin or hair that we decide to do something about it. As an alternative to simply experimenting with different commercial brands, try making your own products, using only natural ingredients. Many of the recipes are very quick and simple to prepare, and you can tailor the product to your requirements more accurately.

Begin by working out your physical profile, including your skin type and hair type. Then you can decide which ingredients will suit you, in order to find a remedy for the problem in hand. Always remember that the success of any home-made product lies in

learning about the different plants and other materials that can be used. Spend time finding out about the herbs and oils that have a reputation for their cleansing, moisturizing and healing properties.

Start with ingredients that you know, probably from cooking or gardening, and keep it simple by trying to stick with what you have immediately available. Then decide what appeals to you, whether it is a fragrance, taste or texture. There are some excellent reference books available (see further reading – pages 249–50), or look at the charts on pages 206–9. These can help you work out the properties of your plant or other raw material, checking them for their suitability to your particular needs.

It is true that bad cooking can ruin the quality of ingredients in food, and so it is with making beauty and health products. Use fresh ingredients wherever possible and choose them from sources that you know. If the plant material is collected from a garden, be sure that it is grown away from the areas fouled by cats and dogs. Try to ensure that the plants are grown organically, that they are free from pesticides and chemical fertilizers. Buy materials from reputable suppliers and if you need to store the supplies, keep them out of direct sunlight and protected from contamination. Fresh herbs should be stored in paper bags until they are used.

cleansing the body

Different cultures have different customs for keeping the body clean, and different methods are used by different generations in every family. There are also varying opinions about what should and should not be involved in the cleansing process.

simple cooking methods

We have tried to make the recipes simple. Some will take longer than others to make, so read the steps before you start so that you know exactly what is involved. On the whole the steps are very basic, allowing recipes to be made in basic conditions, often requiring little equipment. One final point: be careful not to overheat a herbal ingredient as this is likely to harm its effectiveness.

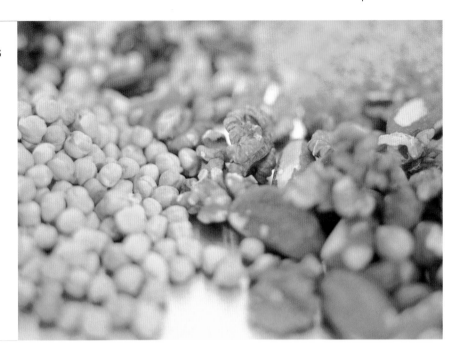

Cleaning the body depends on many factors, including climate and water accessibility, not to mention available materials or religious beliefs. By looking at some of these factors, we can start to appreciate how different cultures have created their own cleansing and beauty routines. It is mainly practical considerations, however, that will determine personal care routines.

There are many interesting examples of adaptability and resourcefulness based on environmental and social conditions. In Japan, for example, a bath is taken not for cleaning but for relaxing, and a shower is used for cleaning. In areas where water and energy are not readily available, the body may be cleansed through the use of different oils or clays. Cleansing also has a metaphorical side; we can reflect whether our own cultures have separated the physical function of the body from that of the spiritual. In the Hindu faith, for example, ceremonial washing is a necessary preparation before praying.

In western society, cleansing has increasingly come to mean getting rid of dirt and bacteria. We need to be cautious, however, in our enthusiasm to kill germs. Bacteria are essential to humans, especially in breaking down waste. Society is beginning to see the evidence of the over-use of antibiotics and antiseptics in the increase of problems involving bacterial infections and other viruses. The more antibiotics and antiseptics are used, the more dependent on them our bodies become, yet the different types of bacteria become more resistant because their instinct to survive leads them to develop new, stronger strains. This combination of the body's weakening immune system and stronger bacterial cells has led to more severe and longer lasting infections, and this has happened despite an increase in the regular use of detergents and disinfectants.

It is worth considering what it means to be clean, and to think about this in the context of how dirty the local environment is. Most cities are polluted with industrial emissions, car exhausts and a whole host of other waste materials that are pumped into the atmosphere. Before you go to sleep at night, it is important to rinse off the grime of the day so as not to allow the skin to absorb any toxic residues. This not only includes environmental pollutants, such as those from traffic and industry, but also body odour – the result of a chemical reaction between the bacteria on the skin and sweat.

And, of course, apart from making yourself clean and smelling fresh, one of the most important reasons to soak in a hot bath or cool off in a shower is to actually feel good: water is a wonderful medium for reviving a tired body or relieving a bad temper.

storing your homemade products

Spend some time getting the right containers for your products. Here are some simple points to consider:

the container: Storing in dark glass and in a cool, dark, dry place is the best option. If you are going to travel, however, pack appropriately in a plastic container. (Refer to Neal's Yard Remedies' shops as a supplier of plastic bottles and jars for just such purposes – see useful addresses on page 248.) If you are using plastic, take care not to store a product containing a high percentage of essential oils as these can cause corrosion. Also, if heat is involved when making a product, allow the product to cool down before pouring it into a plastic container.

the lid: Lids are vital in keeping products as fresh as possible by not allowing any air in – oxidation can lead to premature expiry. Lids with airtight seals, therefore, are ideal. It is advisable, however, to check that the wadding (i.e., the seal on the roof of the lid) is clean and will not affect the product in any way.

the label: Always take time to label the container carefully. Invent a name for your creation – one that will remind you of your reasons for making it. Include the date when the product was made, the ingredients that were used and, perhaps, a batch number for reference. It is also a good idea to keep a book to record the methods that you used.

Try not to spoil a good product with poor presentation: keep it simple, neat and clean.

getting ready

Read the recipe in advance to ensure that you have all the necessary ingredients, not to mention the right quantities of each and the appropriate cooking utensils. If you get into the habit of using fresh herbs then there will probably be extracts that you have already made and stored. Ensure that all storage containers are clean and ready – this includes getting rid of any old labels – before you start making your product. Choosing your containers carefully will make your products more of a pleasure to use as well as increasing their shelf-life.

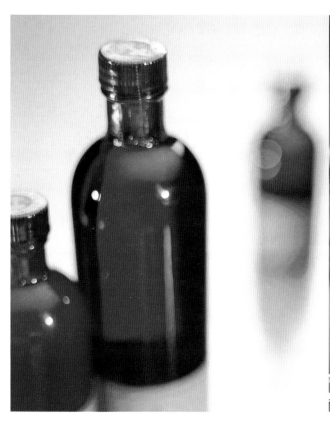
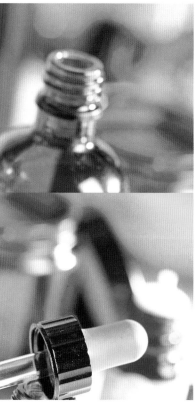

shelf-life

Most products without an infusion
or water component will keep for
several months. To lengthen the
shelf-life of a product further add
an anti-oxidant, such as vitamin C.
Herbal ingredients will expire
quickly in the same way that fresh
vegetables do. Try adding propolis
or benzoin and store them in the
refrigerator. Keep all products out
of the sun and in a cool, dry place.

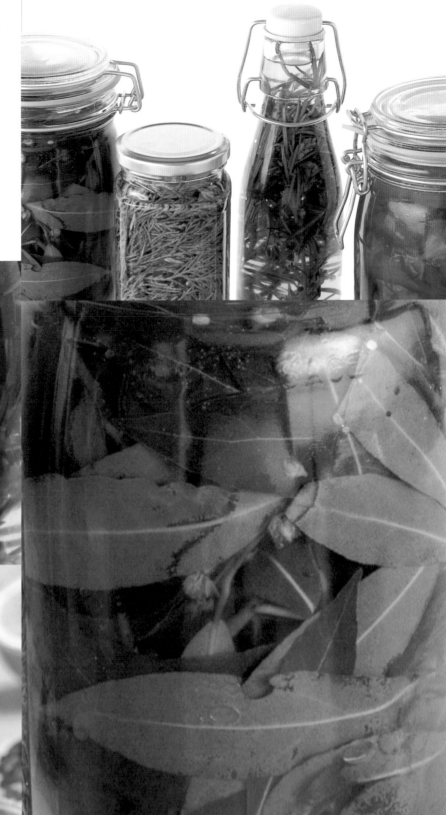

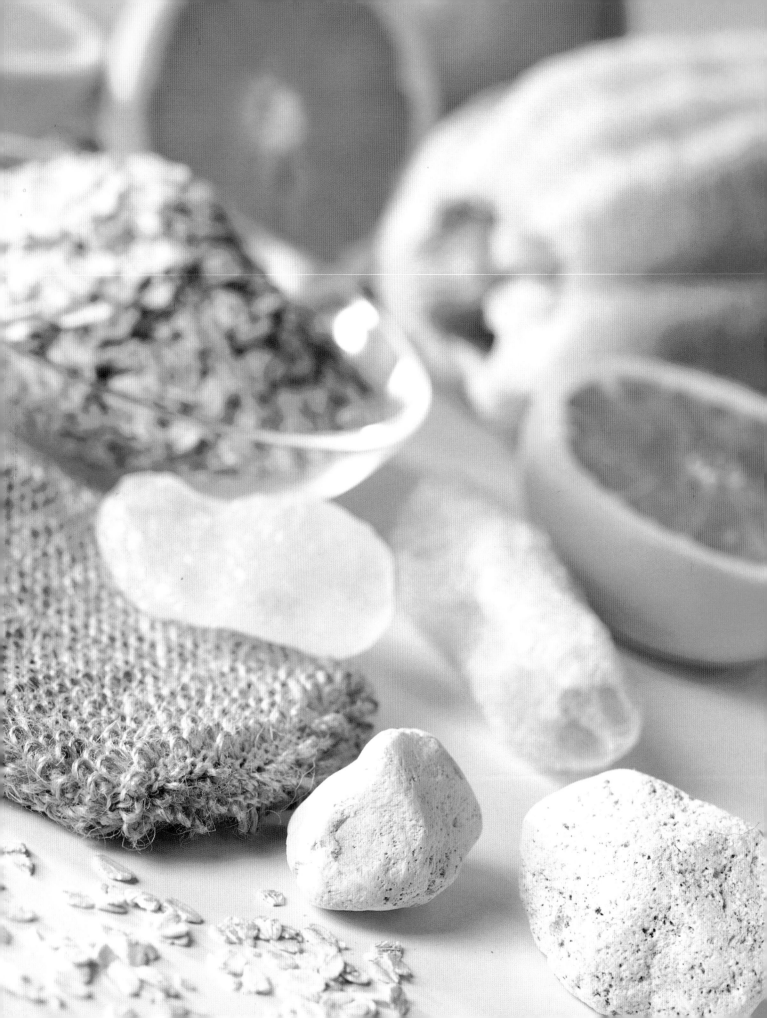

skin & body care

A clear, glowing skin is a sure sign of good health. Diet and hereditary factors play a large part in the way our skin looks, but a regular and careful skin-care routine will pay dividends. The recipes on the following pages will cleanse, moisturize, tone and otherwise pamper your skin, leaving it looking smooth and youthful.

skin care

Our skin is one of the most amazing organs of the body – it has many physiological functions, including protecting us from the elements and holding us together. At the same time, it acts as a guide, providing us with information about the world as well as giving information about us back to the world.

Much of the story our skin has to tell is about our inheritance. Hereditary factors determine a great deal about our skin's colour, type, tendencies and susceptibility to certain skin problems. We can often use this knowledge of our family history in preventative care. For example, if you know your mother had fair skin and was prone to sunburn, and your skin type is basically similar, you can take special precautions.

Inheritance is not the whole story, however; diet and skin-care routines are also important factors in the appearance of the skin. The most important point to remember is that the skin is alive; it is growing new cells and sloughing off old ones all the time, so changes are infinitely possible – for better and for worse. If you nurture your skin and look after it carefully with a regular skin-care regime, the results will be evident for all to see.

The physiological functions of the skin include getting rid of waste matter through the pores (elimination), protecting the body against foreign invaders such as bacteria, viruses and chemical pollutants, regulating body temperature, manufacturing vitamin D from sunlight and providing information about touch and pain. These functions mean that the skin is a good indicator of our general health   signs of prolonged stress or self-neglect will, sooner or later, show up on our skin. Although adopting a good skin-care routine and improving your diet and lifestyle can do much to transform tired, dingy or prematurely ageing skin, if you have a skin disease the best course

of action is to see a natural health therapist who will have experience of and practical suggestions about treating your type of skin condition.

the structure of the skin

The skin consists of two layers: an outer epidermis, where the process of continual skin renewal occurs, and an inner dermis. It is from the deepest region of the epidermis, the basal layer, that new cells are constantly produced. As the cells mature they are pushed closer to the surface by newer cells from below. While the cells migrate to the surface their nuclei are destroyed and replaced by a waterproofing protein called keratin. By the time they reach the *stratum corneum* (outer surface) the cells have been flattened, hardened, closely packed together and almost completely filled with keratin, forming a tough, protective and virtually waterproof layer.

The journey from basal layer to *stratum corneum* takes an estimated 14 days in young people (up to twice as long as we grow older), and approximately the same amount of time will elapse before the cells are sloughed off. Everybody sloughs off millions of dead skin cells every day. In order for this process to work efficiently a fine balance between the production of new cells and the loss of old cells needs to be maintained.

Melanin-producing cells can be found interspersed throughout the basal layer. Melanin is the brown pigment that absorbs harmful ultra-violet rays from the sun and hence provides us with a natural protective screen. Exposure to the sun stimulates increased melanin production, and this results in the skin becoming darker   that is, it becomes tanned. When the melanin is unable to absorb all the ultra-violet rays, because of prolonged and

the structure of the skin

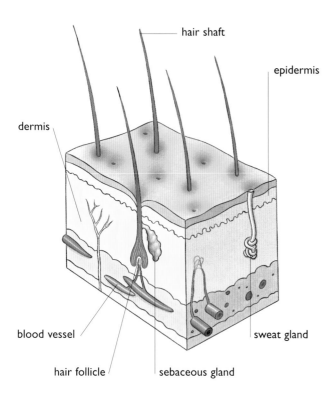

unaccustomed exposure, the skin is damaged and sunburn is experienced.

The inner dermal layer is composed of connective tissue, containing both elastin – the fibres that give the qualities of stretch and suppleness to the skin – and collagen – the fibres that provide strength. The dermis also contains numerous blood vessels.

Sweat glands provide the skin with its excretory function, ridding it of waste products, while also aiding in temperature regulation. Sweat glands can be divided into two types: eccrine glands and apocrine glands. Eccrine glands are distributed throughout the body but are found in higher densities on the soles of the feet and the palms of the hands. They secrete a watery fluid and are thought to react to adrenaline stimulation, which would explain why some people suffer from sweaty palms when they are nervous or anxious.

Apocrine glands occur in hairy parts of the body and only become active when puberty is reached. They are most notably found in the armpit and groin regions, and the distinctive odour associated with these areas is a result of the reaction between bacteria that

naturally and harmlessly occupy the armpit and groin with the secretions from these glands.

Sebaceous glands are another type of gland found in the skin. These are larger on the face, scalp and shoulders. Sebaceous glands secrete an oily substance known as sebum, which keeps the skin and hair conditioned as well as providing antibacterial and antifungal protection.

the ageing process

The skin of small children is smooth, clear and glowing, but as the teenage years are reached evidence of hormonal activity begins to show on the skin, with characteristic blackheads, acne and spots that can cause so much misery to the sufferer. With adolescence past, there is usually a period when we have youthful yet healthy looking skin with the minimum of effort.

From the age of about 25, our skin tends to become progressively more dry as the levels of sebum drop. Then, from the age of about 50, the number of elastin fibres begins to decline radically and our skin starts to lose its natural elasticity and suppleness. Bags start to appear and sagging begins to accelerate. In addition to these signs of ageing, the collagen fibres that are the underlying support structure of the skin become twisted and matted, causing wrinkles and lines.

The good news about collagen damage is that there are steps we can take to minimize it and even remedy damage already done. The main factors affecting collagen damage are exposure to ultra-violet light and the activity of free radicals (see page 19 and the technical glossary – pages 225–39). This is the main reason why exposure to strong sunlight, and especially ultra-violet rays, can cause premature ageing. We can do much to avoid unnecessary damage to our skin by avoiding exposure to the sun's rays or tanning beds, and by using sunscreens and sunblocks.

Free radical activity can be reduced by the use of antioxidants. Externally, the most effective antioxidant is vitamin E and so it makes sense to use a night cream or moisturizer containing it (wheatgerm oil and avocado oil are good natural sources of vitamin E). Internally, antioxidants play a crucial part in our diet and slow down all the signs of ageing, including those apparent in the skin. Important antioxidants in our diet are vitamins

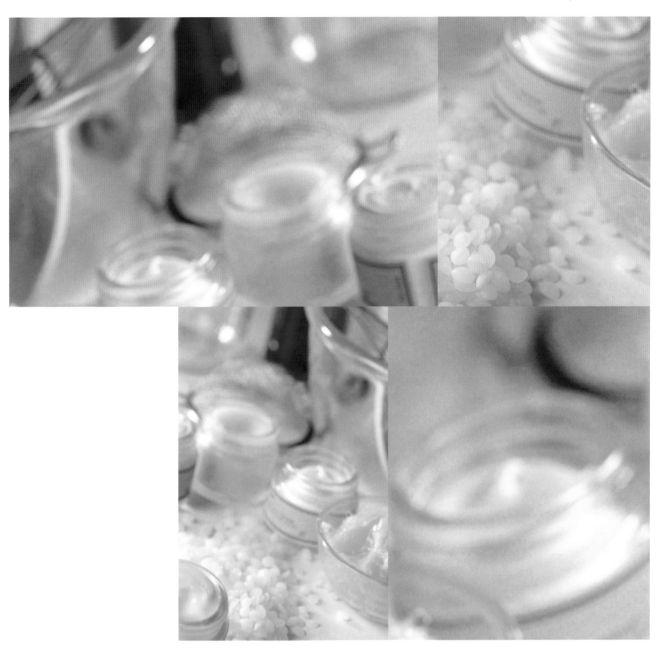

A, C and E, selenium and zinc, many of which are found in fresh fruit and vegetables. Other good things we can do to reduce the effects of ageing are to get plenty of fresh air and exercise, both of which help to oxygenate the cells of the body including the skin.

Smoking is one of the most damaging things you can do to your skin — it not only causes lines to appear around your mouth and blocks the skin's pores with irritating and toxic smoke particles, it also drastically accelerates the release of harmful free radicals. Alcohol can also tend to cause skin damage by exerting a

drying effect and causing rapid dilation of the tiny capillaries in the dermis.

In general, the more you care for your skin and your overall health, the better you will be able to withstand the ravages of the ageing process. A good skin-care routine will pay dividends in years to come, even if it seems a bit of a chore at times. If you have left things until signs of neglect are beginning to appear, starting to use a really good moisturizer and making improvements in your diet, however small, can still make a significant and visible difference.

know your skin type

Knowing what skin type you have is important in helping you to choose which products are the most suitable and beneficial for you. Skin type can alter over time, and sometimes quite quickly; most people find, for example, that their skin becomes more liable to dryness as they get older. If you do find your skin type changing, be prepared to respond quickly and start using different skin-care products.

normal skin

Normal skin is soft, smooth, supple and not prone to eruptions. It should also have a healthy glow. Regular cleansing and the use of a light moisturizer are all that is needed to keep the skin looking clear and healthy. Normal skin, however, is often prone to becoming drier as you grow older. Suitable herbs include elderflower, marsh mallow, rose, marigold and lavender. Essential oils include geranium, lavender, palmarosa and rose.

dry skin

Dry skin tends to be delicate and susceptible to flaking and fine lines. It can feel taut across the face, especially after cleansing. You should never use soap on dry skin; other things that exacerbate dryness are alcohol, exposure to the sun, central heating and wind. Gentle cleansing and careful moisturizing are vital. Herbs that are suitable for dry skin include chamomile, rose, comfrey, marsh mallow and marigold. Essential oils include chamomile, jasmine, neroli, palmarosa, rose and sandalwood.

oily skin

Oily or greasy skin tends to be sallow and shiny and often has open pores. It is prone to blackheads and acne, but it does have the advantage of not wrinkling as easily as dry skin because the oil and grease moisturize it. Thorough yet gentle cleansing is a must for oily skin in order to keep the pores clear and reduce a build-up of sebum. The use of gentle astringent toners may also be helpful. Astringent herbs suitable for oily skin include elderflower, witch hazel, yarrow and lemongrass. Essential oils include cedarwood, cypress, vetiver, patchouli, orange and lemon.

combination skin

The face may have an oily section, usually a panel down the centre including the forehead, nose and chin, and areas of drier skin. You may find it best to treat the centre panel as oily skin and use different products for the drier areas, or use products that are balancing and recommended for normal skin. Balancing herbs include rose, lavender and elderflower. Essential oils include geranium, ylang-ylang, bergamot and lavender.

problem skin

This is skin that is prone to blackheads, acne and spots. It is often oily, although not necessarily so. The most important factors here are diet, to help the skin with its eliminative process, and thorough yet gentle cleansing. If the acne is severe, consulting a professional therapist of natural medicine may be necessary to get the best results. Antiseptic and healing herbs include marigold, eucalyptus, yarrow, comfrey and elderflower. Essential oils include grapefruit, juniper, tea tree, lavender and bergamot. The use of clays for deep cleansing can also be very beneficial.

sensitive skin

This type of skin is usually dry and prone to flaking, itching and redness. There may be a tendency to allergic reactions and also to broken capillaries. Exposure to strong sunlight and drinking alcohol will tend to make things worse. Cleansing should be a very gentle process and soothing and cooling moisturizers should be used. It is advisable to avoid the use of exfoliants, astringent toners and any products containing alcohol or fragrance. Soothing and anti-inflammatory herbs include chamomile, comfrey, marigold, chickweed and marsh mallow. Essential oils include chamomile, Roman chamomile, lavender and rose.

mature skin

As the skin ages it loses elasticity and its ability to retain moisture and the signs of ageing appear, including sagging skin, fine lines and wrinkles. The emphasis of skin care is on nourishing and moisturizing the skin to reduce the effects of the ageing process. Regenerative herbs suitable for mature skin include rose, comfrey, marsh mallow and marigold. Essential oils include frankincense, myrrh, rose, palmarosa, lavender and neroli.

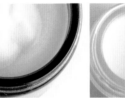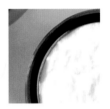

cleansers

The importance of cleansing to create and maintain healthy, clear, youthful and smooth skin cannot be over-emphasized. This is, of course, especially true if you wear make-up which, if left on the skin, will clog the pores and prevent it from breathing. Cleansing also removes dirt, excess sebum and the grime of pollution.

Cleansing should be a gentle as well as a thorough process, otherwise dryness or damage to delicate areas of skin can result. Soap can be very drying and should not really be used on the face. The simplest method of cleansing is to splash tepid water repeatedly over the face and then gently pat dry with a towel.

Many make-up products on the market today are water-resistant and designed to stay on for hours. This can make removing them difficult, but a basic and straightforward way of doing this is to pour a little olive oil or almond oil on to cotton wool and wipe the make-up off. Care should be taken around the eye area not to introduce any make-up into the eyes, as it may cause irritation. The use of a cleansing cream is one of the most effective techniques for removing make-up and any dirt and grime that is trapped in the sebum on your skin. Cleansing creams are a combination of oil and water and help to loosen make-up and other dirt from the skin so that it can be wiped off with cotton wool.

To increase the efficiency of a cleanser, apply a face cloth soaked with warm water to the skin and allow it to sit there for a minute or so before cleansing. This will open the pores and soften the skin, thus enabling the cleanser to penetrate the skin and remove dirt more effectively. Then pour cleanser on to cotton wool and apply it to the face and neck, paying particular attention to the hairline, which is a common area for dirt and debris to build up. Areas of higher sebum secretion, such as the nose and chin, may also require extra care. Remember to choose a cleanser that is suitable for your skin type; if your skin feels taut after using a cleanser, it may be too drying for you.

Once the make-up and grime are off your skin, you can take the opportunity to massage your face to increase the blood flow to the skin and soften it in preparation for other treatments.

As well as daily cleansing of make-up and dirt it is a real treat for your skin to have an occasional deep-cleansing treatment, such as a facial steam or a face pack. If you have oily or problem skin this can be done every couple of days; once a week should be often enough for normal or dry skin. Exfoliating (removing dead skin cells) can also spruce up tired-looking skin; there are plenty of natural ways to do this, the simplest of which is gently rubbing the skin with a 100 per cent cotton face cloth. Exfoliation is not recommended for very sensitive skin.

The chart on the page overleaf is a guide to the essential oils and herbal infusions that are recommended for specific skin types. Use this information when you are creating your own skin preparations.

skin type	essential oils	herbal infusions
normal	geranium, jasmine, lavender, palmarosa, rose	elderflower, marigold, marsh mallow, rose
dry	chamomile, neroli, rose, sandalwood	comfrey, chamomile, marigold, marsh mallow, rose
oily	cedarwood, cypress, lemon, orange, patchouli, vetiver	elderflower, lemongrass, witch hazel, yarrow
combination	bergamot, geranium, lavender, ylang-ylang	elderflower, lavender, rose
problem	bergamot, grapefruit, juniper, lavender, palmarosa, tea tree	comfrey, elderflower, eucalyptus, marigold, yarrow
sensitive	chamomile, helichrysum, lavender, Roman chamomile, rose	chamomile, chickweed, comfrey, marsh mallow
mature	lavender, myrrh, neroli, frankincense, rose	comfrey, marigold, marsh mallow, rose

body care

Most people are not satisfied with their own looks, so it's probably worth remembering that we are more likely to be critical of our own bodies than anybody else. However, it is worth enjoying looking after ourselves. Exercise not only helps us to look good, it makes us feel good, circulating oxygen round the body to re-energize the cells. Pamper yourself, too, by making a special body scrub specifically suited to your skin requirements, or a lotion with carefully chosen essential oils.

body brushing

Body brushing will help your body to eliminate toxins by speeding up lymphatic drainage and stimulating the circulation to the skin. Using a cactus fibre body brush or sisal mitt, brush upwards towards the body on your arms and legs, and in towards the centre of your body across the buttocks, small of your back, upper chest and abdomen. Use a firm, sweeping movement without scratching your skin. Do this for five minutes every morning as part of your cleansing routine. If you suffer from cellulite, body brushing and regular massaging of the area with anti-cellulite oil every day can really help.

deodorants

The aluminium compounds that are used in antiperspirants dry up the epidermis and prevent the sweat leaving the body. By combining with the mucus-like substances found in sweat they form a plug which blocks the exit to the sweat duct. Rather than an antiperspirant, it is far better to use a deodorant which inhibits the bacterial growth in the sweat and masks the odour these bacteria produce. The lemon and coriander deodorant on page 101 reduces the number of bacteria which are actually present under the arms. Alternatively, gently rub the armpits with a quarter of a lemon after the juice has been squeezed out – the lemon pith is an effective deodorant.

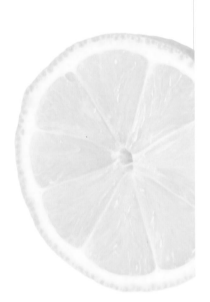

anti-cellulite oil

With regular use, this oil helps to eliminate toxins from fatty tissues of the body and break down cellulite. Massage into the body after a warm bath or shower.

These ingredients are sufficient to make 100 ml (3½ fl oz). It will keep for up to 12 months.

40 ml/2½ tbsp soya oil

40 ml/2½ tbsp almond oil

20 ml/4 tsp wheatgerm oil

5 drops lemon essential oil

5 drops frankincense essential oil

2 drops juniper essential oil

2 drops black pepper essential oil

5 drops sandalwood essential oil

5 drops orange essential oil

2 drops eucalyptus essential oil

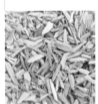
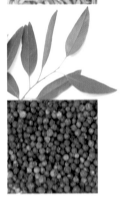

body scrubs

A body scrub is easy to make, easy to use and can be very effective in revitalizing the skin by increasing the circulation and sloughing off the dead skin cells. If you have sensitive skin then body scrubs may be better for your skin than soap.

A wide variety of different food ingredients may be included in an effective body scrub. The chief components will include something abrasive, something cleansing, something nourishing and something to help bind it all together. The following will help as a guide:

abrasive ingredients: clays (e.g., bentonite, kaolin, green clay and fullers earth), ground substances (e.g., pumice, loofah, walnut shells and cherry stones), and ground cereal crops or pulses (e.g., rice, corn, wheat, buckwheat, manioc and aduki beans).

cleansing ingredients: cleansing herbs and oils (e.g., aloe vera and fruits that contain alpha-hydroxy-acids or AHAs, such as grapefruit, lemon, strawberry, papaya, apricots), and the more conventional cleansing cereals (e.g., oats or oatmeal).

nourishing ingredients: avocado, honey, eggs, maple syrup, vitamins, wheatgerm oil, fish oils, banana, yogurt and so on.

binding ingredients: herbal infusions, flower waters, aloe vera, coconut milk, fruit juices and so on.

Always take care to choose ingredients that suit your skin type (see page 88) and add richer and more oily ingredients for dry skin. Try the suggested recipes to start with before you experiment with your own.

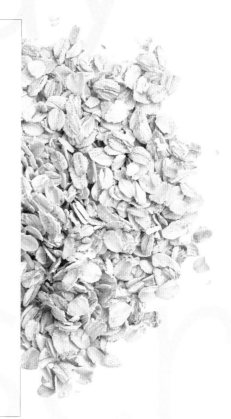

exfoliating body scrub

Oats are highly cleansing, and bran actually penetrates the pores of the skin, removing deeply ingrained dirt and grease. For skin that tends to be oily, use crushed aduki beans and oatmeal. Ground almonds can be added for a more nourishing effect.

20 g/4 tbsp bran
40 g/4 tbsp oats

Place the bran and oats in a muslin (cheesecloth) bag and hang it from the tap so that the bath water runs through the bag. When you are in the bath rub your skin with the bag, paying particular attention to areas of dry, hard skin.

honey and orange body scrub

An exfoliating body scrub, especially good for dry skin. These ingredients are sufficient to make 40 g (1½ oz).

    10 g/1 tbsp kaolin
    30 g/2 tbsp ground rice
    5 ml/1 tsp orange flower water or
        orange blossom infusion
    15 ml/1 tbsp clear honey, warmed
    1 drop orange essential oil
    1 drop geranium essential oil
    1 drop juniper essential oil

Pound the kaolin and ground rice together with a pestle and mortar. Add the orange flower water or infusion and the slightly heated honey to the dry mixture and mix thoroughly until fully combined. Add the essential oils and mix in thoroughly. To use, mix with a small amount of water on the palm of the hand and massage lightly into the skin with small circular movements. Rinse off with warm water. It will keep for up to 2 months.

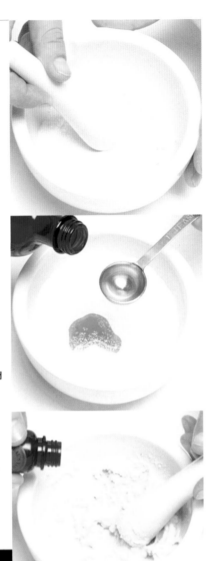

exfoliation

Exfoliation stimulates lymphatic drainage and promotes circulation. It also encourages skin cell production and improves the condition of the skin.

body splash

This is a delicious body splash/spray that will keep you smelling wonderful! These ingredients are sufficient to make 100 ml/3½ fl oz.

    80 ml/5½ tbsp distilled   5 ml/1 tsp orange flower water
        water   2 drops patchouli essential oil
    10 ml/2 tsp aloe vera juice   1 drop geranium essential oil

Combine the ingredients and store in a 100 ml (3½ fl oz bottle). Apply with an atomizer, shaking before use. It will keep for up to 2 months.

elderflower and aloe vera body scrub

An excellent cleansing scrub to exfoliate and stimulate the circulation.

    20 g/3 tbsp elderflowers
    30 ml/6 tsp aloe vera juice
    25 g/2 tbsp rice flour
    3 drops benzoin
    4 tsp organic, plain yoghurt
    4 drops lavender essential oil

Cover the elderflowers in the aloe vera and leave for 15 minutes. Add the flour and mix thoroughly. Then add the benzoin, yoghurt and lavender oil. Apply using firm circular hand movements.

Dead Sea salts

Dead Sea salts are uniquely rich in minerals and can easily be combined with your favourite essential oils or herbs.

To make a simple scrub: put two tablespoons of salts in a soft cotton or muslin bag – sewn up on three sides – then crush the salts using a rolling pin to ensure they are not too abrasive. They can then be added to the bath, in which they will dissolve. Ingredients such as roses and orange peel can also be added to the bag for variation. If oils are added to the salts then they will also fragrance a bath. Try the following, adding a few drops per oil:
* an exotic oil blend could be based on ylang-ylang, palmarosa, and geranium;
* a relaxing yet cleansing blend could be made from lavender, mandarin or marjoram;
* a cleansing wake up for the body and spirit may include oils such as grapefruit and lime.

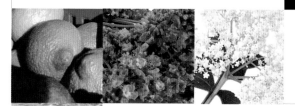

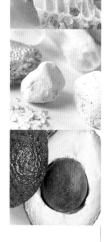

nourishing body scrub

If the body is particularly dry and has a tendency to being scaly, try this recipe using fresh avocado.

    1 ripe avocado
    15 ml/1 tbsp honey
    15 ml/1 tbsp wheatgerm oil
    25 g/3 tbsp ground pumice

    2 drops bergamot essential oil
    or palmarosa essential oil

Mash the avocado, using a fork. Slightly warm the honey and add. Then add the wheatgerm oil and stir the mixture before adding the pumice. Stir in carefully, adding enough to allow the mixture to hold together. The amount required will vary in relation to the size of the avocado. If a fragrance is desired then bergamot will be fresh and cleansing. However, to make this a more exotic mixture, try a blend of the following;

    1 drop each of palmarosa essential oil, rose essential oil, ylang-ylang essential oil
        and vetiver essential oil

body powders

Body powders help the skin to remain supple and prevent chafing. They should be dusted lightly over the skin, once the body has dried off after washing, to absorb any excess moisture.

lavender and tea tree powder

A body powder combining the antibacterial properties of propolis with the powerfully antiseptic essential oils of lavender and tea tree.

20 g/3 tbsp cornstarch
20 drops propolis tincture
5 drops lavender essential oil
5 drops tea tree essential oil

Sift the cornstarch evenly on to a plate. Mix the propolis and essential oils together and spray on to the cornstarch using a fine mist atomizer pump. Take care not to saturate the powder or else it will become lumpy. Store in an old talc dispenser or empty ground pepper shaker. It will keep for up to 6 months.

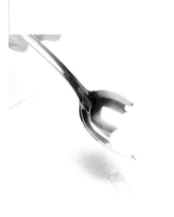

geranium and orange powder

20 g/3 tbsp cornstarch
5 drops geranium
   essential oil
5 drops orange essential oil

Sift the cornstarch evenly on to a plate. Mix the oils and spray on to the cornstarch using a fine spray atomizer pump. Store in an old talc dispenser or empty ground pepper shaker. The powder will keep for up to 6 months.

calendula powder

This is a body powder for delicate and sensitive skin.

20 g/2 tbsp kaolin
5 drops calendula tincture
5 drops lemon essential oil

Sift the kaolin evenly on to a plate. Mix the tincture and essential oil and spray on to the kaolin, using an atomizer pump. Store in an old talc dispenser or empty ground pepper shaker. It will keep for up to 6 months.

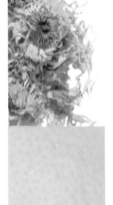

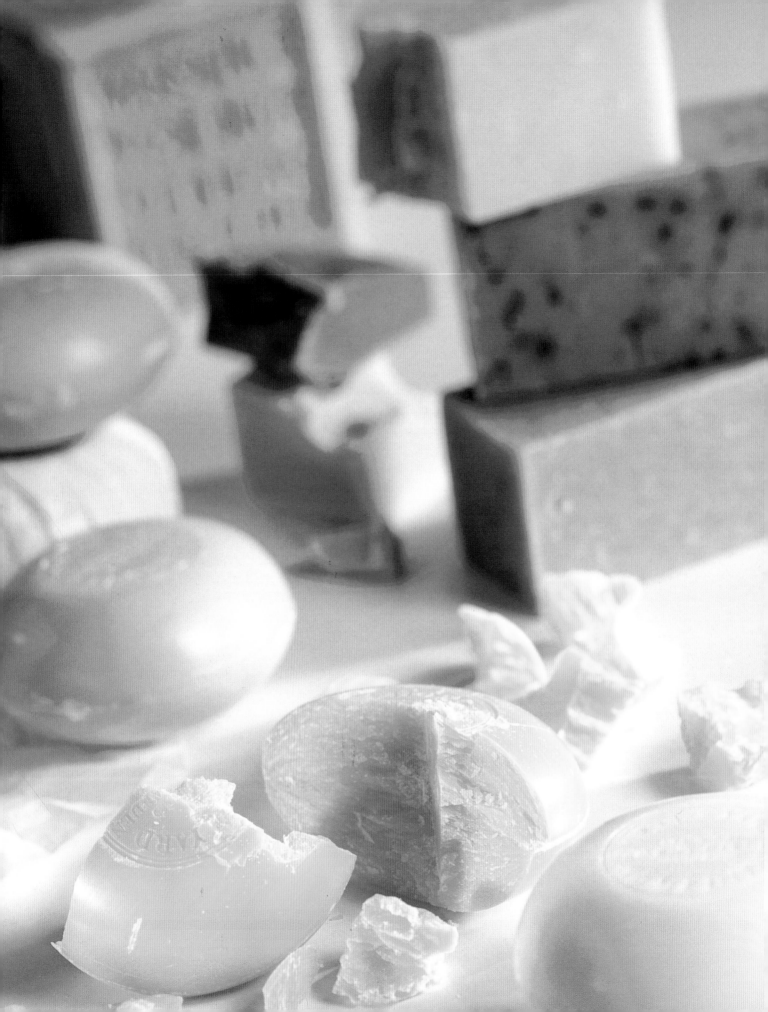

soap

Soaps have been made for thousands of years. Excavations from Ancient Rome have revealed that soap made from goat's tallow and wood ash was used to wash fibres and cloth. In later centuries soap was used in the treatment of diseases before it came to be associated purely with personal cleanliness. In France, the well-known Marseilles block was made in the thirteenth century from animal tallow and olive oil. Today traditional societies still make soap from fats and oils available. In some places, oil for soaps is derived from locally produced plant oils, but in other areas the fat is used from the processing of animals.

the chemistry of soap

The raw materials required to produce a modern hard soap are fats and oils, and some form of alkali (lye), such as caustic soda (sodium hydroxide). Saponification refers to the process by which soap is produced. The oils are split into two major parts: fatty acids and glycerine, and then the sodium or potassium part of the alkali joins with the fatty acid part of the oil; this produces the 'salt' of the fatty acid – also known as soap.

Caustic soda can be purchased from a chemist or hardware shop. Make certain that you buy 100 per cent sodium hydroxide. It is very corrosive and must be handled with great care – always wear protective plastic gloves and goggles. Be sure to follow any safety instructions and store in a safe, airtight container.

making the soap

The basic rule for making soap is to ensure that the balance of lye and oil is correct. Often it will take some experimenting to get this balance right. The type of oil used is also important. The correct combination of these two factors will ensure that the soap hardens, lathers and has the right acid/alkaline balance, as measured on the pH scale: 1 being the most acidic, 7 being neutral and 14 being the most alkaline. The skin is slightly acidic with a pH value of around 6.5, but soap is often found to have a pH of up to 10 or 10.5. As this is so alkaline, it can be an irritant to sensitive skin.

Fats and oils have specific saponification values and it is necessary to ensure that the correct oil or balance of oils are used. Different oils will require different amounts of sodium hydroxide; the quality of one oil will also cause a variation.

It should be possible to buy a pH testing kit, such as litmus paper, at a garden centre. Testing the pH value of your home-made soap will enable you to see whether it is sufficiently neutral and not too alkaline to use, although this is not essential.

There are many different soap bases that you can make, although none are as easy to make as some of the other recipes in this book because of the variation in raw materials. If this process seems too daunting, then ready-made soap bases are available. These only need to be heated and mixed with other ingredients to make your own creations. You will need to follow the manufacturer's instructions on the packet.

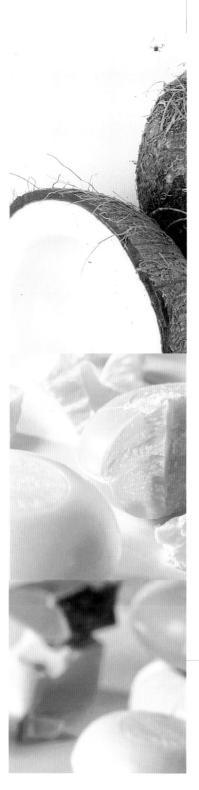

basic castile soap

Makes at least 20 x 100 g (3½ oz) bars. You can then add a variety of different essential oils to your bars. Try some of the suggestions on page 97 as an ideal starting point.

> 2.45 kg/5½lb olive oil
> 188 g/6½ oz coconut oil
> 188 g/6½ oz palm oil
> 750 ml/1⅓ pints mineral water
> 375 g/13 oz caustic soda (lye crystals)

It is strongly advised that good quality plastic gloves and goggles are worn when making this recipe as caustic soda can be quite corrosive.

Weigh out the oils and put them in a stainless steel pan over a low heat until they have melted. Heat the mixture until the temperature reaches 140°F (60°C). To make the lye mixture, warm the mineral water until it is lukewarm, pour into a glass or stainless steel bowl, and mix in the caustic soda until the crystals have dissolved. Leave to cool. Add the lye mixture to the hot oil and stir with a wooden spoon until thoroughly mixed. Using a metal whisk, beat the mixture for approximately 20 seconds. The consistency should now be similar to that of thick custard so that if a line is drawn on the surface it will remain.

To fragrance the soap base, divide the base mixture into the required quantities. For example, if four varieties of soap are wanted, separate the mixture into four different bowls and add the other ingredients as required. Pour or spoon the mixture into pre-greased, stainless steel moulds or dishes, cover with a cloth and leave to set for 24 hours.

Wearing plastic gloves, remove the partially hardened soap from the moulds and cut into bars using a cheese wire or knife. Arrange on trays and leave to dry out and harden fully. This will take several weeks and during this time the pH value of the soap will drop, becoming more neutral, and hence milder. You may find that a whitish residue appears on the surface of the soap. This can easily be scraped off if desired. The soap will continue to dry out for several months, depending on the weather, but the reduction of the pH value will slow down and remain stable after a few weeks.

Use the following ideas as a basic guide to fragrancing and personalizing your soap. Once you have mastered the technique, you may prefer to make your own combinations. Make sure that you do not include more than 5 per cent additions to the soap base (i.e., that all additional ingredients amount only to 5 per cent of the total weight of the soap). All the quantities suggested here are to add to 400 g (14 lb) of soap base.

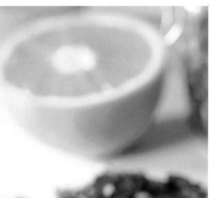

wake-up bar

4 drops lemon essential oil

10 drops grapefruit essential oil

5 drops lemongrass essential oil

18 drops lime essential oil

zest of 1 orange

relax and soak bar

1 tbsp crushed, dried rose petals

30 drops lavender essential oil

16 drops rose absolute

5 drops marjoram essential oil

1 tbsp red clay, if desired

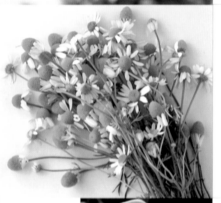

freshen-up bar

1 tsp neem oil

5 drops propolis tincture

30 drops lemon essential oil

40 drops palmarosa essential oil

2 teabags green tea (optional)

soft and delicate bar

10 ml/2 tsp calendula
    macerate

2 tsp dried chamomile flowers

25 drops chamomile
    essential oil

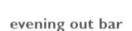

garden clean-up bar

1 tbsp green clay

3 crushed spirulina tablets

1 tbsp bran or oatmeal

20 drops rosemary essential oil

evening out bar

10 ml/2 tsp avocado oil

3 tsp ylang-ylang essential oil

12 drops geranium essential oil

12 drops clary sage essential oil

5 drops rose absolute

2 drops vanilla

moisturizing skin oils

The following recipes all make 100 ml (3½ fl oz/scant ½ cup). All you need do is blend the essential oils with the base oils. Store in dark glass bottles away from sunlight. They will keep for up to 30 months.

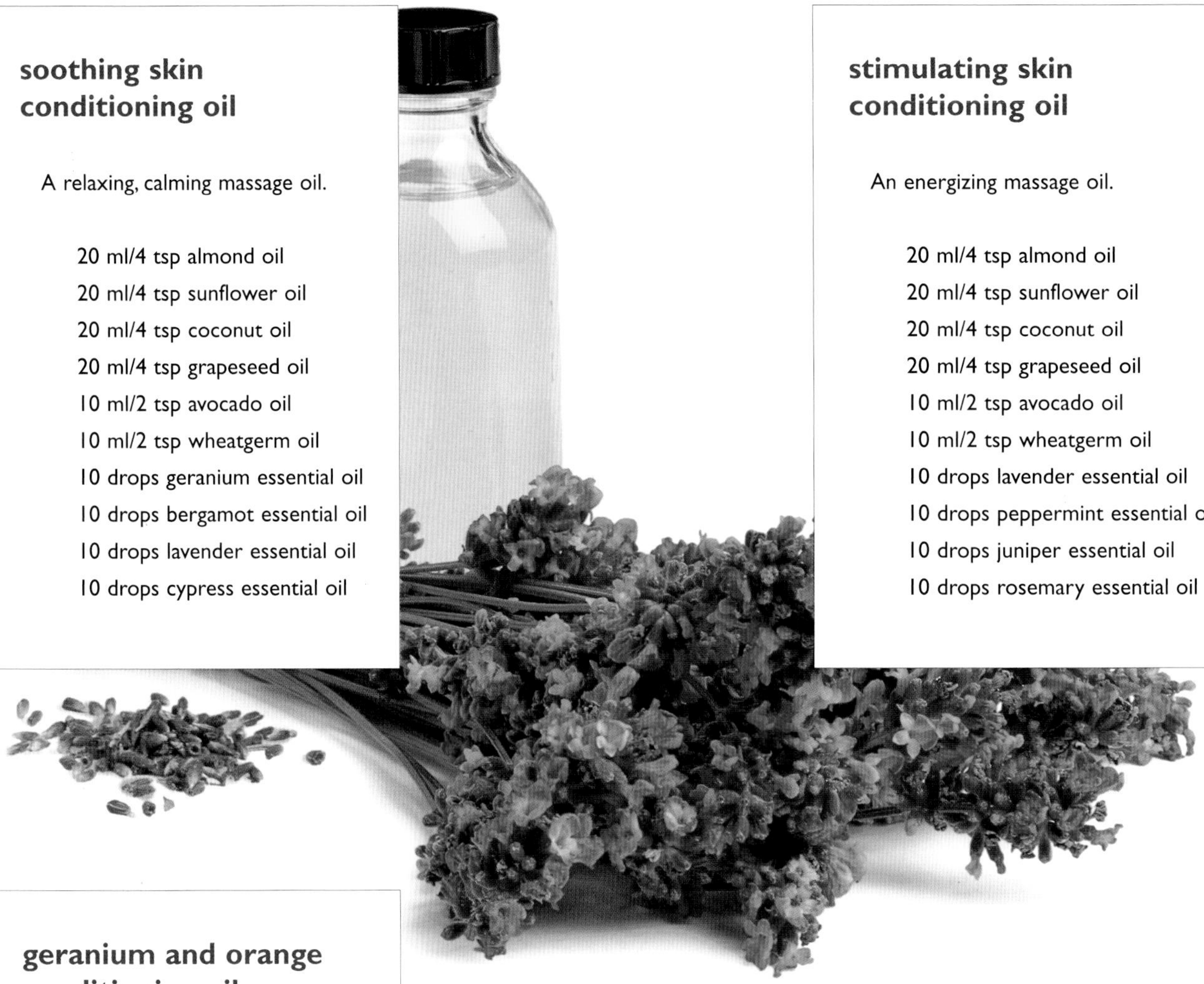

soothing skin conditioning oil

A relaxing, calming massage oil.

20 ml/4 tsp almond oil
20 ml/4 tsp sunflower oil
20 ml/4 tsp coconut oil
20 ml/4 tsp grapeseed oil
10 ml/2 tsp avocado oil
10 ml/2 tsp wheatgerm oil
10 drops geranium essential oil
10 drops bergamot essential oil
10 drops lavender essential oil
10 drops cypress essential oil

stimulating skin conditioning oil

An energizing massage oil.

20 ml/4 tsp almond oil
20 ml/4 tsp sunflower oil
20 ml/4 tsp coconut oil
20 ml/4 tsp grapeseed oil
10 ml/2 tsp avocado oil
10 ml/2 tsp wheatgerm oil
10 drops lavender essential oil
10 drops peppermint essential oil
10 drops juniper essential oil
10 drops rosemary essential oil

geranium and orange conditioning oil

A light, fragrant massage oil, suitable for all skin types.

40 ml/2½ tbsp soya oil
40 ml/2½ tbsp almond oil
20 ml/4 tsp wheatgerm oil
20 drops geranium essential oil
20 drops orange essential oil

body smoothing and moisturizers

Many people aspire to look like the models portrayed in the media and often maintain false expectations about their bodies. But if we don't conform to these ideals then we have to find ways of feeling good about how we look – especially with no clothes on! Undoubtedly our bodies look and feel better if we eat sensibly and lead a healthy, active lifestyle. It will also help to focus on cleansing and toning your body – try making a body moisturizer to help smooth and soften the skin.

body toning moisturizer

3 tsp apricot oil

30 ml/2 tbsp raspberry
leaf infusion

10 g/2 tsp emulsifying wax

2 drops black pepper
essential oil

3 drops ginger essential oil

2 drops lemon essential oil

Heat the apricot oil in a bowl set over a saucepan of boiling water (bain marie). Heat the emulsifying wax and raspberry leaf infusion gently in a pan until the emulsifier has dissolved in the infusion. Slowly add the infusion to the oil mixture, stirring constantly. When the mixture has cooled, add the essential oils.

body moisturizer for dry and ageing skin

2 g/$\frac{1}{2}$ tsp cocoa butter

1 tsp calendula oil

2 tsp wheatgerm oil

30 ml/2 tbsp water

10 g/2 tsp emulsifying wax

2 drops frankincense
essential oil

1 drop neroli essential oil

Heat the cocoa butter, calendula oil and wheatgerm oil in a bain marie. Gently heat the emulsifier and water in a pan until the emulsifier has dissolved. Slowly add the water mixture to the oil mixture, whisking it together for about 10 seconds. When the mixture has cooled, add the oils.

skin conditioning moisturizer

5 ml/1 tsp lanolin

5 ml/1 tsp avocado oil

5 ml/1 tsp evening primrose oil

30 ml/2 tbsp chickweed and
chamomile infusion

10 g/2 tsp emulsifying wax

Melt the lanolin, avocado oil and evening primrose oil in a bowl set over a saucepan of boiling water (bain marie). Put the chickweed and chamomile infusion and emulsifying wax into a pan and heat gently until the emulsifier has dissolved. Slowly add the infusion to the oil mixture, whisking it together for about 10 seconds.

luxury body moisturizer

2 g/$\frac{1}{2}$ tsp cocoa butter
and shea nut butter mix

1 tsp avocado oil

30 ml/2 tbsp rose petal infusion

10 g/2 tbsp emulsifying wax

2 drops rose essential oil

3 drops geranium essential oil

Melt the cocoa butter and shea nut butter mix with the avocado oil in a bowl set over a saucepan of boiling water. In a pan, gently heat the rose petal infusion and emulsifying wax until the wax has completely dissolved in the infusion. Slowly add the infusion to the oil mixture, whisking it together for about 10 seconds. When the mixture cools down, add the oils.

special treatments

To make these treatment oils simply blend the essential oils into the base oils. Unless otherwise mentioned, the recipes make 100 ml (3½ fl oz). To protect the essential oils from sunlight, store them in dark glass bottles.

anti-parasitic oil

This oil contains parasiticide essential oils and can be used to prevent and/or get rid of parasites living on the skin, such as scabies. Simply mix together and apply using an atomizer spray.

100 ml/3½ fl oz almond oil
10 drops palmarosa
    essential oil
10 drops lavandin or lavender
    essential oil
10 drops wild thyme
    essential oil
10 drops rosemary essential
    oil
10 drops lemon essential oil

spray-on insect repellent – essential oil blend

Where the skin is hot or sensitive, replace half the lavender flower water with aloe vera.

1 drop cinnamon essential oil
1 drop lemongrass essential oil
2 drops orange essential oil
2 drops wild thyme essential oil
4 drops lavender essential oil
4 drops pine essential oil

4 drops eucalyptus citriodora
    essential oil
5 drops citronella essential oil
100 ml/3½ fl oz lavender
    flower water

Mix the essential oils with the flower water. Shake well before use and apply with an atomizer spray. It will keep for 6 months.

after-insect bite soother

This is a soothing, cooling and calming product to use on skin that has been bitten. Spray on the affected area using an atomizer or simply dab on with cotton wool. As a dispersant has not been added, it is important to shake well before use to ensure even dispersal of essential oils through the product.

1.5 ml/30 drops
    plantain tincture
1.5 ml/30 drops
    calendula tincture
5 ml/1 tsp aloe vera juice
2 ml/4 tsp witch hazel

1.5 ml/30 drops yarrow
    tincture
1.2 ml/24 drops lavender
    essential oil
0.3 ml/6 drops tea tree
    essential oil

Combine the tinctures and aloe vera juice in the witch hazel. Add the essential oils. Store in a dark glass bottle, with an atomizer, out of direct sunlight. Will keep for up to 6 months.

spray-on insect repellent

These ingredients are sufficient to make 25 ml (1 fl oz).

1 drop sandalwood
    essential oil
2 drops citronella
    essential oil

3 drops eucalyptus
    citriodora essential oil
25 ml/5 tsp lavender
    flower water

Add the essential oils to the lavender flower water and store in a dark, glass bottle. Shake before use and spray on the skin using an atomizer. It will keep for 6 months.

deodorant stone

A deodorant stone is a crystal specially grown from potassium sulphate. It works by inhibiting bacterial growth.

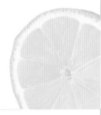

lemon and coriander deodorant

A refreshing and effective deodorant. These ingredients are sufficient to make 100 ml/3½ fl oz.

  90 ml/6 tbsp witch hazel
  10 ml/2 tsp vegetable glycerin
  2 drops clove essential oil
  2 drops coriander essential oil
  5 drops grapefruit essential oil
  2 drops lavender essential oil
  10 drops lemon essential oil
  5 drops lime essential oil
  5 drops palmarosa essential oil

Mix the witch hazel and vegetable glycerin together. Add the essential oils and mix. Shake well before use. Store in a dark glass bottle, preferably with an atomizer spray, for up to 6 months.

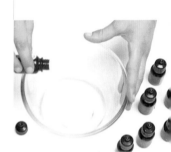

bay and lemon deodorant

Deodorant stones are an ideal alternative to aluminium-based deodorants. However, some people prefer a spray-on liquid. This recipe uses the stone for its antibacterial properties, which combine well with essential oils and aloe vera.

  1 deodorant stone
  1 litre/4 cups water
  5 ml/1 tsp aloe vera juice
  10 drops bay laurel essential oil
  5 drops sandalwood essential oil
  10 drops lemon essential oil
  3 drops eucalyptus essential oil

Smash the deodorant stone into pieces and place them in the water; boil until dissolved. Allow the mixture to cool and add the aloe vera juice, then mix in the essential oils. Store in a glass bottle with a fine spray atomizer. Will keep for up to 3 months.

peppermint and bergamot deodorant

A refreshing and fragrant deodorant. As a dispersant has not been added it is important to shake well before use to ensure even dispersal of essential oils through the product.

  5 ml/1 tsp vegetable glycerin
  40 ml/2½ tbsp witch hazel
  40 ml/2½ tbsp lavender flower water
  4 drops peppermint essential oil
  10 drops bergamot essential oil
  1 drop cypress essential oil
  7 drops lemon essential oil
  8 drops grapefruit essential oil

Combine the vegetable glycerin in the witch hazel. Add the essential oils and mix. Store in a dark glass bottle with a fine spray atomizer. Will keep for up to 6 months.

sun products

The sun tanning oils, moisturizers and other treatments on these pages are nourishing and conditioning to the skin. Simply blend all the oils together and store them in dark glass bottles. Prolonged exposure to the sun's rays can be dangerous, however, even when protective lotion is applied. It is strongly advised that protective lotions and oils are constantly re-applied and that people spend no longer than 30 minutes in the sun during the hottest part of the day.

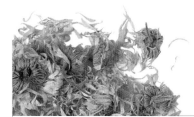

calendula and St John's wort soothing oil

Calendula heals and soothes the skin, while St John's wort acts by calming stimulated nerve tissue, and is often used in after-sun skin-care products. Never use in the sun because St John's wort is photosensitizing.

5 ml/1 tsp calendula oil
5 ml/1 tsp St John's wort oil
2 drops lavender essential oil

Mix the ingredients together and store in a dark glass bottle for up to 6 months.

sesame sun oil

Sesame oil provides only a low degree of protection against the sun's rays, so it is most suitable for dark skin, but this oil will nourish dry skin. The ingredients will make 100 ml (3½ fl oz). It will keep for up to 12 months.

40 ml/2½ tbsp sesame oil
40 ml/2½ tbsp coconut oil
20 ml/4 tsp grapeseed oil
40 drops petitgrain essential oil
5 drops lavender essential oil

aloe vera cooler

This is an excellent lotion for taking the heat out of sunburnt and damaged skin. Aloe vera soothes and softens the skin and calendula is added for its healing properties.

10 ml/2 tsp aloe vera juice
15 drops calendula tincture

Mix the ingredients together and store in a dark glass bottle for up to 6 months.

The recipes on this page may be used to heal and condition sunburnt skin – but remember that you should try to avoid overexposure to the sun in the first place.

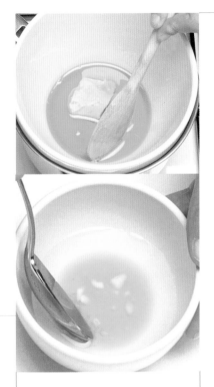

lime and coconut sun oil

This oil offers no protection and is only suitable for dark skin which tans very easily, or for use after exposure to the sun. These ingredients will make 60 ml (4 tbsp). It will keep for up to 12 months.

    10 ml/2 tsp wheatgerm oil
    20 g/¾ oz cocoa butter
    50 ml/3⅓ tbsp coconut oil
    5 drops benzoin tincture
    10 drops lime essential oil

Combine the oils, cocoa butter and tincture in a bowl and mix well.

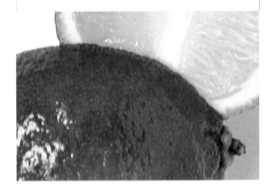

soothing ointment for sunburnt skin

Another way of applying treatment to sunburnt skin is to add the essential oils and tinctures to an ointment base, which is slowly absorbed into the skin. It will keep for up to 30 months.

    1 drop chamomile blue*
        essential oil
    4 drops lavender
        essential oil
    15 drops calendula
        tincture
    25 g/1 oz ointment base

Combine the oils and tincture and add to the ointment base.

cocoa butter body lotion

A soothing and moisturizing body lotion suitable for skin which has been exposed to the sun and also to use as a general skin conditioner. This recipe makes a 100ml (3½ fl oz) bottle.

    15 g/½ oz cocoa butter
    1 tsp lanolin
    75 ml/5 tbsp wheatgerm oil
    45 ml/3 tbsp water
    5 ml/1 tsp clear honey
    5 tsp emulsifying wax
    5 drops benzoin tincture
    5 drops sandalwood
        essential oil
    5 drops helichrysum
        essential oil
    5 drops ylang-ylang
        essential oil

Melt the cocoa butter, lanolin and wheatgerm oil in a bowl set over a pan of water. Heat the water and dissolve the honey and emulsifying wax in it. Add the water mixture to the oil mixture one tablespoon at a time, whisking. Add the benzoin tincture and essential oils. Shake before use. Store in a glass bottle in the refrigerator for up to 3 weeks.

*Chamomile blue is an excellent anti-inflammatory oil, which is good to use on sensitive skin.

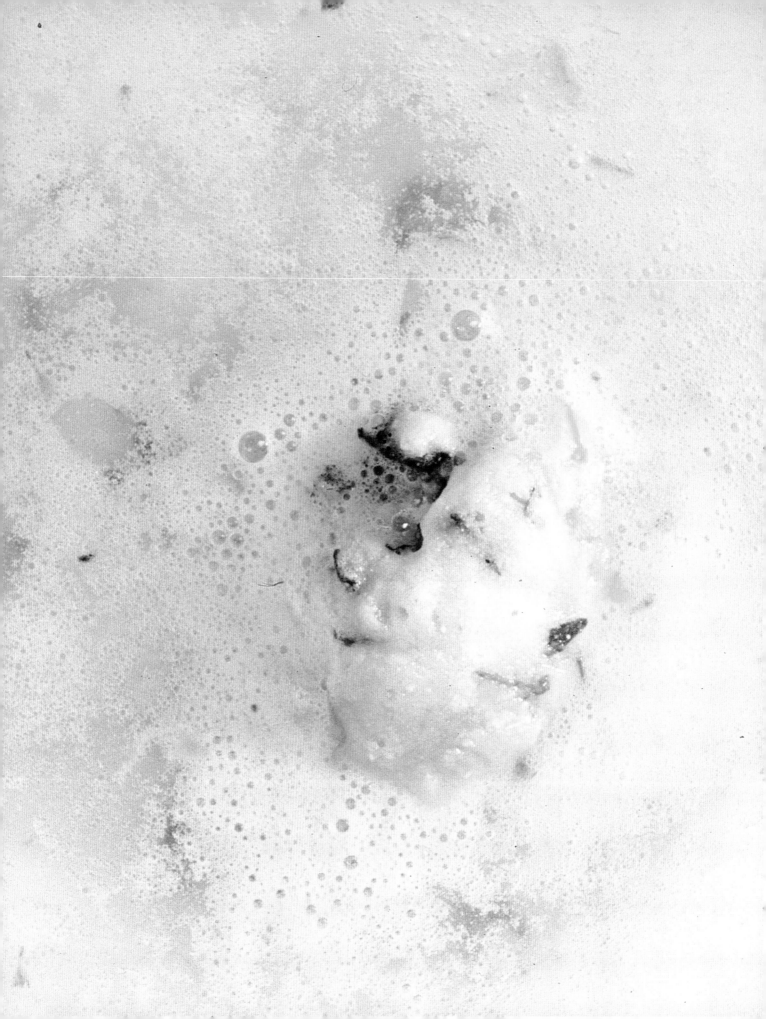

bath bombs

Opinion is divided as to whether an invigorating shower or a bath is best. If you have a shower as well as a bathtub the ideal is to sluice off all those dead cells, bacteria and pollutants before you luxuriate in a hot bath – which of course you can always share if you're concerned about using so much water! Choose a blend of essential oils to fragrance the bath, or add in one of the following recipes. Fill the bath and take time to relax – try candlelight for a truly soothing environment.

These balls of fizz are a fantastic way of livening up bathtimes. Either use them to add a kick start to your morning by combining refreshing and stimulating citrus essential oils, indulge in a sensual hedonistic recipe and turn your bath into a fragrant jacuzzi, or treat the kids to a fun, yet ultimately calming experience before bedtime. The three recipes given here are just an indication of the wide range of bath bombs that can be created. They will keep for up to 2 months.

citrus burst

80 g/3 tbsp sodium
  bicarbonate
15 ml/1 tbsp citric
  acid
4 drops grapefruit
  essential oil
4 drops lemon
  essential oil
1 drop lime
  essential oil
1 drop rosemary
  essential oil

sensual

80 g/3 tbsp sodium
  bicarbonate
15 ml/1 tbsp citric acid
4 drops mandarin
  essential oil
4 drops sandalwood
  essential oil
1 drop ylang-ylang
  essential oil
1 drop petitgrain
  essential oil
pinch of rose petals

kids

80 g/3 tbsp sodium
  bicarbonate
15 ml/1 tbsp citric acid
7 drops mandarin
  essential oil
2 drops orange
  essential oil
1 drop lavender
  essential oil

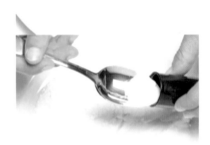

Mix the sodium bicarbonate and citric acid together on a plate. Sprinkle the essential oils on to the sodium bicarbonate mixture. Use the mixture as a powder sprinkled directly into the bath, or press it firmly into shaped moulds such as old camera film cases, ice-cube trays and pastry cutters. Add the powder or block to the bath just before you step in.

If you want to add some colour to your bath bomb, add a dash of carrot oil to give an orange colour, or avocado oil for a green tint. You might also like to add finely chopped herbs such as mint, or flowers including lavender or calendula.

Make your bath bomb mixture into a present – simply press the mixture into a round ball and wrap it in aluminium foil.

milk baths

Milk supplies us with a high content of vitamins, minerals and calcium. It is easily absorbed by the skin and is just as effective used externally. Bathing in milk leaves the skin feeling conditioned and moisturized, but as the smell of milk in the bath can be unpleasant, it is best combined with essential oils.

To get the best from your milk bath, use it immediately it is prepared. Pour it into a ready-run bath just before you step in, then lie back and enjoy it.

cleopatra's beauty bath

These ingredients are sufficient for one bath.

100 ml/3½ fl oz/scant
  ½ cup full-fat milk
  (cow's, sheep's or
  goat's)
5 ml/1 tsp clear honey
5 drops jasmine absolute
5 drops ylang-ylang
  essential oil

Heat the milk gently in a saucepan and add the honey. Take off the heat and add the essential oils. Use immediately by adding to a ready-run warm bath.

tropical coconut milk bath

For one nourishing and relaxing bath, pour 45 g (3 tbsp) powdered coconut milk into a ready-run warm bath, lie back and think of palm trees. A good variation on this is to leave a vanilla pod and a tonka bean in the coconut powder to create a tropical fragrance.

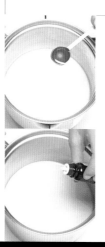

kids' milkshake bath

This is a great recipe for children with sensitive skin. These ingredients are sufficient for one bath.

100 ml/3½ fl oz/scant
  ½ cup full-fat milk
  (cow's, sheep's or
  goat's)
5 ml/1 tsp natural food
  colouring

Mix the milk with the food colouring in a bowl and then pour into a warm bath.

essential oils for baths

relaxing: 5 drops lavender essential oil and 5 drops ylang-ylang essential oil
refreshing: 5 drops bergamot essential oil and 5 drops grapefruit essential oil

essential oil baths

Adding essential oils to the bath is a wonderfully pleasurable and very popular way of using them. The warmth of the water encourages relaxation and also enables the essential oils to penetrate the skin. The oils should only be added to the water once the bath has been run and immediately before you step in, as the heat will encourage their evaporation.

It is important to remember that only the essential oils that are non-irritant, such as Roman chamomile and lavender, should be added directly to the bath. Just add 4–6 drops of essential oil and swirl the water around before stepping in.

All other essential oils should be diluted first in a carrier because they will not fully disperse in the water and their molecules may well come into direct contact with the skin and mucous membranes which can cause irritation and sensitization (see the safety details for each oil in the glossary of essential oils, pages 164–205). Suitable carriers include base oils, specially prepared bath oil bases, which have a dispersant added, and full-fat milk.

To prepare a bath using a carrier, mix 4–6 drops of essential oil to an egg-cupful of milk or 10 ml (2 tsp) of oil, add the mixture to the bath and swirl the water before stepping in. Good base oils to use are soya, almond and grapeseed.

For a rather more nourishing effect, add a teaspoon of evening primrose oil or jojoba oil. Oil blends can also be mixed with sea salts before adding to the bath.

stimulating:
Bergamot, coriander, cypress, grapefruit, juniper, lemon, lime, peppermint, pine, rosemary.

uplifting:
Bergamot, clary sage, geranium, jasmine, mandarin, melissa, neroli, frankincense, orange, palmarosa, rose.

relaxing:
Chamomile, clary sage, geranium, lavender, marjoram, neroli, rose, sandalwood, vetiver, ylang-ylang.

deep cleansing:
Cypress, grapefruit, juniper, lemon, tea tree.

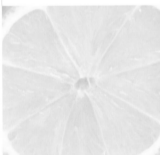
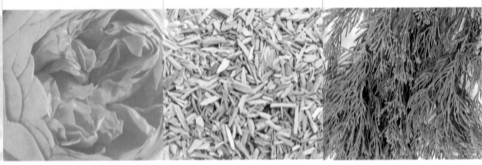

herbal infusions

anti-cellulite bath infusion

With a combination of a careful diet, massage, exercise and dry brushing it is possible to banish cellulite. Adding this diuretic and stimulating infusion to the bath will also help.

½ tsp bladderwrack

1 tsp celery seeds

2 tsp sea salt

2 drops juniper essential oil

2 drops black pepper essential oil

2 tsp fennel seeds

500 ml/18 fl oz/2¼ cups water

2 drops fennel essential oil

2 drops eucalyptus essential oil

Make an infusion from the bladderwrack, fennel and celery seeds and the water. Mix in the salt and add the essential oils. Use immediately by adding it to a ready-run warm bath.

seaweed and arnica bath infusion

This combines an infusion of mineral-rich seaweed with arnica tincture and essential oils of lemon, pine and juniper to create a refreshing and revitalizing bath.

½ tsp bladderwrack

1 tsp comfrey leaf

2 tsp juniper berries

500 ml/18 fl oz/2¼ cups water

2 heaped tsp sea salt

5 drops arnica tincture

2 drops pine essential oil

2 drops lavender essential oil

2 drops lemon essential oil

2 drops juniper essential oil

Make an infusion from the bladderwrack, comfrey, juniper berries and water. Add salt and stir, then add the arnica tincture and essential oils. Use immediately by adding to a ready-run warm bath.

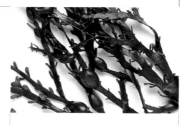

rose and rosehip infusion

This infusion makes a good tonic for dry and sensitive skin.

500 ml/18 fl oz/2¼ cups water

2 tsp dried rose petals/buds

1 tsp dried rosehips

1 tsp salt

5 ml/1 tsp cider vinegar

5 drops calendula tincture

8 drops rose essential oil

2 drops geranium essential oil

Make an infusion using the rosehips, rose petals and water. Strain. Add the rest of the ingredients. Use immediately by adding to a ready-run warm bath.

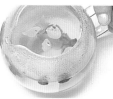

water

When a recipe calls for water, use filtered, bottled or distilled water or water that has been boiled and allowed to cool.

lemongrass and bay leaf infusion

This infusion is suitable after a period of any sporting activity or over-exertion.

2 tsp bay leaves
1 tsp rosemary
500 ml/18 fl oz/2¼ cups water
5 drops lemongrass essential oil

Make an infusion of the bay leaves and rosemary and the water. Add the lemongrass essential oil. Use immediately by adding to a ready-run warm bath.

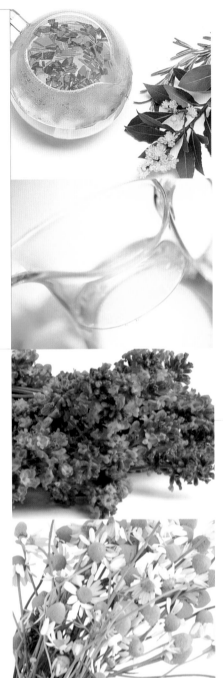

aloe vera and lavender infusion

This is cooling and soothing, perfect for sensitive skin which has been exposed to the sun.

2 tsp lavender flowers
2 tsp chamomile flowers
500 ml/18 fl oz/2¼ cups water
30 ml/2 tbsp aloe vera juice
10 drops lavender essential oil

Make an infusion of the lavender, chamomile and water. Add the aloe vera and lavender essential oil. Use immediately by adding to a ready-run warm bath.

sitz baths

A sitz bath is an excellent way of treating haemorrhoids, thrush, pruritis, stitches following childbirth and so on. Half-fill a large bowl or small bath with warm water. Use the same method of dilution as for baths and sit in the water for 10 minutes. Adding tea tree oil to a sitz bath is the classic treatment for thrush.

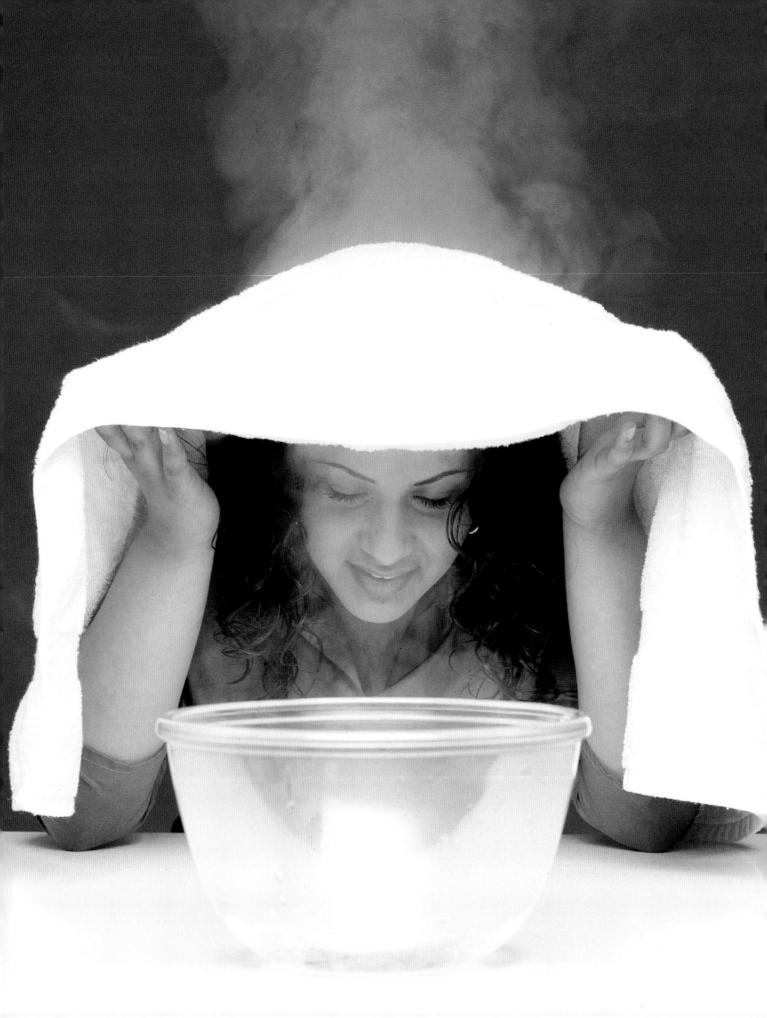

the face

facial steams

Steaming the face is an excellent way of deep-cleansing the skin. The steam opens the pores of the skin, allowing the active constituents of the herbs and oils used to be really effective. **Note:** Facial steams are not recommended if you have thread veins or very delicate skin.

Either fill a bowl with boiling water and add the required essential oils or pour boiling water over a handful of herbs. Place a towel over your head and the bowl and remain there for 5 minutes. Do be careful, though, not to persist if you are finding it uncomfortable. Too much heat can be damaging, as can inhaling the oils if you find them overpowering – so be gentle! Only add 1 drop of oil in a bowl of water until you become confident that the effects are beneficial. Remember to close the pores after this cleansing process by using an astringent toner.

facial steam blend

Excellent for treating blackheads, acne and problem skin. Use as a facial steam twice a week for six weeks for best results. It also makes an excellent deep-cleansing facial steam for any skin type on an occasional basis.

4 drops bergamot essential oil
2 drops chamomile essential oil
4 drops geranium essential oil
4 drops grapefruit essential oil
2 drops juniper essential oil
2 drops patchouli essential oil

Combine in a 10 ml (2 tsp) dropper bottle and add 3–4 drops to a bowl of hot water for a facial steam. You can also add the essential oils to 30 ml (2 tbsp) grapeseed oil and apply to the skin as a facial tonic oil.

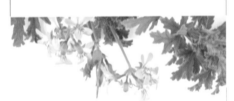

washing ball

A washing ball is an unusual idea, resembling a small ball of dough. It has a gritty consistency, which is very different from the smooth lather we are used to from soap. However, it does cleanse the face without dehydrating the skin, and regular use will result in a smooth complexion.

125 g/4 oz/5 tbsp raisins
125 g/4 oz/15 tbsp ground almonds
2 slices soft brown bread

Depending on the size, finely chop the raisins. Mix the almonds with the raisins. Finely crumble the bread and add to the mixture. Alternatively, use a blender to mix all of the above ingredients. Roll the mixture into between six and ten balls and use instead of soap.

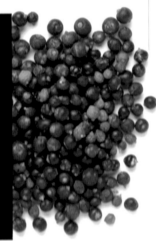

simple cleansing suggestions

- The cream base on page 42 can be used instead of soap.
- Plain live yogurt can be used as a cleanser. Apply with cotton wool to remove dirt before toning and moisturizing the face – very good for problem skin.
- Sweet almond oil can be used to take off all make-up including eye make-up.

cleansers

chamomile and elderflower face scrub

A gentle and cleansing scrub for sensitive skin.

- 25 g/10 tbsp (heaped) chamomile flowers or 10 chamomile teabags
- 25 g/10 tbsp (heaped) elderflowers or 10 elderflower teabags
- 10 ml/2tsp aloe vera juice
- 2 tbsp plain yoghurt

Make an infusion using a cupful of boiling water and half the quantity of herbs. Cover and leave to one side. Using a mortar and pestle, grind the remaining herbs to a fine powder. If you are using teabags, open them and use the contents without grinding. Combine with the aloe vera and stir in the yoghurt. Add sufficient infusion to make a thin paste. To use, apply to the face and gently rub for exfoliation and deep cleansing. Use the remaining water to wash off the mixture and tone the skin.

rose and honey face scrub

A fragrant scrub to cleanse and refresh normal skin.

- 25 g/3 tbsp dried rose petals
- 10 g/2 tbsp dried lavender flowers
- 1 drop lavender oil
- 1 drop rose oil
- 2 tsp clear honey

Make an infusion using half the roses and a cupful of boiling water. Cover and leave to one side. Using a mortar and pestle grind the remaining rose petals and lavender flowers until they have reached a powdery consistency. Combine the powdered herbs with the oil and honey, and then add enough rose infusion to form the mixture into a soft paste. To use, apply to the face and gently rub in a circular motion to cleanse the skin.

cleansing lotion

A simple lotion base for very sensitive skin.

- 25 g/2½ tbsp organic oats
- mineral water
- 1 egg yolk
- 50 ml/3½ tbsp almond oil

Put the oats into a bowl, pour on enough water to cover and leave for at least 1 hour. Whisk the egg yolk in a blender, adding a drop of oil at a time. Once all the oil has been added the mixture should be a thick emulsion. Strain the oats, squeezing all the water into a bowl to make the oatmilk. Add slowly to the egg mixture to thin it to the consistency of a lotion. This recipe can be fragranced by adding an oil, such as lavender, before the oatmilk is included.

a simple yoghurt cleanser

Live yoghurt is a traditional cleanser for the face. It is cooling, gentle and refreshing. Use once a week to maintain a clear complexion.

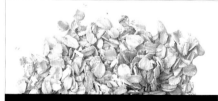

oatmilk

Oatmilk can be made by soaking oats in mineral water, then straining them through muslin (cheesecloth). This makes a softening and soothing water to use for cleaning the face, and is particularly good for very sensitive and delicate skin.

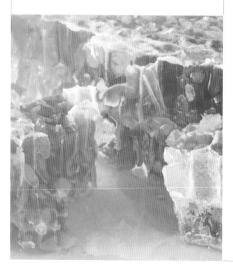

face packs and masks

These face packs are made using fresh fruit and are therefore quite messy, so make sure you have plenty of towels ready to protect your clothes. All these recipes are sufficient for one treatment.

avocado and honey face pack

A nourishing and regenerating facial for rejuvenating tired or mature skin.

I ripe avocado
5 ml/I tsp clear honey
5 ml/I tsp lemon juice
5 ml/I tsp plain yogurt

Combine all the ingredients in a bowl and mash into a paste, using a fork. Leave in the refrigerator for 30 minutes. Apply the pack to your face and leave on for 10 minutes. Gently remove with cool water, then pat dry with a clean towel.

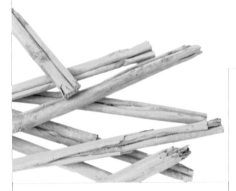

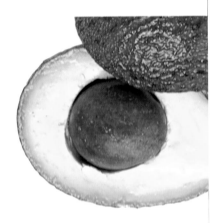

apple and cinnamon face pack

An antiseptic mask for oily or problem skin.

I ripe apple, peeled and
    grated
½ tsp single (light) cream
5ml/I tsp clear honey
I tbsp ground oats
½ tsp ground cinnamon

Combine all the ingredients in a bowl and mash into a paste, using a fork. Apply the pack to your face and leave on for 10 minutes. Gently remove with cool water, then pat dry with a clean towel.

banana face pack

A rich and nourishing face pack for dry skin.

I egg yolk
10 ml/2 tsp almond oil
I ripe banana

Combine all the ingredients in a bowl and mash into a paste, using a fork. Apply the pack to your face and leave on for 10 minutes. Gently remove with cool water, then pat dry with a clean towel.

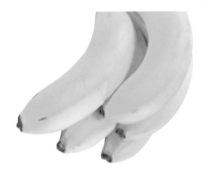

grapefruit mask

A skin-toning facial treatment, naturally rich in alpha-hydroxy-acids (AHAs), suitable for all skin types.

1 grapefruit
1 small pot plain yogurt

Peel the grapefruit, break the flesh into segments and remove the seeds and pith. Blend enough yogurt with the fruit to make a paste. Leave the mixture for 1 hour in the refrigerator. Apply the pack to your face and leave on for 10 minutes. Gently remove with cool water, then pat dry with a clean towel.

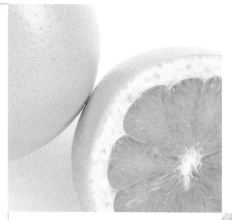

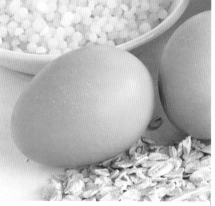

strawberry and oat exfoliating mask

A gentle exfoliating face pack to cleanse and tone the skin. These ingredients are sufficient for one treatment.

20 g/2 tbsp ground oats
3 large ripe strawberries
5 ml/1 tsp single (light) cream

Grind the oats to a fine powder, using a pestle and mortar or blender. Mash up the strawberries, using a fork, and mix with the oats. Add enough cream to make a paste. Apply the pack to your face and leave on for 10 minutes. Gently remove with cool water, then pat dry with a clean towel.

lavender and witch hazel mask

This face mask unblocks and tightens pores and absorbs excess sebum. These ingredients are sufficient for one treatment.

2 tsp fuller's earth
10 ml/2 tsp witch hazel
1 egg, lightly beaten
2 drops lavender essential oil

Mix the fuller's earth with the witch hazel to make a paste. Add the beaten egg and mix in the essential oil. Apply the pack to your face and leave on for 10 minutes. Gently remove with cool water, then pat dry with a clean towel.

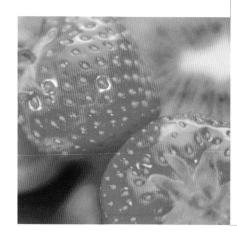

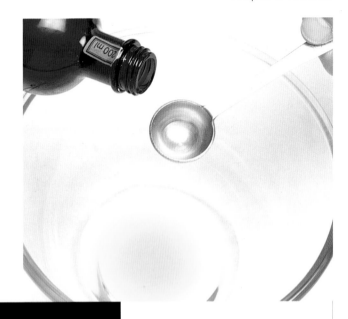

clay mask 1

This is suitable for most skin types, except very dry skin. The ingredients are sufficient for one or two treatments. It will keep for up to 3 months.

30 ml/2 tbsp aloe vera juice
5 ml/1 tsp witch hazel
5 ml/1 tsp clear honey
5 g/½ tbsp kaolin
10 g/1 tbsp bentonite
1 drop lavender essential oil

Mix together the aloe vera juice, witch hazel and honey. Slowly add the kaolin and bentonite, stirring constantly. Force the mixture through a sieve (strainer). Add the essential oil and mix in thoroughly. Gently apply the mask over the face, avoiding the eyes. Leave on for 10 minutes, then wash off with warm water.

variations

Flower waters may be substituted for the witch hazel in either mask, according to your skin type:
• **problem skin:** lavender flower water
• **oily skin:** witch hazel
• **mature skin:** rosewater
• **normal skin:** orange flower water

clay mask 2

Try this slightly different recipe if you have more oily skin, or suffer from blackheads. These ingredients are sufficient for one or two treatments. It will keep for up to 3 months.

30 ml/2 tbsp aloe vera juice
5 ml/1 tsp witch hazel
5 ml/1 tsp fresh grapefruit juice
15 g/1½ tbsp kaolin
5 g/½ tbsp bentonite
1 drop lemon essential oil

Mix together the aloe vera, witch hazel and grapefruit juice. Slowly add the kaolin and bentonite, stirring constantly. Force the mixture through a sieve (strainer). Add the essential oil and mix. Gently apply the mask over the face, avoiding the eyes. Leave on for 10 minutes, then wash off with warm water.

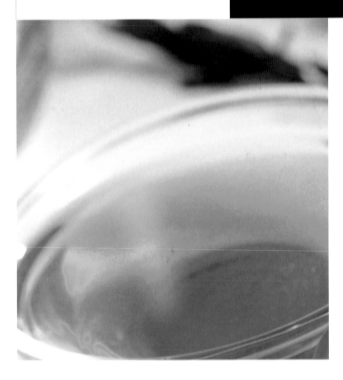

toners

Toners are used to cool and refresh the skin. They also remove any remaining traces of dirt and grease left from your cleanser. They are useful for oily skin because many of them are astringent, and help to reduce sebum levels and refine open pores.

In former times, toners were often flower waters, such as rosewater or lavender water, the by-product of essential oil distillation. These days flower waters are often manufactured by mixing essential oil with water, using a dispersant. Many skin toners contain a small amount of alcohol, which is fine if you have oily skin but may be rather drying for very dry or sensitive skin.

infusions as toners

Many herbal infusions can be used as skin toners when cooled. See the chart on page 88 to find the right herb for your skin type.

lavender and witch hazel

Make a lavender and witch hazel infusion. The antiseptic and astringent properties make it particularly appropriate for oily or problem skin.

parsley water

Soak fresh parsley (use organic if possible) in still mineral water overnight. This parsley water can be used to tone the skin and is particularly good for cleansing the skin of blackheads.

lemon and glycerin

This mixture has a slightly astringent and strengthening effect on the capillaries; use it if you have thread veins. These ingredients will make 20 ml (4 tsp). It will keep for 3 months.

20 ml/4 tsp vegetable glycerin
juice of 1 lemon
1 drop neroli essential oil
1 drop rose absolute

Mix the vegetable glycerin with the lemon juice and add the essential oils. Apply twice a day to thread veins.

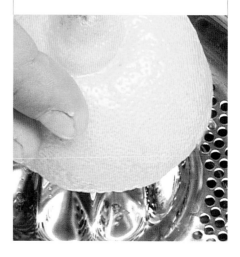

refreshing spritzer

This is a beneficial face or body spray. These ingredients are sufficient to make 100 ml (3½ fl oz). Keep it in the refrigerator when not in use and replace every 2 days.

2 tsp (heaped) fresh mint
2 tsp (heaped) fresh dill
1 tsp (heaped) fresh parsley
85 ml/3 fl oz/⅓ cup mineral water

Using the herbs above, make a strong infusion (see page 38). Add the mineral water to the infusion and pour the mixture into a bottle with a spray atomizer attachment.

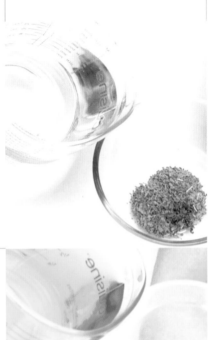

refreshing face spray

A spray that is particularly good for dry skin. If your skin tends to be greasy, use witch hazel instead of orange flower water. These ingredients are sufficient to make 100 ml (3½ fl oz). It will keep for up to 2 days in the refrigerator.

85 ml/3 fl oz/⅓ cup distilled water
10 ml/2 tsp aloe vera juice
2 ml/½ tsp orange flower water
1 drop propolis tincture
1 drop neroli essential oil
1 drop rosemary essential oil

Combine the ingredients and store in a bottle. Shake before using with an atomizer spray.

lemon and aloe vera toner

A refreshing and healing toner suitable for all skin types. Either apply using cotton wool after cleansing or use throughout the day as a cooling and stimulating spray. A dispersant has not been added so it is important to shake well before use to ensure the essential oils are evenly mixed through the liquid. The quantities given here will make 100 ml (3½ fl oz).

80 ml/5 tbsp lavender flower water
10 ml/2 tsp witch hazel
5 ml/1 tsp aloe vera juice
14 drops bergamot essential oil
4 drops lemon essential oil
4 drops petitgrain essential oil
4 drops lavender essential oil
2 drops rosemary essential oil
2 drops black pepper essential oil

Simply combine all the ingredients. Store in a glass bottle, preferably with an atomizer spray, out of direct sunlight for up to 6 months.

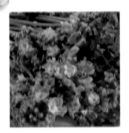

moisturizers

Moisturizers are probably the most popular cosmetic product, and they are certainly a very important part of any skin-care routine. A good moisturizer should rehydrate the skin and keep it feeling supple without making it feel greasy or preventing the skin from being able to breathe. It can also help to protect the skin by providing a barrier against pollutants and irritants, and the latest generation of moisturizers often have a sunscreen added to protect the skin from the harmful effects of the sun.

Moisturizers need to combine an oil for emollient properties, which help to keep the skin supple, and water for moisturizing, rehydrating properties. In order to keep the oil and water combined an emulsifier will be needed. The simplest emulsifiers are beeswax and emulsifying wax, and we use these in the following recipes.

Moisturizers are formulated to penetrate the surface of the skin, so they are the ideal way to deliver therapeutic ingredients to it. This is true whether they are made of highly technological ingredients or natural ingredients such as herbs and essential oils.

restoring pH

If your skin has been dehydrated by using soap, you can restore the pH balance by splashing your face daily with 5 ml (1 tsp) cider vinegar diluted in 600 ml (1 pint/2½ cups) water. You could make an extraction of elderflowers in the vinegar for an extra cleansing effect.

lavender and lemon moisturizer

A moisturizer with antiseptic and healing properties suitable for oily or problem skin. This recipe makes a 40 g (1½ oz) jar.

- 1 tsp beeswax (granules or grated)
- 5 g/1 tsp cocoa butter
- 45 ml/3 tbsp grapeseed oil
- 10 g/3 tsp emulsifying wax
- 30 ml/1 fl oz/2 tbsp lavender infusion
- 10 drops lemon essential oil

Heat the beeswax, cocoa butter and base oil in a bowl over a saucepan of boiling water. Dissolve the emulsifying wax in the lavender infusion. Slowly add the infusion to the oil mixture, using a fast whisk action for about 10 seconds. When the mixture cools down, add the essential oil. Store in a dark glass jar in the refrigerator. It will keep for up to 2 months.

avocado moisturizer

A rich and nourishing moisturizer for dry skin. This recipe makes a 40 g (1½ oz) jar.

- 5 g/1 tsp beeswax (granules or grated)
- 5 g/1 tsp cocoa butter
- 15 ml/½ fl oz/1 tbsp avocado oil
- 30 ml/1 fl oz/2 tbsp almond oil
- 10 g/3 tsp emulsifying wax
- 30 ml/1 fl oz/2 tbsp marsh mallow infusion
- 5 drops sandalwood essential oil
- 5 drops bergamot essential oil

Heat the beeswax, cocoa butter and base oils in a bowl set over a saucepan of boiling water. Dissolve the emulsifier in the marsh mallow infusion. Slowly add the infusion to the oil mixture, using a fast whisk action for about 10 seconds. When the mixture cools down, add the essential oils. Store in a dark glass jar in the refrigerator. It will keep for up to 2 months.

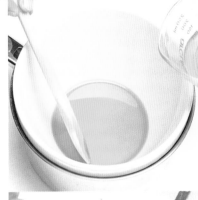
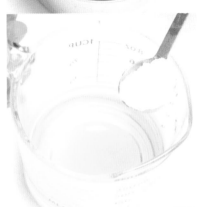
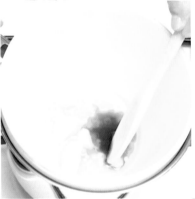

geranium and apricot moisturizer

A light and balancing moisturizer for normal or combination skin. This recipe makes a 40 g (1½ oz) jar.

- 5 g/1 tsp beeswax (granules or grated)
- 5 g/1tsp cocoa butter
- 15 ml/½ fl oz/1 tbsp apricot kernel oil
- 30 ml/1 fl oz/2 tbsp grapeseed oil
- 2 tsp emulsifying wax
- 30 ml/1 fl oz/2 tbsp rose petal infusion
- 10 drops geranium essential oil

Heat the beeswax, cocoa butter and base oils in a bowl set over a saucepan of boiling water. Dissolve the emulsifying wax in the rose petal infusion. Slowly add the infusion to the oil mixture, stirring constantly. When the mixture cools down, add the essential oil. Store in a dark glass jar in the refrigerator. It will keep for up to 2 months.

rose facial oil

This is an exquisite oil suitable for delicate skin. Apply nightly for a luxurious and rejuvenating facial massage. It also makes a delightful conditioning oil when applied to damp skin. This recipe makes a 30 ml (1 fl oz) bottle.

- 10 ml/2 tsp evening primrose oil
- 20 ml/4 tsp grapeseed oil
- 2 drops rose essential oil
- 2 drops patchouli essential oil
- 2 drops geranium essential oil

Blend the base oils and essential oils together. Store in a dark glass bottle. It will last for up to 6 months.

eye care

Our eyes reveal so much about us that it is worth spending a little time each day to give them special attention. The stresses and strains of modern life – especially staring at computer and television screens – can result in sore, puffy and tired eyes, but here are some recipes to soothe and refresh, as well as ways of cleansing away make-up and everyday grime.

We tend to take our eyes for granted, although they are one of the most vital of our organs. They deserve to be looked after for they convey much of who and how we are to the world around us.

The best recipe for the eyes is of course to look after your general health. Remember, too, that eyes need rest. With the increasing use of computer screens at work and television at home, eyes are subject to extra strain which can result in puffiness and soreness. Exercise can help to alleviate puffiness, while sleep and a balanced diet of fresh and whole foods will be good for your eyes and for your general well-being. Drink lots of water and avoid salt, caffeine and alcohol.

Tired or strained eyes can be soothed by being bathed in herbal infusions. Chamomile is often used, but even more effective is an infusion made with the leaves of *Euphrasia officinalis*, commonly known as eyebright. The astringent and anti-inflammatory properties of this herb have made it a traditional treatment for eye irritations, including conjunctivitis and the soreness caused by fatigue or being in a smoky atmosphere. In another traditional recipe for eye infections, eyebright is combined with golden seal (*Hydrastis canadensis*) to make a soothing eye bath.

The skin around the eyes is especially delicate. Always take great care when you are removing eye make-up. A little almond oil on cotton wool will quickly remove most make-up, or try the eye make-up remover cream on page 122. Whenever you make and use any preparations for your eyes, be especially scrupulous about sterilizing the equipment you use. Eye infections can be transmitted very quickly and cleanliness at all times is absolutely essential.

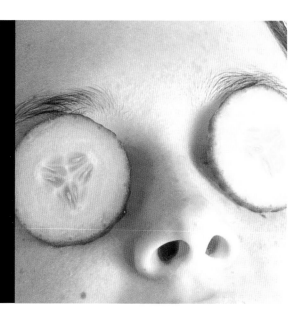

relieving tired eyes

If your eyes feel tired or have bags under them try lying back, closing your eyes and applying one of the following:

dry, sore eyes: cotton wool pads soaked in aloe vera juice

hot, sore eyes: slices of cooling cucumber

puffy eyes: slices of potato

tired eyes: used chamomile teabags (preferably organic); other herbs that will help include witch hazel, calendula and elderflower

refreshers

eye baths

Eyes can benefit from bathing, but make sure your hands are washed and that any equipment you use is free from dirt or contamination.

Prepare a herbal infusion (see page 38) with the appropriate herbs (see below). Herbal infusions must be made fresh daily.

Strain through muslin (cheesecloth) or an unbleached coffee filter to ensure that no irritating herb particles are present. Use an eye bath or an eggcup that has been sterilized with boiling water. Tip your head back, holding the eye bath to your eye. Clean the eye bath in between bathing each eye to avoid spreading any infection.

eye bags

Eye bags look and feel rather like eyemask-shaped beanbags and it is a simple sewing job to make them up. The linseed is very cooling to the skin, a property that cotton wool does not have, and it will absorb the essential oils.

100 g/3½ oz/5 tbsp linseeds
2 drops neroli essential oil
2 drops lavender essential oil

Choose some very soft fabric that you feel would be comfortable placed over your eyes. A close-weave cotton such as lawn is probably best. Cut out two shapes that will cover both eyes. Stitch together all the way around the edges, leaving a small gap through which you pour the linseed to which a mixture of 2 drops each of neroli and lavender essential oils have been added. Close up the gap. Lie down, place the bag over your eyes and relax. When the fragrance has faded, just open up the bag and add some more drops of essential oils.

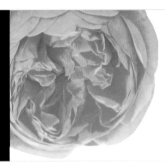

herbs for eye baths

tired eyes: rose petals
strained eyes: eyebright and chamomile
conjunctivitis: eyebright and marigold

eye wash for conjunctivitis

The conjunctiva is the mucous membrane that covers the eyeball and lines the lids. Inflammation of this membrane, characterized by a watery bloodshot look and a feeling of discomfort, is known as conjunctivitis. The infection can easily be spread from one eye to the other so care should be taken.

1 tsp (heaped) dried eyebright
1 tsp (heaped) dried marigold
1 tsp (heaped) dried elderflower
1 litre/1¾ pts mineral water

Place the dried herbs in the water and boil for 5 minutes. Allow the liquid to cool slightly, then pour through fine muslin (cheesecloth) or unbleached coffee filter paper. The liquid can either be left to cool and used as an eye wash or, while it is still warm, used in a compress. Soak pieces of cotton or muslin (cheesecloth) in the liquid, wring out, then place over the closed eyelids. Leave in place for 15 minutes. This process should be repeated 3–4 times a day. If symptoms persist after 3 days seek medical advice.

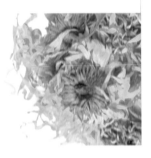

gels and lotions

eye gel

This is a wonderful gel to help
tighten the skin around the eyes
and reduce puffiness. However,
great care must be taken when
using products around the eyes.
Do not put this cooling and toning
gel into the eyes, or where it can
seep in. These ingredients will make
65 ml (2$\frac{1}{2}$ fl oz/4 tbsp). Store in
the refrigerator and do not use
longer than a week after making it.

20 ml/4 tsp cornflower
infusion
20 ml/4 tsp calendula infusion
$\frac{1}{4}$ tsp carrageen
20 ml/4 tsp distilled water
5 ml/1 tsp euphrasia tincture

Make the cornflower and
calendula infusions as directed
on page 38. Mix the carrageen
with the distilled water until
fully dissolved. Add the infusions
to the distilled water along with
the tincture and allow to set.

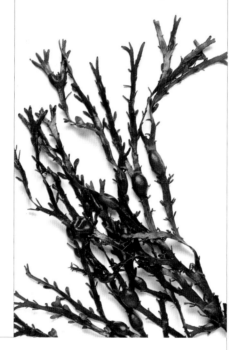

eye make-up remover

To remove make-up, gently wipe
the eyes with a little almond oil
on cotton wool. Alternatively, try
the following cream, which uses
chamomile infusion to soothe.
The ingredients given here will
make approximately 100 ml
(3$\frac{1}{2}$ fl oz/7 tbsp).

5 g/1 tsp beeswax
(granules or grated)
$\frac{1}{2}$ tsp shea nut butter
$\frac{1}{4}$ tsp cocoa butter
10 ml/2 tsp almond oil
40 drops aloe vera juice
70 ml/14 tsp chamomile infusion
10 ml/2 tsp emusifying wax

Heat the beeswax, shea nut
butter, cocoa butter and almond
oil together until melted. Add the
aloe vera juice to the chamomile
infusion, mix in the emusifying wax
and heat the mixture. Check the
temperatures of the oil mix and the
infusion mix. When both are 70°C
(158°F), mix them together with a
hand whisk. Allow to cool before
pouring into a dark-coloured glass
bottle. The cream will keep for up
to 3 weeks in the refrigerator.

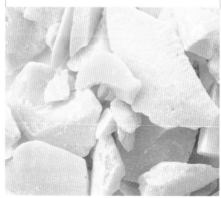

mouth and ear care

After our eyes, people tend to notice our mouths. Smooth lips and gleaming teeth will make a friendly smile doubly welcoming, and the confidence that comes from the certainty that our breath is fresh and sweet will affect our whole demeanour. Use natural ingredients in your daily routines, and notice the difference.

lavender and lemon mouthwash

An antiseptic and healing mouthwash for sore gums that will also freshen the breath. These ingredients are sufficient to make 90 ml (3 fl oz/6 tbsp). It will keep for up to 6 months.

15 ml/3 tsp lavender tincture
15 ml/3 tsp calendula tincture
50 ml/10 tsp vegetable
   glycerin
2 drops lemon essential oil
2 drops orange essential oil
5 drops peppermint
   essential oil

Blend all the ingredients together and pour them into a bottle. Shake the bottle and dilute 1 teaspoon in a little water to rinse around the mouth.

variations

If the gums are bleeding, try adding raspberry tincture. Echinacea, myrrh or golden seal tinctures are good for infections. (In each case replace the lavender tincture.)

peppermint toothpaste

A simple toothpaste for regular use. Fennel or lemon essential oil can be used instead of peppermint, if you prefer. If your teeth are aching add clove, which will help anaesthetize the pain. These ingredients are sufficient for one treatment.

1 tsp sodium bicarbonate
5 ml/1 tsp vegetable glycerin
3 drops peppermint
   essential oil

Mix the sodium bicarbonate with the vegetable glycerin. Add the essential oil.

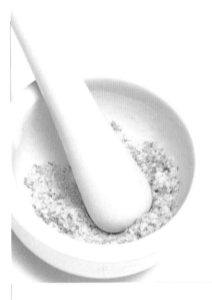

sage and myrrh toothpowder

An excellent remedy for sore and bleeding gums. These ingredients are sufficient for one treatment.

1 g/½ tbsp sage
5 g/1 tsp salt
5 drops myrrh essential oil

Grind the sage and salt together, using a mortar and pestle. Add the essential oil, preferably spraying through an atomizer. Brush on to your teeth and gums, using a toothbrush. Do not swallow.

lip balms

mandarin lip balm

The balm will keep for up to 6 months.

5 g/1 tsp beeswax
70 g/2¾ oz cocoa butter
1 tsp coconut oil
5 drops St John's wort tincture
5 drops calendula tincture
10 drops mandarin
   essential oil

Melt the beeswax, cocoa butter and coconut oil in a bowl over a saucepan of hot water. Add the tinctures and then the essential oil. Pour into a jar before the mixture begins to harden.

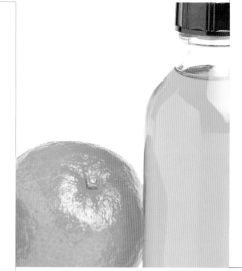

grapefruit conditioning lip balm

A moisturizing and naturally antiseptic lip balm for dry or sore lips. It will keep for up to 6 months.

1 g cocoa butter
9 g shea or cocoa butter
10 drops grapefruit
   essential oil

Melt the cocoa and shea butter over a bowl of hot water. Add the essential oil and pour into jars. Leave to set. This may take up to 12 hours, depending on room temperature.

moisturizing herbal lip balm

In this recipe, sesame oil has been used to moisturize and hydrate the delicate skin of the lips, helping to protect them against the sun; wheatgerm oil is high in vitamin E, which is an antioxidant and acts as a natural preservative; carrot oil is high in vitamin C; and myrrh essential oil is good for dry and chapped skin.

20 g/4 tsp beeswax (granules
   or grated)
50 ml/10 tsp sesame oil
5 ml/1 tsp carrot oil

14 ml/scant 3 tsp wheatgerm oil
1 drop myrrh essential oil
2 drops lemon essential oil

Put the beeswax, sesame, carrot and wheatgerm oils into a saucepan and heat slowly. Stir the mixture until all the beeswax has melted. Remove the mixture from the heat and allow to cool slightly. Add the essential oils, pour the mixture into a container and allow to set.

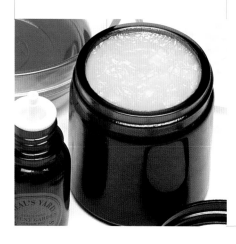

special treatments

earache

The following will help to relieve earache, but do seek professional assistance if the pain becomes extreme or is persistent.

Use garlic macerate or mullein macerate (see page 40), putting a few drops of the warmed oil on to a piece of cotton wool and placing it gently inside the ear. Remember not to put anything into the ear that is not clean, nor anything too small which will be difficult to remove. Do not put anything into your ear if your eardrum is perforated.

ear/body piercing

There are a number of antibacterial and antiseptic herbs and oils that can be used after piercing. Make an infusion from echinacea or golden seal, and dab on to prevent infection. Alternatively, dab on a drop of lavender or tea tree essential oil.

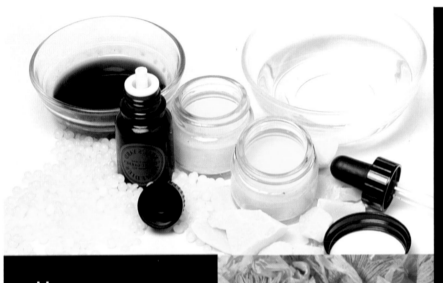

toothache

Apply clove essential oil to a cottonwool bud and hold on to the tooth. Teething pain can be soothed by rubbing the gums with marsh mallow root decoction, or by allowing the baby to chew on a piece of orris or marsh mallow root. Teething problems can be relieved by giving Chamomilla granules 6X (a homoeopathic remedy) as required.

cold sores

Apply tea tree essential oil to the skin at the first sign of a cold sore developing. Continue to use until the cold sore has dried up. Dab on calendula tincture to dry up and heal a cold sore. For the last stage of the cold sore, apply calendula ointment.

hand creams

Many people do not realize until too late that the hands can give away the age quicker than a carefully protected face. For centuries, women have been creating hand creams and using skin whiteners to conceal age spots and loose skin. A little time spent in putting on hand cream and taking care to wear gloves when washing up or gardening will make a great difference. Here are a few recipes for hand care that are fun to make and wonderful to use.

rose and almond hand cream

This is a beautifully rich hand cream. An infusion of chamomile or elderflower can be substituted for the rosewater. The recipe makes two 40 g (1½ oz) jars.

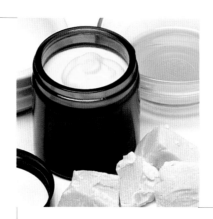

8 g/1½ tsp cocoa butter
5 g/1 tsp beeswax
    (granules or grated)
30 ml/2 tbsp almond oil
45 ml/1½ fl oz/3 tbsp
    rosewater
10 g/3 tsp emulsifying wax
10 drops rose absolute

Melt the cocoa butter, beeswax and almond oil over a bowl of hot water. Heat the rosewater slightly and dissolve the emulsifying wax into it. Stir the rosewater and emulsifying wax into the oily mixture very slowly and continue stirring until the cream cools. Add the rose absolute and stir. Store in a jar in the refrigerator. It will keep for up to 2 months.

chamomile and oat moisturizing hand scrub

A good alternative to soap for sensitive hands. These ingredients are sufficient to make 40 g (1½ oz).

30 ml/2 tbsp vegetable glycerin
15 g/½ oz/2 tbsp cornflour (cornstarch)
5 ml/1 tsp chamomile flower water
2 tsp finely ground oats
2 tsp finely ground rice

Heat the vegetable glycerin over a bowl of hot water. Slowly add the cornflour (cornstarch), stirring constantly to make a paste. Take off the heat and slowly add the chamomile water, still stirring. Stir in the ground oats and ground rice. Store in a jar and use in the same way as liquid soap. It will keep for up to 2 months.

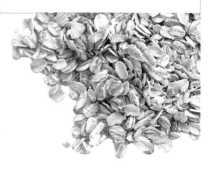

orange and frankincense hand cream

This is another rich cream, suitable for dry, work-worn hands. The recipe makes two 40 g (1½ oz) jars.

8 g/1½ tsp cocoa butter

5 g/1 tsp beeswax (granules or grated)

10 ml/2 tsp almond oil and wheatgerm oil, mixed

45 ml/1½ fl oz/3 tbsp orange flower water

10 g/3 tsp emulsifying wax

10 drops orange essential oil

5 drops frankincense essential oil

Melt the cocoa butter, beeswax and almond and wheatgerm oil over a bowl of hot water. Heat the orange flower water slightly and dissolve the emulsifying wax into it. Stir the orange flower water mixture into the oily mixture very slowly. Stir until the cream cools, then add the essential oils and stir. Store in a jar in the refrigerator. It will keep for up to 2 months.

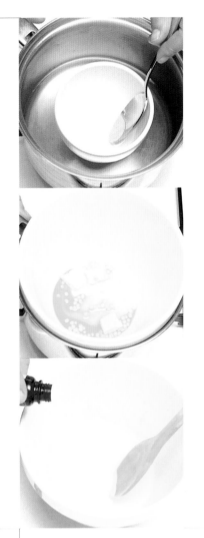

ayurvedic nail formula

To condition and strengthen the nails.

15 ml/½ fl oz/1 tbsp almond oil

2 drops sandalwood essential oil

2 drops cypress essential oil

2 drops lavender essential oil

Blend all the oils together and store in a bottle. To use, heat the bottle of blended oils in a bowl of hot water. Apply daily to the nails on cotton wool buds. It will keep for up to 6 months.

myrrh nail strengthener

Use this nail strengthener daily. The quantities are sufficient for one treatment.

25 ml/1½ tbsp horsetail infusion

15 g/1 tbsp lanolin

10 drops myrrh

Hold the nails in a bowl containing the horsetail infusion and leave for at least 5 minutes. Mix together the lanolin and myrrh and rub thoroughly into the nails. Wash off any excess.

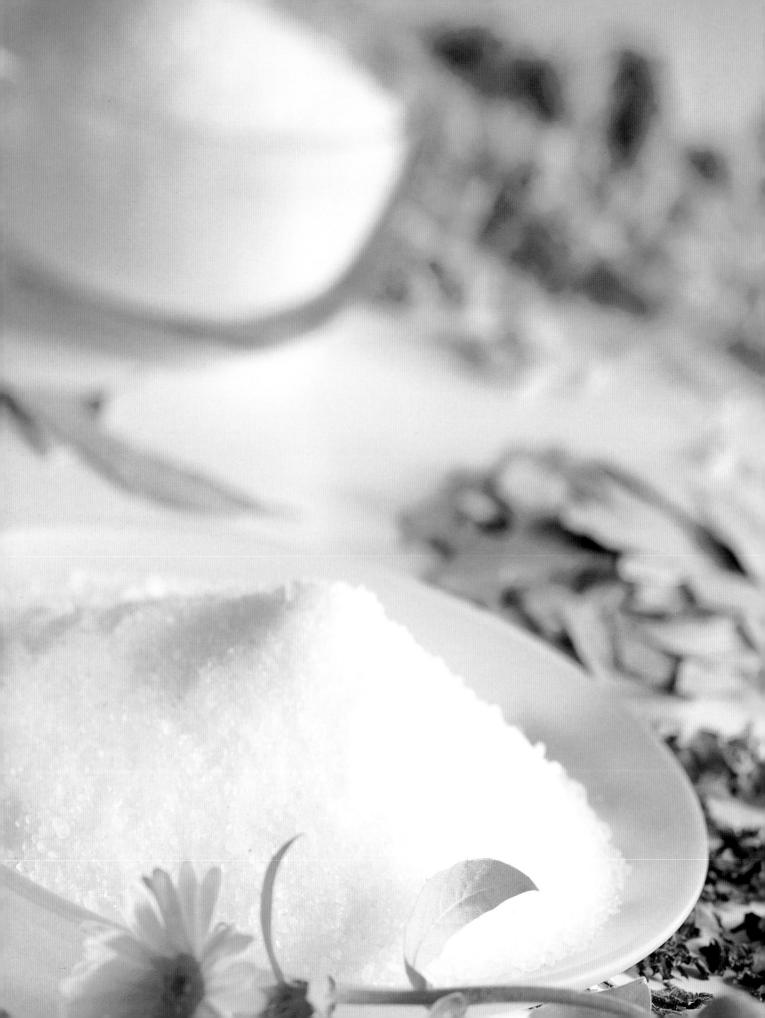

foot care

They may not be on show, but our feet deserve the same care as our hands. Use special baths to refresh and revive tired feet, soften dried skin with soothing creams, and take action now to avoid problems later. Use all manner of herbs and your favourite essential oils in the following recipes to create healing and invigorating lotions, balms and creams.

Many of us complain that our feet are killing us, but we expect them to put up with us walking for miles in shoes that are often ill-fitting or unsuitable in some way. Then we try to ignore any problems, hoping they will just go away.

Give your feet a treat and prepare a foot bath. There's nothing better than soaking tired and aching feet when you get home after a long day – a washing-up bowl half full of warm water is easy enough to arrange. Dead Sea salt or sea salt is refreshing and cleansing. Add infused herbs such as marsh mallow, witch hazel, rosemary, thyme, comfrey and calendula. Also try essential oils of lavender, eucalyptus, tea tree, rosemary, peppermint, geranium, thyme, Tagetes. Use tincture of arnica for bruised and aching feet, while Epsom salts will help revive them.

With 250,000 sweat glands covering the soles of the feet it is no wonder that they may feel a little on the damp side from time to time! The distinctive odour often associated with the feet results from the reaction between bacteria (naturally and harmlessly found in this area) and sweat. Washing the feet with soap and wearing cotton socks to reduce sweating will help, as will some of the suggestions in this section, especially the Lavender and Lemon Foot Deodorant and the Blackcurrant and Lemon Foot Powder on page 133. They have all been tried with varying results!

Corns develop due to repeated pressure and trauma, commonly forming either between or over the joints of the toes. To alleviate them, soak your feet in a bowl of warm water with 6–8 drops of *Tagetes* essential oil added. Remove the build-up of hard skin using myrrh and mandarin foot scrub, or use a pumice stone directly on the corn.

Athlete's foot is a common foot complaint which is caused by a fungal infection. The top layers of affected skin continually peel away, revealing a red, inflamed and very itchy patch of skin. Flare-ups, when painful blisters may appear, can often be linked with warm weather and damp feet, so it is important to keep your feet cool and dry.

Strict foot hygiene is essential. After washing the feet, make sure that they are dried completely. Pay particular attention to the skin between the toes, as the most common site of infection is between the fourth and fifth toes. Wear only socks made from natural fibres and when possible give your feet a break from wearing shoes altogether.

blister buster

Combine infusions of comfrey and witch hazel and dab on to the affected area regularly with cotton wool to heal blisters.

foot massage

Reflexology is a method of healing that appears to have originated in China. To massage your feet, begin by sitting comfortably, holding one foot. Using mainly your thumbs but also your fingers, work your way around the whole surface of the foot, applying a good pressure, bit by bit, to each area.

First work your way over the sole of the foot from the toes to the heel. Then work on the top of the foot up to and including the ankle, where the reflexology points for other parts of the body are situated. Massage one foot completely before doing the other. Make sure that your hands remain in contact with the foot throughout the massage.

Any tender spot can be said to represent tension, or possibly illness, in the corresponding organ. The chart below shows the organs of the body associated with the different parts of the foot. Apply a steady pressure for 30 minutes to the painful spot, working gently around it and coming back to it again and again until any pain has been worked through. If you are performing reflexology on someone else, remember to be gentle, especially when massaging sensitive parts of the foot, and responsive to any signs of pain or excessive tenderness.

---

foot massage oil

To make the massage base, combine 90 ml (3 fl oz/ 6 tbsp) of almond oil with 10 ml (2 tsp) of wheatgerm oil. Add one of the suggested combinations of essential oils listed below:

morning blend: 8 drops basil, 5 drops orange, 10 drops sandalwood, 5 drops myrrh, 2 drops peppermint

evening blend: 5 drops lavender, 10 drops ylang-ylang

restorative blend: 5 drops tea tree, 10 drops lavender

---

reflexology chart

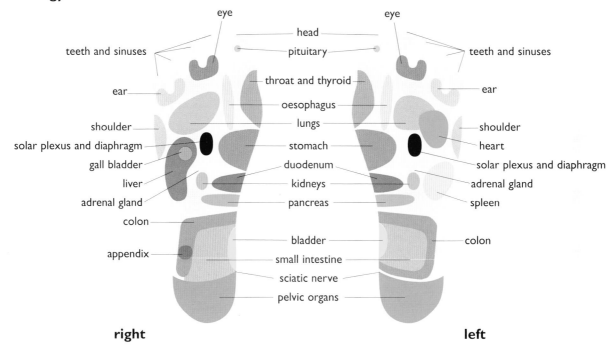

right   left

foot baths and balms

mulled winter warmer

This is a warming and deeply relaxing foot bath which slowly increases circulation to cold feet. Rosehip and hibiscus tea bags can be used as a convenient alternative to the loose herbs.

  1 tbsp dried rosehips
  2 tbsp dried hibiscus
  1 tsp cloves
  1 tsp juniper berries
  3 bay leaves, crushed
  1 tbsp orange peel,
    fresh or dried
  3 drops ginger essential oil

Place all the ingredients in a muslin (cheesecloth) bag and gently stir them in a bowl of boiling water. When the liquid has cooled enough for the skin to bear, immerse your feet.

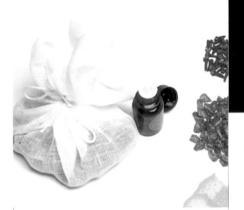

refreshing foot fizz

Create your own foot spa.

  2 drops essential oil
  100 g/3 tbsp sodium
    bicarbonate
  15 ml/½ fl oz/1 tbsp
    citric acid

For the essential oil, choose between combinations of lemon and lime, geranium and orange, and peppermint and black pepper. Dissolve all the ingredients together in hot water in a large bowl for the feet.

verrucas

Try these local remedies; if they fail to help, seek professional advice.
garlic macerated oil: dab on daily
fresh dandelion sap: squeeze the milky sap found inside the dandelion stalk on daily
thuja tincture: dab on daily
tea tree essential oil: dab on daily

mustard foot bath

This is a wonderful bath for cold winter evenings. It warms you up and helps to prevent colds and flu.

  75 g/5 tbsp mustard powder
  2 tbsp dried spearmint
  600 ml/1 pt/2½ cups water
  5 drops eucalyptus citrodora
    essential oil

Make an infusion using the mustard, spearmint and water. Add the eucalyptus oil. Use immediately by adding to a foot bath filled with warm water.

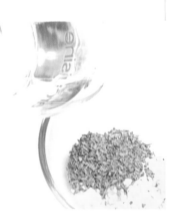

double mint foot cream

A cooling and refreshing cream which will gently soften and soothe the skin. The ingredients are sufficient to make 100 g (3½ oz).

10 g/2 tsp cocoa butter
10 g/2 tsp beeswax
30 ml/1 fl oz/2 tbsp almond oil
15 ml/½ fl oz/1 tbsp
   wheatgerm oil
30 ml/2 tbsp/1 fl oz
   spearmint infusion
10 g emulsifying wax
10 drops peppermint
   essential oil

Heat the cocoa butter, beeswax and base oils together in a bowl over a saucepan of water until the ingredients have melted. Warm the infusion and dissolve the emulsifying wax in it. Take the oily mixture off the heat, slowly add the infusion and stir until cool. Add the essential oils and store in a glass jar in the refrigerator. It will keep for at least 2 months.

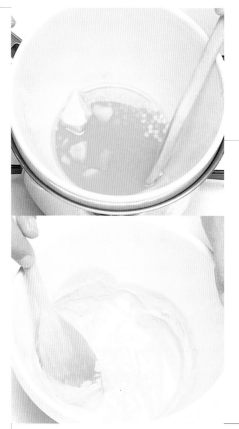

foot bath for hot feet

To 1 tablespoon of Dead Sea salts add 10 drops of peppermint essential oil. Dissolve in hot water in a bowl for the feet. Also try grapefruit or tea tree essential oils.

chilli not chilly

A quick and easy way to warm cold feet is to add cayenne and mustard powder to talcum powder. Both these herbs are rubifacients, which means they stimulate local circulation to the skin and hence add heat. When using before going to bed it is a good idea to wear socks so the powder does not get into the bedding.

tea tree and thyme foot balm

An antiseptic and healing cream, particularly good for treating athlete's foot. It will last for 6 months if stored in an airtight jar. When you are cleaning the bowl afterwards, heat it to melt excess balm and wipe away with kitchen roll – do not wash it down the drain. These ingredients are sufficient to make 40 g (1½ oz).

10 g/2 tsp beeswax (granules or grated)
45 ml/1½ fl oz/3 tbsp almond oil
15 ml/½ fl oz/1 tbsp wheatgerm oil
5 ml/1 tsp marsh mallow tincture
5 ml/1 tsp comfrey tincture
5 drops thyme essential oil
5 drops tea tree essential oil

Heat the beeswax and almond oil in a bowl set over a saucepan of boiling water until the beeswax has melted. Add the wheatgerm oil and the marsh mallow and comfrey tinctures and stir. Remove from the heat and cool slightly. Add the essential oils and mix thoroughly. Pour into a glass jar and allow to set.

special treatments

myrrh and mandarin foot scrub

Not only does this scrub remove hard skin effectively, it also softens and protects the delicate skin left behind. The easiest way to crush the pumice stone is to pound it using a pestle and mortar. Both the size of the crushed pumice particles and the overall quantity used depend on how sensitive the soles of your feet are – you may find that with successive batches you are able to tolerate more. These ingredients are sufficient to make 40 g (1½ oz).

- 10 g/2 tsp cocoa butter
- 10 g/2 tsp beeswax (granules or grated)
- 45 ml/1½ fl oz/3 tbsp apricot kernel oil
- 30 ml/1 fl oz/2 tbsp marsh mallow infusion
- 10 g/3½ tsp emulsifying wax
- 15 g/1 tbsp crushed pumice stone
- 12 drops myrrh essential oil
- 8 drops mandarin essential oil

Heat the cocoa butter, beeswax and apricot kernel oil together in a bowl set over a pan of water until all ingredients are melted. Warm the marsh mallow infusion and dissolve the emulsifying wax in it. Take the oily mixture off the heat. Slowly add the infusion to the oily mixture and stir until cool. Add the pumice stone and the essential oils to the cream and mix thoroughly. It will keep for up to 6 months.

lavender and lemon foot deodorant

Witch hazel is an effective astringent, which decreases the flow of secretions from the sweat glands. Lavender kills the bacteria, while lemon acts as a deodorizer. These ingredients are sufficient to make 30 ml (2 tbsp).

- 30 ml/2 tbsp witch hazel
- 5 drops lavender essential oil
- 5 drops lemon essential oil

Blend the witch hazel with the essential oils, pour into an atomizer and spray regularly on to clean feet. To ensure an even mix, shake before each application. It will keep for up to 2 months.

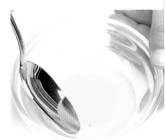
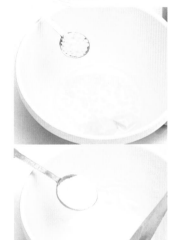

blackcurrant and lemon foot powder

This foot powder not only absorbs the secretions but aims to decrease excess sweat production itself, hence treating the source of the odour. After washing and drying your feet thoroughly, sprinkle on the powder and gently rub it in. This powder can also be dusted into footwear for added protection.

- 1½ g/1 tbsp dried sage
- 5 g/2 tbsp blackcurrant leaves
- 10 g/1 tbsp kaolin
- 5 drops lemon essential oil

Grind the sage and blackcurrant into a fine powder, using a pestle and mortar. Add the kaolin and mix thoroughly, then add the lemon essential oil. Store in an old talcum powder dispenser or an empty ground pepper shaker. It will keep for up to 2 months.

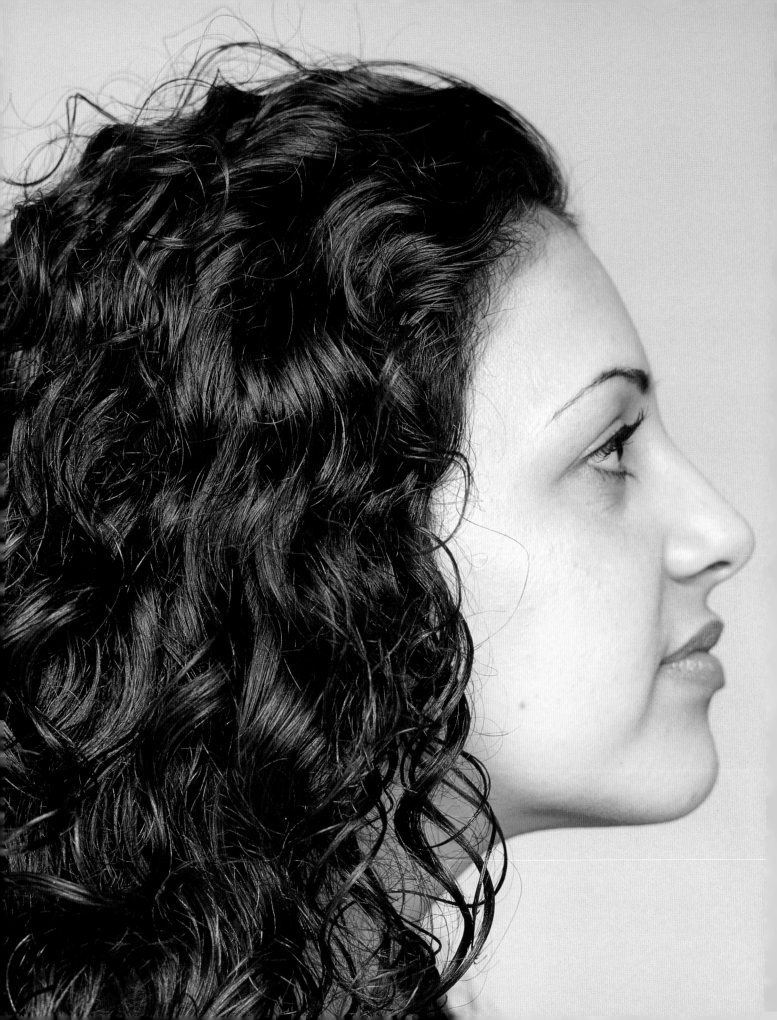

hair care

Beautiful hair can be one of our best assets and by spending time to make our hair look good, it can lift our spirits and help us to feel positive about the day and ourselves. We all want to have healthy hair that is shiny, bouncy and has a good colour. Remember that looking good comes from within, and this is particularly reflected in the condition of your hair. Good hair health is due to three main factors: your general physical state, environmental conditions and how well you care for your hair.

As a result, the condition of your hair can be a very good indicator of your general health. The hair will reflect whether you are stressed or eating well, your hormonal balance, circulation, illness etc. So if you want to improve your hair then you could start with being kind to yourself! Get enough rest and generally do not expect too much from your body, give yourself a diet that will nourish and strengthen your whole system and this, in turn, will impact on the vitality of your hair.

Your hair will not always look the same or need to be treated in the same way week in, week out. Your hair will change according to the changes you go through.

A good way to start a healthy hair regime is to eat what is good for you. The general consensus of opinion is that you should:

- ensure a high intake of fruit and vegetables
- choose foods that are high in natural fibre
- reduce intake of fatty foods

These are the three main principles for a good diet that will help you to be healthy and look good. Of course they are very broad guidelines. For hair growth and shine ensure that you include oils in your diet that are high in polyunsaturates, such as sunflower, safflower, wheatgerm, soya bean and corn oils. These, along with green vegetables, contain essential fatty acids, linoleic and alpha-linoleic, which are necessary for healthy growth and body repair. They are also found in evening primrose oil and borage or star flower oil. If your hair is really dry and brittle, then try 6 weeks of taking the tissue salt Silica 6X (a homoeopathic remedy) twice daily. This

can help strengthen both the nails and hair. Zinc and other vitamins or minerals may also be of benefit (see table on pages 20–1).

It has been said many times before, but smoking will definitely be to the detriment of healthy hair as it depletes the body of vitamins, so give it up! Your hair will also smell better and not discolour.

Try to replace your caffeine-based drinks (coffee, tea, chocolate, cola and so on) with herb teas and lots of spring or filtered water on a daily basis. Blood-cleansing herbs such as cleavers, burdock and dandelion can be taken if the body feels sluggish and the hair is lank and lifeless. Nettle tea is a very good tonic herb and is especially good to take in the spring.

environmental changes

The condition of your hair will vary according to the time of year, most notably in winter and summer. In the winter, the scalp is tighter and the hair grows at a slower rate. Central heating can be a problem, as it causes drying and can make the hair dull and more static. In the summer, the sun has a damaging and drying effect: the hair may become bleached and lose its vitality. Swimming can also damage the hair, either because of the chlorine or the salt in the water. Take care to protect your hair from unnecessary damage by keeping it covered when swimming and using a balm or oil to prevent moisture loss in the hot sun.

hair types
normal hair

What do we mean by normal hair? It means something different to everybody – hair varies enormously. For example, north and south Europeans require very different treatments according to whether their hair is blonde, dark or auburn, grey, straight or wavy, and in each category there is undoubtably a type considered normal. Afro-Caribbean hair, Asian hair, and so on – again, there is normal standard for each type and all require something different. Read the other categories to select the one that best describes your hair condition. Lists of useful herbs and essential oils are provided to treat your hair type.

greasy hair

This condition occurs when the sebaceous glands over-secrete. It can be due to hormonal changes or other health conditions. Drink lots of water and get enough exercise to improve your circulation, which will in turn improve the condition of your hair. The condition may be made worse by too frequent washing as this will affect the acid/alkaline balance of the scalp. Try to ensure that you leave at least 48 hours between each wash. Wash gently, with mild or diluted shampoo. Make astringent lotions or rinses for the hair that will tighten the scalp. Always rinse using cold water. If you use a hair dryer use it on a cool setting to ensure that you do not further stimulate the sebum flow.

Herbs: elderflower, lemon balm, mint, rosemary, sage, yarrow and bay. One or more of these can be used as an infusion to dilute a shampoo. Alternatively, macerate these herbs in cider vinegar and add 2–3 tablespoons to your final rinse. Try adding tinctures of these herbs to your shampoo or conditioner – see pages 141–3.

Essential oils: bergamot, cedarwood, cypress, geranium, grapefruit, juniper, lemon, lime and petitgrain. Use oils sparingly to benefit from their astringent properties. Add 2–3 drops in total for one application of shampoo base or conditioner.

Using beer will help hair to set. Add it to the final rinse and use to hold the hair in place.

dry and treated hair

When hair is dry there is not enough sebum secretion. The hair will lack shine and become brittle and split. Dry and fine hair will need to be cut regularly as the ends are brittle and easily broken. After washing, it is best to let your hair dry naturally. If you use a hair-dryer, however, use it on a cool setting and keep it a good distance away from the head. When brushing hair, hold the head to the side and rotate the brush (a bristle brush is best). In this way you will close the shaft of the hair, which will make it shine.

Add some nourishing oils to your shampoo, either by using a herbal macerate or by adding a few drops of any of the following oils: evening primrose oil, borage, sunflower, jojoba and almond.

Herbs: calendula, chamomile, marsh mallow and comfrey can all be macerated in the oils listed above or used as infusions and added to shampoos or conditioners to add softness. Avoid using tinctures as the alcohol will dry out the hair further. Make a seaweed or horsetail infusion to nourish your hair and provide a good strengthening tonic. You can use these infusions either in the final rinse after washing or diluted as a hairspray.

Essential oils: frankincense, palmarosa and sandalwood are all known to be very helpful for dry skin conditions. Geranium, chamomile, rose, patchouli and vetiver are other essential oils to try. The oils may be added to shampoos and conditioners, or you can put a few drops into some flower water and use it as a hair spray, ensuring the mixture is well shaken before use.

Condition dry hair with rich foods, such as egg yolk, avocado and yogurt (see recipes on pages 142–3). Try mixing egg yolk and honey together for a moisturizing hair mask. Leave for two hours before washing off.

A good treatment for dry hair is to mix a few drops of essential oil into melted coconut oil, almond or olive oil and apply it directly on to the ends of the hair or even to the whole head and scalp. This will help prevent the ends from splitting and be a nourishing treat for the hair and scalp generally. This is particularly good for Afro-Caribbean hair, which can be very sensitive, fine and easily broken. Afro-Caribbean hair can lack elasticity, so another way to retain the moisture is by using herbal infusions, which you can add to a hair balm and apply before going out for the evening.

To remove an oil treatment, apply a mild shampoo directly to the hair and emulsify by mixing it in well, then add warm water and rinse off. The treatment should leave

hair type	essential oils	herbal infusions
normal	cedarwood, lavender, orange, rosemary	rose, rosemary, thyme
greasy	bergamot, cedarwood, cypress, geranium, grapefruit, juniper, lemon, lime, petitgrain	bay, elderflower, lemon balm, mint, rosemary, sage, yarrow
dry	chamomile, frankincense, geranium, palmarosa, patchouli, rose, sandalwood	calendula, chamomile, comfrey, horsetail, marsh mallow, seaweed
damaged	frankincense, lavender	calendula, coltsfoot, comfrey, horsetail, seaweed
dull	melissa, rosemary	ginseng, horsetail, nettle, rosemary, sage
fine	geranium	calendula, oat straw, seaweed
dark	rosemary, thyme	nettle, rosemary, thyme
fair	Roman chamomile	chamomile, mullein flowers
grey	sage	rosemary, sage
frequent wash	geranium, lavender, rosemary	coltsfoot, elderflower, horsetail, seaweed
children	Roman chamomile	chamomile, rose
dandruff	cedarwood, patchouli, rosemary, sage, tea tree, thyme	lavender, nettle, peppermint, rosemary, sage, thyme

your hair feeling nourished and bouncy. To soften dry hair, use a little moisturizer or hair balm after drying the hair; lightly apply the moisturizer or balm to the ends of the hair to help close the hair shaft and create a protective film around it. If you have short hair, using a greater quantity of hair balm should improve the overall look of your hair and give it lots of shine.

dry scalp

A dry or flaking scalp may be caused by several things, for example stress or eczema. Depending on the condition of the scalp, effective treatments include macerating rosemary herb in either olive oil, almond or jojoba oil and then adding shea nut butter or any of the essential oils recommended for dry hair. Shea nut butter can also be used on its own. Part your hair and apply with a brush or your finger tips. Gently massage the whole scalp, paying particular attention to the area behind the ears. Leave on for as long as possible before washing off. To help with scalp dryness in babies, apply a little organic almond oil and rub gently.

dandruff

This is a condition caused by yeast over-production and results in unsightly white flaking of the skin on the scalp.

Herbs: peppermint, thyme, rosemary, lavender and nettles. Make a maceration of these herbs, apply to the scalp and leave for as long as possible before washing off with very mild or diluted shampoo. A final rinse with an infusion may also help.

Essential oils: cedarwood, patchouli, sage, tea tree, thyme and rosemary. Use individually or combine with an almond oil base and apply as with the maceration above.

head lice

The standard commercial treatments for head lice contain organo-phosphates. These have well-publicized side effects and are known to be environmentally unfriendly. Fortunately, it is possible to make your own mixture (see page 147). This will be much safer but it will take time to make and careful combing with a nit comb will be required to remove all the eggs (nits). Neem, a well-known traditional insecticide, is now fairly widely available. If you can locate some, use it instead of almond oil as the base for essential oils. Alternatively, you may find coconut oil easier to use: it has the advantage of not dripping when you put it on. Finish the treatment with an antiseptic rinse (see page 147). As an extra deterrent you could add neem leaf infusion to the rinse, but beware of the smell!

Herbs: neem, quassia and pyrethrum.

Essential oils: rosemary, tea tree, lavender, geranium and eucalyptus.

thinning hair

This is a problem that many people suffer from. It can arise from a variety of causes, including hormonal changes, illness, stress or ageing. Whatever the cause, thinning hair is always disturbing. In fact, everyone loses a certain amount of hair all the time. If it becomes excessive, massage the scalp morning and evening to stimulate the circulation and relax the head. Drinking plenty of water will help, and rosemary tea will also help stimulate the circulation. Make a mixture of bay and rosemary herb infusion and use as a final rinse after washing or put on the scalp as a treatment by mixing with base oil such as coconut oil or almond oil. Always use a very mild or diluted shampoo and use cold water for the final rinse to increase the circulation and tone the scalp. When brushing thinning hair hold the head down.

caring for your hair

It is not difficult to make big changes to the way your hair looks. One of the easiest ways is by getting a good haircut. If you do not feel confident about what you need, your hairdresser should be able to advise you, and remember that regular cutting is good for the hair (hair grows about an inch every 6–8 weeks).

There is a huge variety of hair products on the market. If you do not have a favourite brand that you regularly buy it can be difficult to choose. There are, however, a number of simple ways to deal with any changes or problems and there are some recipes (from page 141 onwards) that will give you the opportunity to create simple and natural products of your own.

why make your own hair products?

Making your own hair products is good for several reasons. First, it gives you total control over exactly what you are putting on your hair. Second, most of the ingredients are available from the kitchen cupboard so

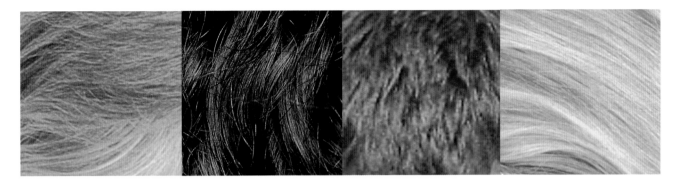

the products are generally quick and cheap to prepare. And third, home-made hair products will in general be better for the environment.

the recipes

Balancing a desire to use natural products against effective hair cleansing and conditioning is not easy, but the recipes in this section have been devised to achieve the best possible compromise. In addition to the herb-based shampoos and conditioners, there are recipes for natural ways to colour the hair and add highlights and some special suggestions for combating hair loss.

There are dozens of hair-care products on the market today and selecting an appropriate one is often a difficult process that can be avoided by making your own at home. A typical routine for developing and maintaining beautiful hair consists of shampooing, conditioning, scalp massage and the use of treatments and finishing products. Few of us, however, have the time to perform all of these tasks on a regular basis, and we generally, therefore, limit hair care to washing and conditioning.

When you are making your own hair-care products, it is useful to know how each type of preparation works. The primary aim of shampooing is, of course, to remove dirt from the hair. This dirt consists mainly of bodily secretions, but atmospheric dust and pollutants and residues from hair-grooming preparations also need to be cleaned away. An effective shampoo removes grease and water-soluble dirt without stripping away all the natural oiliness of the hair. The active cleansing ingredient in shampoos is known as a surfactant, which functions by removing the dirt from the hair surface and dispersing it in the

washing solution so that it is not redeposited on the clean hair or scalp. Surfactants are commonly known as detergents.

The earliest shampoos contained soap, but today they are generally based on non-soap detergents. Detergents are a synthetically produced group of chemicals and, although they are often based on a natural material, such as coconut oil or palm kernel oil, they are generally highly modified. This causes one of the most difficult formulation dilemmas for those of us committed to producing a highly natural product. A shampoo based on soap would create dull and damaged-looking hair when used over a long period unless much time and effort were taken to condition the hair. Modern shampoos offer a convenience and effectiveness that is difficult to match with totally natural products.

In formulating the Neal's Yard Remedies range of shampoos we have tried to come up with the best compromise. Detergents are used but are balanced by herbs and natural oils, which provide their natural benefits. It is not the ultimate solution, but it is one that allows us to offer our customers convenience while at the same time producing a shampoo containing a large percentage of natural raw materials.

The recipes presented in this section are great for those of us with the time to spend using them correctly. The shampoo bar is a fabulous travelling companion, but make sure that you condition your hair well after use because soaps can be drying on the hair. When you use the dry shampoo base, section your hair before applying it in order to avoid too much clumping of dry materials.

Home-made shampoos contain a large proportion of water. This means that they need to be made and stored with care to avoid microbial contamination. It is probably best to make up the shampoo on the day you intend to use it.

If you do not have much time to spare but would like to make your own products, you can start with some ordinary shampoo and add your own herbal infusions and essential oils. This will dilute the detergent, so you will have a shampoo that foams less but is much milder on your hair. As a rough guide the following ratio is recommended:

50 per cent ordinary shampoo –
    e.g., 50 ml/3¼ tbsp
45 per cent herbal infusion –
    e.g., 45 ml/1½ fl oz/3 tbsp
4 per cent natural oils (jojoba, coconut) –
    e.g., 4 ml/1 scant tsp
0.2–1 per cent essential oils –
    e.g., 0.2–1 ml/4–20 drops

Whichever product you decide suits you, remember to pay attention to what your hair is telling you. If it starts to look lank and dull, make some changes to your favourite formula to achieve a better result. Hormonal and environmental factors will influence the feel and look of your hair, and you may find that a formula that once worked well for you has to be adapted.

Hair conditioner is much easier to achieve naturally than shampoo, and the range of materials is also greater. The active ingredients in commercial conditioners are known as cationic surfactants. After shampooing, hair is often left without sufficient natural oil, and conditioners aim to repair this. The cationic surfactants in conventional conditioners are attracted to damaged hair where keratin has been affected and a negative charge has built up. This results in overall improvement to the condition of the hair.

Using a herb rinse is a great way of achieving the same results as conventional conditioners with home-made ones. Use the chart on page 137 to select the herb that is suitable for your hair type. Make an infusion (see page 38) and add to it some fresh fruit juice, glycerin and lecithin.

Before synthetic detergents were invented, rinses of lemon juice or cider vinegar were used to improve the shine and feel of the hair after washing. Both materials are acidic, help to soften the water and have an astringent effect on the hair, shrinking the cuticles and making the shaft smoother. If your hair tends to be greasy, use a water-based product; if it is dry, choose an oil-based one. The recipes provided here give both options.

There are some excellent, easily available conditioning bases, which can be used on their own or combined with other ingredients, including beer, eggs, milk and natural vegetable and nut oils such as jojoba and coconut.

Many of the recipes in this section may be adapted to suit your own hair type. The essential oils and herbal infusions on page 137 may be substituted for ingredients listed where appropriate.

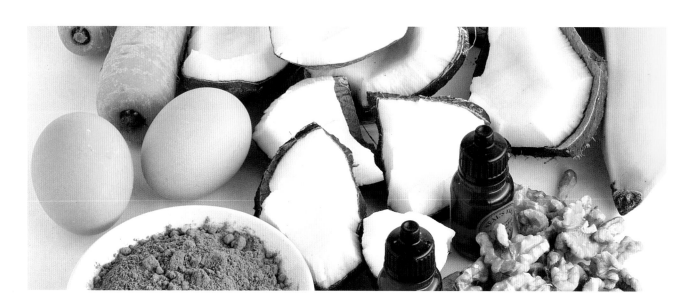

shampoos

soapwort hair cleanser

250 ml/8 fl oz/1 cup water

25 g/7 tsp (heaped) soapwort

25 g/10 tbsp herbs: rosemary and sage mix for
   dark hair, or chamomile flowers for fair hair

10 drops of rosemary or bay essential oil

Using fresh plants if possible, make an infusion by boiling and pouring the water on to the herbs, cover and leave to stand for a couple of hours. Strain, add the oils and then pour into a bottle. Apply by massaging into the hair, so that the whole head is covered before rinsing off. There is no lather but the hair is left feeling soft and cleaned. Store in the fridge for up to 6 days. Shake well before use.

yo-jojoba and a bottle of rum

An excellent pre-shampoo treatment and hair tonic. These ingredients make enough for one treatment.

5 ml/1 tsp rum

5 ml/1 tsp jojoba oil

5 ml/1 tsp liquid lecithin

4 drops essential oil of your choice

Blend all the ingredients together, then massage over your head and scalp. Wrap a towel around your head and leave for 1 hour. Wash out, using a mild shampoo with lemon juice added.

dry shampoo base

A dry shampoo to freshen up and cleanse your hair when you are in a hurry. See the chart on page 137 for a guide to the use of herbs. These ingredients make enough for one treatment.

1 tsp orris root

2 tsp arrowroot

2 tsp dried herbs

Mix all the ingredients together and grind to a fine powder in a mortar and pestle. Rub the powder into wet hair and then rinse out.

sage shampoo bar

This handy shampoo bar is useful for travelling. It is most effective on short hair. These ingredients will make about six bars.

1 tsp dried sage

300 ml/½ pt/1¼ cups water

½ bar almond soap

45 ml/3 tbsp vegetable glycerin

10 drops lemon essential oil

Make an infusion (see page 38) using the sage and water, and strain it. Grate the soap and add it to the sage infusion. Heat until all the soap has melted. While the mixture is still hot, add the vegetable glycerin. Remove from heat. Add the essential oil, pour the mixture into baking tins and leave uncovered to set. Use the bars as soap. They will keep for 3 weeks in the refrigerator.

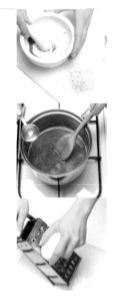

conditioners

carrot and avocado hair treatment

This is a nourishing treatment for dry and neglected hair. Use jojoba oil as the base for the carrot macerate. These ingredients are sufficient for one treatment.

> 10 ml/2 tsp carrot
>   macerated oil
> 1 ripe avocado

Prepare the macerated oil with grated carrot according to the recipe on page 40. Mash the avocado, then blend it with the oil to make a paste. Apply the mixture to the hair and scalp and leave for 1 hour. Wash off, using a mild shampoo with added lemon juice.

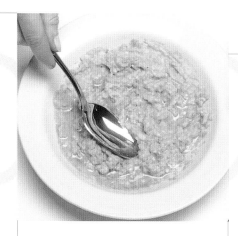

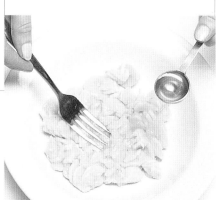

coconut conditioner

This recipe is easy to make and is suitable for all hair types, depending on the essential oils used. See the chart on page 137 for a guide to the use of essential oils. These ingredients will make 100 g (3½ oz). It will keep for up to 12 months.

> 100 g/3½ oz jar coconut oil
> 20 drops essential oil

Melt the coconut oil by standing the jar in a bowl of hot water. Add the essential oils and stir before it re-sets. To use, melt a little of the oil in the palm of your hand and massage it into the hair and scalp. Leave on for at least 2 hours and then shampoo off. Applying the shampoo to your hair before rinsing with water makes the oil easier to remove.

banana and grapeseed hair treatment

A simple-to-make, deep conditioning treatment for dry hair. These ingredients are enough for one treatment.

> 1 ripe banana
> 10 ml/2 tsp grapeseed oil

Mash the banana, using a fork, then mix with the oil to make a paste. Massage into the hair and scalp, cover the hair with clingfilm (plastic wrap) and leave for 30 minutes. Wash out, using a mild shampoo with added lemon juice.

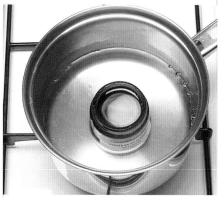

beer rinse for fine hair

Beer is a traditional tonic for adding shine and body to fine hair. The smell of it fades when the hair dries. These ingredients are sufficient for one treatment.

I pint beer
150 ml/¼ pt/⅔ cup
   cider vinegar

Blend the beer with the vinegar. Pour over your hair several times as the final rinse after shampooing, and then allow the hair to dry naturally.

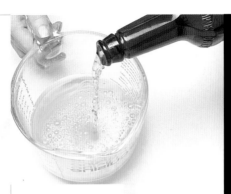

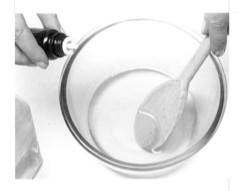

cider vinegar treatments

Cider vinegar can be used to rinse and condition the hair and to restore the pH balance of the scalp. For extra effect, herbs such as rosemary, bay, sage and eucalyptus can be macerated in the vinegar. See the chart on page 137 for a guide to the use of herbs.

apple and thyme rinse

A hair and scalp tonic, particularly good for treating dandruff. These ingredients are sufficient for one treatment.

10 drops wild thyme
   essential oil
100 ml/3½ fl oz/7 tbsp apple
   juice/apple cider vinegar

Blend the thyme essential oil with the apple juice or vinegar. Massage the mixture into your scalp and leave for up to 5 minutes. Rinse your hair with water and then shampoo it.

quick treatments

- To treat dry hair, massage olive oil into the hair, paying particular attention to the ends if they are split, and wrap the hair in a warm towel. Leave for 1 hour and rinse out using a mild shampoo with added lemon juice.

- For a conditioning treatment, beat an egg and then rub it into the hair. Rinse out using an infusion of chamomile flowers. Use cool water, or the egg will set!

- Clay mixed with water to form a paste can be used instead of shampoo. Rhassoul is a special type of mud from Morocco, which is used specifically for this purpose.

- For extra shine and vitality, rub sweet almond oil into your scalp and hair. Leave in for 2 hours, then rub in natural yogurt and leave for a further 30 minutes. Wash out using a mild shampoo.

- If your hair is chlorine damaged, massage corn syrup into your scalp and hair. Leave for 30 minutes, and then wash out using a mild shampoo with added lemon juice.

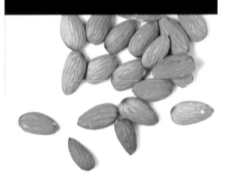

hair dyes and highlighters

Before you use any natural hair dye, it is important to cover the skin around the hairline with ointment base to avoid any discolouration. When working out the length of time to leave the dye on the hair, the porosity of the hair and the colour required must be taken into consideration – the times given here are just a rough guide, and the effects are not guaranteed. Always condition the hair after applying colourant to rebalance the pH.

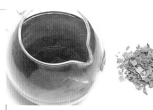

chamomile highlighter

For blonde hair. These ingredients are sufficient for one treatment.

7 g/4 tbsp dried
chamomile flowers
100 ml/3½ fl oz water

Infuse the dried chamomile with water, allowing it to stand for 20 minutes before straining. Apply to the hair, leave on for 20 minutes and rinse out.

walnut rinse

This is a rinse for dark hair. These ingredients are sufficient for one treatment.

100 ml/3½ fl oz/7 tbsp water
2 tsp walnut leaves
1 teabag (black tea)

Decoct the water with walnut leaves and the tea bag. Allow to stand for at least 30 minutes. Apply to the hair and leave for 30 minutes. Rinse out, then shampoo and condition the hair.

sage and black tea

For grey hair. For the first couple of treatments apply to the whole head. Thereafter, this mixture can be used to touch up the roots every couple of weeks. These ingredients are sufficient for one treatment.

4 tbsp dried sage leaves
100 ml/3½ fl oz water
1 teabag (black tea)

Decoct the water with the sage and teabag. Allow to stand for 30 minutes. Apply to the hair, leave for 30 minutes. Rinse out, then shampoo and condition the hair.

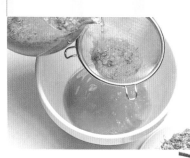

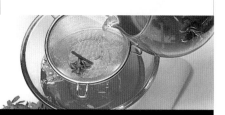

infusions

Other herb infusions (see page 38) can be used as a final rinse after washing the hair. If you are using fresh herbs, they should be picked early in the day, before the sun is hot, because the heat of the sun causes any essential oil to evaporate from the leaves.

henna

Henna will colour the hair varying shades of red, depending on the country in which it was grown. Use hot water to make a paste with the powder and apply it, as hot as possible, to the hair, taking care to cover the roots. How long it should be left will depend on the freshness of the henna, your own hair and the heat of the water. Always test it on a small section of hair first to avoid unwanted results. Be careful not to stain your hands when you are using it, and remember that henna will stain bowls and washbasins, too.

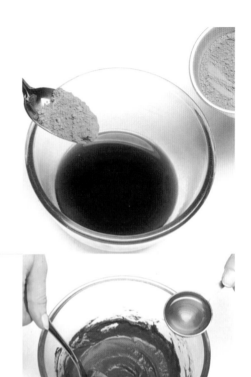

henna rinse

In the following recipe, tea will give a bright red; for a darker red, use coffee. These ingredients are sufficient for one treatment.

    1 teabag (black tea) or 1 tsp ground coffee
    100 g/3½ oz henna
    15 ml/1 tbsp olive oil
    250 ml/8 fl oz/1 cup water

Make a cup of tea or coffee and add the henna. Mix in the olive oil and add more water (if necessary) to make a smooth paste. Apply immediately to the hair, then cover with clingfilm (plastic wrap), silver foil and a warm towel. Leave on for 2–3 hours, then rinse, shampoo and condition the hair.

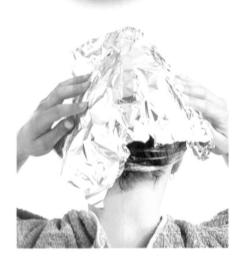

special treatments

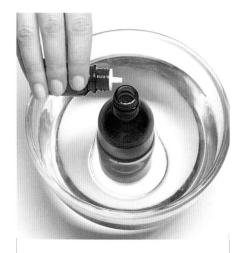

stimulating hair oil

This is a particularly useful treatment for hair loss. These ingredients are sufficient to make about 10 ml (2 tsp). It will keep for up to 12 months.

> 2 drops basil essential oil
> 2 drops rosemary essential oil
> 10 ml/2 tsp avocado oil

Mix the essential oils with the base oil (in this case avocado). Heat the bottle before use in a bowl of hot water. Massage the mixture into the scalp for at least 30 minutes. Repeat regularly for the best results.

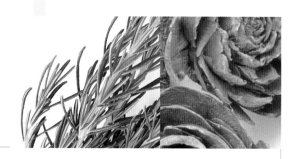

rosemary and cedarwood hair treatment

The Neal's Yard Remedies rosemary and cedarwood hair treatment has received glowing praise in the past for helping hair to grow. It is very easy to make yourself. These ingredients are sufficient to make 100 g (3½ oz). The treatment will keep for up to 30 months.

> 100 g/3½ oz jar coconut oil
> 20 drops rosemary essential oil
> 10 drops cedarwood essential oil

Melt the coconut oil by standing the glass jar in a bowl of hot water. Add the essential oils and mix thoroughly. To use, warm some oil by rubbing it in the palm of your hand, and then methodically work it through your hair, concentrating on massaging the scalp. Wrap a warm towel around your head and leave for 30 minutes. Remove the oil by applying shampoo before adding water. Rinse and repeat if necessary.

head lice rinse

You can replace the quassia used here with neem, a herb known for its insecticidal properties. However, it does not smell very inviting! These ingredients are sufficient for one treatment.

  30 g/1 oz/5 tbsp quassia chips
  600 ml/1 pt/2½ cups water

Either soak the quassia in water overnight or decoct it for 10 minutes. Use this mix to wash down bedding, coat collars and so forth. It is also a good idea to use it as a weekly preventative hair rinse during a period of louse infestation at school.

treatment for head lice

This is an excellent treatment for lice. All bedding and clothes must also be washed to remove any eggs (see head lice rinse in next column). These ingredients are sufficient to make 100 ml (3½ fl oz). The treatment will keep for up to 12 months.

  20 drops geranium essential oil
  20 drops lavender essential oil
  20 drops rosemary essential oil
  20 drops tea tree essential oil
  100 ml/3½ fl oz/7 tbsp almond or coconut oil

Add the essential oils to the almond or coconut oil. Depending on hair length, massage 10–15ml (2–3 tsp) through the hair and all over the scalp. Cover the head and leave for 4 hours. Massage the shampoo thoroughly through the hair before rinsing with water. Comb the hair with a fine-toothed comb. Repeat after 48 hours, and then again after 8 days.

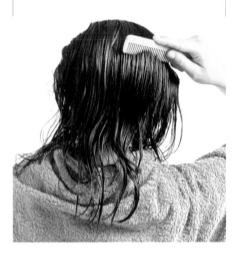

baby care

The proliferation of equipment and toiletries targeted at babies is a sure sign of our consumerist age. Babies need very few products, and will only use a little of each product. Products for babies should be as simple as possible, without fragrance, colourants or unnecessary chemical additives. All ingredients should be organically produced where possible. The majority of the ingredients selected for the recipes that follow are available organically.

baby powder

A fine, light powder to dry and soothe your baby's skin.

> 20 g/3 tbsp cornflour (cornstarch)
> 5 drops propolis tincture
> 2 drops Roman chamomile
>   essential oil

Sift the corn starch evenly on to a plate. Mix the propolis tincture and Roman chamomile essential oil and spray on to the cornflour (cornstarch) using a fine mist atomizer pump. Take care not to saturate the powder, or it will become lumpy. Store in an old talc dispenser or an empty ground pepper shaker. It will keep for up to 6 months.

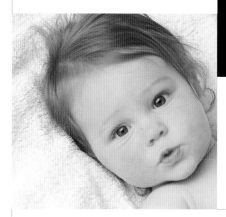

nappy rash

The simplest barrier cream to prevent nappy rash is zinc and castor oil – buy one without any added fragrance or additional preservatives.

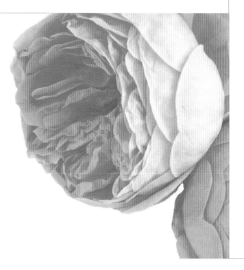

baby massage oil

A mild and soothing massage oil especially created for delicate skin. It should be noted when blending an oil to use on a baby that the dilution of essential oils must not exceed 1 per cent of the total volume (e.g., only 1 ml per 100 ml/3½ fl oz). Always keep oil away from the eyes. It will keep for 12 months.

> 8 drops lavender essential oil
> 6 drops Roman chamomile essential oil
> 6 drops rose absolute
> 100 ml/3½ fl oz sunflower oil

Add the drops of essential oils to the sunflower oil base. Store in a glass bottle out of direct sunlight.

cradle cap

A common yet harmless scalp condition of young babies thought to be the result of over-active sebaceous glands. It varies in appearance from light white flakes to thick yellow crusting which may develop over the majority of the scalp or be confined to specific patches.

Either:
Combine equal parts of calendula and chamomile macerates, as directed on page 40, and follow the steps below.

Or:
Use almond oil.

Gently rub the chosen product over the baby's scalp and allow to soak in well. Wash the flakes away with water.

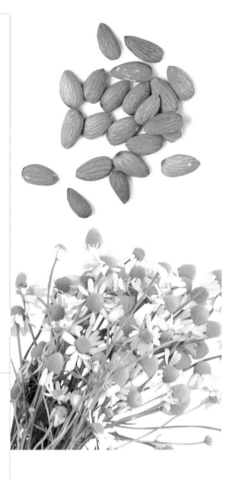

mandarin baby bath oil

Mandarin is a wonderfully scented oil, with calming and soothing properties and no toxicity, which make it excellent for baby products. As a dispersant has not been added, this blend will sit on the surface of the bath water ensuring contact when your baby is placed in and taken out of the water. It will keep for 12 months.

10 drops mandarin essential oil
100 ml/3 fl oz sunflower oil

Simply combine the mandarin essential oil with the sunflower. Use about 10 ml (2 tsp) of the blend per bath. Store in a glass bottle out of direct sunlight.

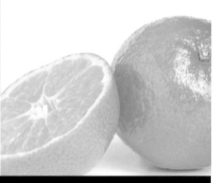

teething

Usually starting at around 6 months old, teething is often a trying time for all concerned – the gums become inflamed and sore and it can be very painful.

A classic treatment is the chewing of marsh mallow root in place of a teething ring, which has the added advantage of being a demulcent and a healer. Another comforting treatment is to add two drops of marsh mallow tincture to one tablespoon of honey and gently massage over the gums. Honey is soothing and mildly antiseptic and also tastes good to ease fretting minds!

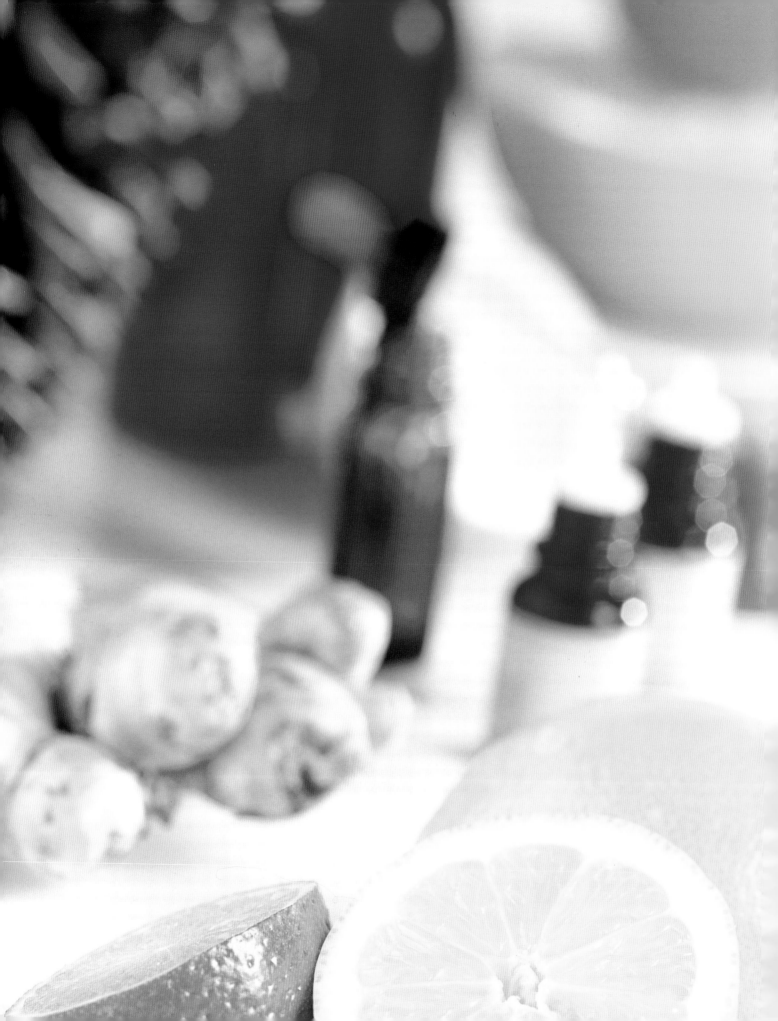

glossary of essential oils

4

The following glossary

explains how essential oils

work and the many ways in

which they can be applied.

There are portraits of 42

commonly used oils, each

with a profile of its own

characteristic combination of

properties, both therapeutic

and psychological.

what are essential oils?

It is the essential oils within plants that give them their characteristic smell and flavour. When we smell the delightful fragrance of jasmine flowers in the early evening, open a cedarwood box and inhale its woody smell or add the zest of a lemon to a drink, it is the essential oil that we are enjoying.

Any part of a plant may contain its essential oil – flowers, leaves, fruit, stems, wood, bark, seeds, resin, berries or roots. However, not all plants contain significant amounts of essential oils, and where this happens the purpose or function of those plants is not yet fully understood. It is thought that the oils' fragrance may attract or repel insects and other animals. Essential oils also have anti-viral and anti-fungal properties for the plant and can be understood as part of the plant's immune system. Other functions of essential oils within plants may be as plant 'hormones' and act as an internal transport system (as with blood in animals).

methods of extraction

An essential oil may be extracted from the plant material by one of four different methods. These methods are described below.

distillation

Most of the essential oils that we use are produced by a process known as distillation. The plant material is placed in a container and boiling water, or steam from a boiler, is passed through the plant matter and then forced into an outlet pipe that carries away the vapours produced. The vapour passes through a pipe which runs through a jacket of flowing cold water (the condenser) and then drips into a second vessel that acts as a receiver for the condensed liquid.

During this process the boiling water or steam softens the tissues of the plant material and causes the release of the essential oil. This vapourizes and passes along with the steam through the vapour pipe, then

both vapours condense to liquid in the area of the condenser. The mixture of liquid essential oil and water then flows into the receiving vessel. Oil and water have different densities, so once they are in the receiving vessel they separate. The essential oil rises to the top, where it is drawn off, filtered and poured into containers ready for dispatch. Some essential oils are partially soluble in the distillation water and in these cases the water may be recovered to use as a 'flower water' or distillate; rose-water or orange-flower water is obtained in this way.

Some essential oils are contained within hard, dense plant tissues, and this material has to be broken up or powdered before the essential oil can be released during distillation. Cedarwood, for example, is distilled from wood chips and sawdust collected from the sawmills where the wood has been cut for timber.

Stills used for essential oil production may be relatively small, such as those moved around the lavender fields in France on a trailer, or massive commercial machinery housed in large industrial buildings. Some ancient stills were made of terracotta; modern stills are usually stainless steel.

expression

Citrus oils are obtained from oil glands found in the outer rind of the fruit and are generally not distilled but expressed. Expression used to be carried out by hand, rasping the peel against an abrasive surface and collecting the resulting liquid. Modern methods of expression vary from crushing the entire fruit, with subsequent separation of the oil from the peel and juice, to machine abrasion of the outer rind. Examples of essential oils that are usually produced by expression include sweet orange, bergamot, grapefruit and lemon; lime oil is usually distilled as this produces a finer product.

absolutes

The essential oil found in jasmine flowers is too delicate to be produced by distillation – the heat tends to destroy the odour. In the past, a process known as enfleurage was used to extract the fragrance from flowers such as jasmine; it was a well-known industry in the Grasse region of France. It entailed placing the freshly picked flowers on to wooden-framed glass plates called chassis, upon which a layer of specially prepared fat had been spread. The chassis were stacked up overnight until the fat became saturated with the essential oil from the flowers. The fragrant enfleurage fat, known as pommade, was treated by extraction with alcohol to produce an absolute.

These days, most absolutes are not produced by such a romantic or craft-based method as enfleurage, but are made by solvent extraction. In this process the plant material is placed in a container with a volatile solvent, usually hexane. Blades are fitted to the inside of the drum and the contents are thoroughly mixed so that the solvent penetrates the plant tissue. The solvent will dissolve out the essential oil, not to mention waxes, chlorophyll and any resinous matter. The extract is then placed in another vessel for the solvent recovery stage. The vessel is gently heated until the highly volatile solvent vapourizes off, leaving a residue known as the concrète or resinoid. In the final stage of production, the concrète is subjected to pure alcohol which separates the absolute from the residual wax. The alcohol solvent is then recovered, and the finished absolute is packed ready for dispatch.

Rose is most usually available as an absolute because of its high cost. While it is possible to produce rose oil by steam distillation, the yield tends to be relatively low and the resulting essential oil is very expensive indeed.

nitrogen extraction and carbon dioxide extraction

These methods of extracting essential oils have the advantage of not using heat, as in distillation, or solvents. Instead, the process is carried out under very high pressure using gas. It may be that we will see an increasing use of essential oils produced by gas extraction as we become more familiar and confident with such methods.

the chemistry of essential oils

A single essential oil will usually be made up of hundreds of different chemical components. Each individual component will bring its own set of properties to the oil, so the total result is a very complex substance. All the constituents of an essential oil are organic, that is, their molecular structures contain carbon.

The chemical components of a typical essential oil generally occur as a combination of major, minor and trace constituents. An example of a major constituent is menthol, which makes up about 40 per cent of peppermint oil. Typically, the number of major constituents is relatively small; the number of minor constituents is larger and the number of trace elements very large. It is the presence and combinations of these constituents that give each essential oil its characteristic smell. Some are so strong-smelling that even if they are not a major constituent they will still contribute greatly to the smell of the oil. Citral, for example, occurs in lemon oil as a minor constituent, and yet because the major constituents of lemon oil are relatively weak, it is the 'lemony' citral that we experience when we smell the essential oil.

Trace constituents may be so minute in an essential oil that their presence is expressed as so many parts per million. Nevertheless, some trace constituents are detectable by the human nose, and may still impart an important therapeutic value to the oil. An example of this is the constituent thioterpineol, which is a trace component of grapefruit oil, and is one of the most powerful-smelling substances known.

The majority of essential oil components fall into two categories: hydrocarbons, or terpenes, and oxygenated compounds.

terpenes

Terpenes are composed of hydrogen and carbon atoms only, and are based on the chemical building block known as an isoprene unit. One important feature of terpene molecules is that they rapidly combine with oxygen from the air. This process starts off a chain reaction known as oxidation which unfortunately alters the odour and therapeutic properties of the affected essential oil for the worse. What this means is that essential oils rich in terpenes will oxidize and deteriorate in a short space of time. Lemon is an example of an essential oil rich in terpenes which will spoil quickly once exposed to air; the shelf life of lemon oil, once opened, is only about six to twelve months.

There are two families of terpenes: monoterpenes and sesquiterpenes. Monoterpenes are particularly prone to rapid oxidation, and tend to have a weak smell. They are very common in essential oils, one example being orange oil, in which they are a major constituent. Sesquiterpenes are less widely found in essential oils but tend to impart a strong smell to an oil. They are less prone to rapid oxidation. An example of a sesquiterpene is caryophyllene, which has a pungent, dry, woody odour and is a major component in clove oil.

oxygenated compounds

The oxygenated compounds of essential oils belong to a number of different chemical families. Important examples are: alcohols, which are in fact a group of terpene derivatives (for example, geraniol, found in geranium oil); phenols, which are frequently skin irritants (thymol, found in thyme); aldehydes, which are quite widely found in essential oils and also tend to be skin irritants (citral, found in lemongrass); esters, which often have a strong fruity odour (linalyl acetate, found in bergamot oil); lactones (bergapten, found in bergamot oil); and ketones, which are stable compounds not readily metabolized by the body (camphor, found in rosemary oil).

What most of the oxygenated compounds have in common is that they are less prone to oxidation than the monoterpenes, and they tend to have a relatively strong smell. It is primarily the odour of the oxygenated compounds, and to a lesser extent the sesquiterpenes, that gives an essential oil its smell. It is, of course, the combination and presence of all these terpenes and oxygenated compounds that impart the therapeutic and, at times, hazardous properties to an essential oil.

quality

It is because a single essential oil is composed of hundreds of constituents – each one possibly interacting with any of the others – that it is so difficult to replicate an essential oil synthetically. A pure essential oil is like a fine musical symphony, composed of hundreds of individual notes, and yet only in combination pleasing to the senses and beneficial to a person. With modern technology, it is not hard to synthesize several of the major components of an essential oil such as jasmine and combine them so that the smell is somewhat similar, yet the overall effect and benefit to an individual is insignificant compared to pure jasmine. A plastic rose may remind us of the real thing, but its experience will always be disappointing compared to that of a true rose because it will not have the touch, the texture and the scent that the true rose has, let alone the presence.

Synthetic or 'nature identical' oils are produced because they are cheaper than pure essential oils and also because they are more consistent. The manufacture of essential oils was developed to supply the food industry with flavours and the perfume industry with fragrances. The flavour and fragrance market requirements are for a raw material that is cheap and exactly the same every year and not prone to variations as growing conditions change from harvest to harvest. It is only in recent years that aromatherapy has become popular and aromatherapists have begun to demand essential oils guaranteed to be pure and natural for their therapeutic use.

It is very difficult as an individual customer to determine that an essential oil from a supplier is totally pure and natural. Most 'adulterated' essential oils will not be an easily identified synthetic copy, but a blend of a true essential oil with an amount of a 'nature identical' material added to increase the volume and thereby reduce the cost. A relatively more expensive essential oil will be bulked out by adding a similar-smelling, much cheaper oil, such as the addition of cheaper cananga oil to more expensive ylang-ylang. Finally, some essential oils may already be diluted by the addition of a base oil, such as almond. This may be promoted by some companies as a method of offering some of the very expensive oils, such as rose, at a more affordable price.

The best guarantee of quality is to buy your essential oils from a supplier who has a good reputation and a genuine interest in the therapeutic properties of its range. Back-up material that should be available on request could include the country of origin of a particular oil, the variety (Latin name), batch number and year of production.

Companies supplying essential oils will take certain measures to ensure the quality of their oils. They can visit the producers on a regular basis, which is practical for some oils such as the European ones, but less so for those from, say, Madagascar. There are also quality tests which are becoming increasingly accurate in determining the purity of an essential oil. Simple tests include visual inspection and checking the odour, specific gravity and refractive index. Larger companies will also carry out gas liquid chromatography (GLC) on all batches of an essential oil. During a GLC, the vapour of a small amount of an essential oil is separated out into its individual components. The results of this separation are recorded by the instrument as a series of peaks on a sheet of paper, with each peak corresponding to a single constituent. The GLC analysis taken from a new batch of oil, say lavender oil, will then be compared against a standard lavender oil analysis to check that the number and ratio of constituents is acceptable.

No amount of testing, including even GLC analysis, is a total guarantee of purity, but the more steps that a company takes to establish quality, the more likely it is that a pure and natural essential oil is being offered.

Pesticides and herbicides are frequent contaminants of essential oils. If used on the crop during its cultivation, they will be carried through the expression or distillation process. This is a huge problem that has developed out of modern agricultural practices. The amount of pesticide and herbicide residue in essential oils is about the same as that considered acceptable in foods. Fortunately, however, most pesticides and herbicides are not as readily absorbed into the system through human skin, when applying a massage oil, for example, as they are when eating contaminated food.

One positive step that can be taken here is to buy essential oils that are wild-crafted or organically produced. Some companies do supply a range of essential oils that are certified as organically produced by the Soil Association in the UK, or other organic organization of the country of production. Buying these oils means not only that you are getting an essential oil uncontaminated by synthetic fertilizers and biocides, but you are also supporting the move towards sustainable agriculture and healthier produce.

storage

The factors that will cause an essential oil to deteriorate are light, heat and oxygen. The best essential oil for therapeutic purposes is the freshest one. Sunlight is particularly damaging, and is capable of catalysing the reactions that cause deterioration. For this reason, essential oils should be stored in coloured glass bottles and preferably kept in the dark. Do not keep essential oils, or even made-up massage oils, in plastic containers as there tends to be a chemical reaction between the plastic and certain essential oil components that will spoil the odour and therapeutic properties of the oil.

Essential oils should be stored in a cool place. An unheated room is adequate for many oils, but oils rich in terpenes, such as citrus and pine, are particularly prone to deterioration through heat and should be stored in the refrigerator. All essential oils will keep for longer in the refrigerator, although some of the resinous oils, such as cedarwood, and the absolutes, such as rose, will tend to become rather viscous at lower than room temperature and will have to be removed from the refrigerator for a while before they can be poured. If there are young children in the house, a child-proof lock should be attached to the door of the refrigerator.

It is better to buy small quantities of essential oils regularly, but if you wish to buy a larger quantity it is advisable to pour it into a number of small bottles (about 10 ml) for storage. This is because each time a bottle is opened more oxygen enters the bottle, accelerating the process of oxidation.

The shelf-life will vary from oil to oil and according to the conditions under which it is stored. The following guidelines apply to essential oils that are stored under cool, dark conditions: essential oils rich in terpenes, such as citrus oils, pine and rosemary, will deteriorate most quickly and should be used within 6–12 months of purchase; cedarwood, patchouli, sandalwood, vetiver and other resinous essential oils will keep for up to 3 years; and most other essential oils should be used within 2 years.

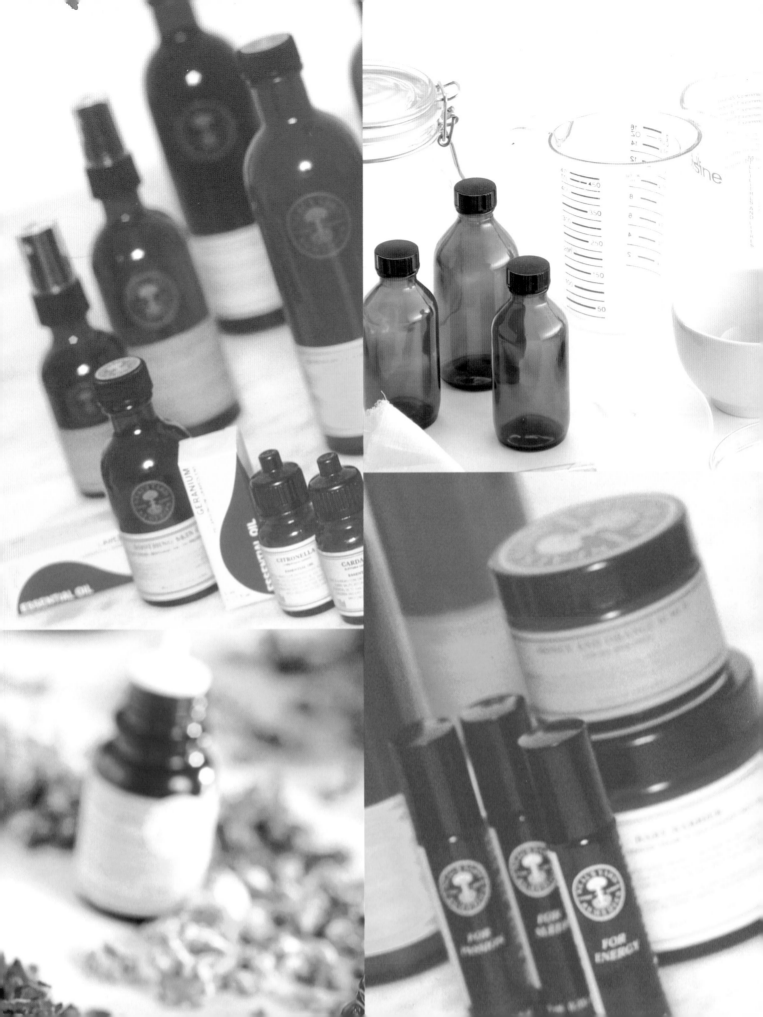

methods of application

The symbols described on the following pages appear throughout the essential oil profiles as a quick reference to the way in which the individual oils may be used. Once you have become familiar with the symbols, you will find it easy to flick through the oil profiles to find the appropriate oils for your needs. For example, if you would like to use an oil to fragrance a room, or for a massage blend, simply look through the oils section to find which oils carry the appropriate symbols, and decide which of those oils is best suited to your particular needs.

massage

Massage is one of the most popular ways of using essential oils and is the method favoured by professional aromatherapists. With an aromatherapy massage you get the benefit of the massage itself as well as the benefits of the essential oils. Massaging a blended oil into your own skin can be very beneficial too, and may easily be made part of a daily skin and health care routine.

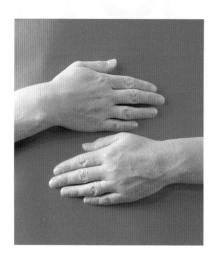

To create a massage oil you will need to dilute the essential oils into a base or carrier oil (see page 59). A therapeutic massage oil usually contains 1–3 per cent of essential oil to base oil. For practical purposes, it is assumed that there are just over 20 drops of essential oil to 1 ml. This means that to 100 ml (3½ fl oz/scant ½ cup) of base oil, 20–60 drops of essential oil (or of combined essential oils) are added. If you make up enough massage oil to last for several applications, store it in a dark-coloured glass bottle and use it within 6–12 months. You may substitute a lotion base for the carrier oil if you prefer.

To make enough blended oil for just one massage, pour approximately 10 ml (2 tsp) of base oil on to a saucer and add 4–6 drops in total of your chosen essential oil or combination of oils.

There are many massage courses available that will help you to learn the different techniques of massage. If you practise first on yourself, and then on a friend or partner, you will become more confident about using your hands, and discovering what is pleasurable and beneficial. It is important for the recipient to feel warm and comfortable during a massage, and you should ensure that your hands are warm before touching the skin. Concentrate on any areas that are causing discomfort – for example, rub the oil into the abdomen to relieve period pains or colic. Covering the skin with a towel or cloth after the massage helps to keep the recipient warm and also encourages absorption of the essential oils.

baths

Adding essential oils to the bath is a wonderfully pleasurable and very popular way of using them. The warmth of the water encourages relaxation and also enables the essential oils to penetrate the skin. The oils should only be added to the water once the bath has been run, as the heat will encourage their evaporation.

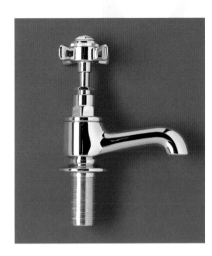

Only the essential oils that are absolutely non-irritant, such as Roman chamomile and lavender, should be added direct to the bath; add 4–6 drops of essential oil and swirl the water around before stepping in. Most essential oils should be pre-diluted in a carrier because they will not fully disperse in the water and their molecules may well come into direct contact with the skin and mucous membranes. Suitable pre-diluting substances include base oils, specially prepared bath oil bases which have a dispersant added, and full-fat milk. To prepare a bath using a carrier, mix 4–6 drops of essential oil in an eggcupful of milk or 10 ml (2 tsp) of base oil, add the mixture to the bath and swirl the water before stepping in.

Sitz baths A sitz bath is an excellent way of treating haemorrhoids, thrush, pruritis, stitches following childbirth, and so on. Half-fill a large bowl or small bath with warm water. Use the same method of dilution as for baths, and sit in the water for 10 minutes. Tea tree oil in a sitz bath is the classic treatment for thrush.

Hand baths and foot baths To make a hand or foot bath add 4–6 drops of essential oil to a washing-up bowl full of hot water. Place your hands or feet in the bowl and soak for 10 minutes.

Hand baths can be a part of a skin care routine, a way of treating pain and swelling of the hand joints, or just a very quick and easy way to create a general reviving effect. Foot baths are excellent for treating problems such as athlete's foot, for alleviating foot pain and swelling, and for helping to relieve discomfort in other parts of the body through the reflexology points found on the foot. A lavender footbath after a day on your feet is one of the most blissful experiences imaginable!

compresses

Compresses may be either hot or cold. A hot compress is an effective way of treating many local complaints, such as skin infections, including abscesses and boils, and muscular or joint problems, including arthritis, rheumatism, sprains, strains, backache and so on.

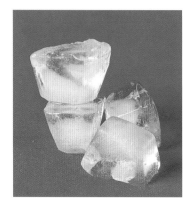

To make a hot compress, pour hot water into a bowl and then add the essential oil. When treating a small area, such as a single boil, an eggcupful of hot water and 2 drops of essential oil will suffice; for a larger area, use a large bowl of water and 6–8 drops of essential oil. Place a cotton cloth in the water, ensuring that the cloth comes into contact with the essential oils on the surface, then squeeze out the excess water from the cloth and immediately put it on the painful or infected area. Keep the area warm by wrapping it in clingfilm (plastic wrap) and wrap a towel around the clingfilm. This process may be repeated after 20 minutes; keep the compress in place for about 1 hour. A hot compress made with ginger essential oil combined with cypress, juniper, pine and lavender is wonderfully warming and relieving for rheumatism or arthritis.

A cold compress may be preferred for certain types of headache and also if the area already feels over-hot and inflamed. To make a cold compress, pour cold water into a bowl and add some ice cubes. Put 4–6 drops of essential oil into the water and then dip in the cotton cloth, wring it out and place it over the affected part. An ice pack (or a pack of frozen vegetables) can then be placed over the cloth to keep the area cold.

room sprays

Room sprays can be used to disinfect and deodorize a room, repel insects and fumigate a sickroom. To make a room spray, half-fill a plant spray with water, add 40–60 drops of essential oils of your choice, shake the mixture well, then spray it liberally around the room.

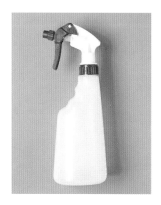

Essential oils with good antiseptic properties, such as cedarwood, eucalyptus, lavender and tea tree, are ideal to use in sprays to fumigate rooms, while lemon, lemongrass and citronella can be used in a spray to repel insects. Most essential oil can be used to fragrance a room, but the citrus oils are particularly refreshing. After using the plant spray it is advisable to pour any remaining liquid into a glass container for storage and thoroughly wash and rinse out the spray. This will prevent corrosion.

burners & vaporizers

These can be used to deodorize or fumigate a room, or simply to create a special atmosphere. If you sit near to the burner or vaporizer it can also be a useful way of inhaling the vapours and benefiting from the therapeutic properties of the oil.

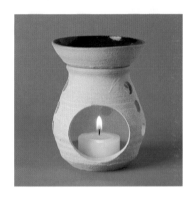

Essential oil burners that use either a candle or electric power to heat the oils are on sale; put a little warm water on to the 'hot plate' and then add a few drops of essential oil. Vaporizers are especially good for a child's room as they have a fan inside that disperses the vapour rather than using a source of heat.

inhalations

A steam inhalation is an excellent way of treating coughs, colds and sore throats and of deep-cleansing the skin. Put very hot water into a bowl and add 3–4 drops of essential oil. Then lean over the bowl, place a large towel over your head and the bowl to create a tent to contain the steam, and inhale the vapours.

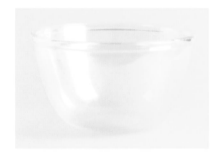

Steam inhalations should be used with caution by people with epilepsy or asthma as they can be rather overpowering. Children under 10 years old should not lean over the bowl; instead, place the bowl on a table near the child and use a towel or similar to waft the steam gently towards them.

A quick and easy method of inhalation is to add 2–3 drops of essential oil to a tissue, and hold this near to the nose every few moments to inhale the vapours.

saunas

Essential oils make a wonderful addition to saunas. Simply add 20–40 drops of an essential oil or oils to the pitcher of water that is used to splash the coals during a sauna. Cypress, eucalyptus and pine essential oils are particularly appropriate for use in the sauna.

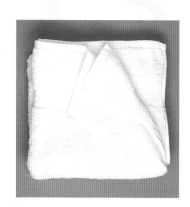

gargles & mouthwashes

Gargles are a good way to treat sore throats and hoarseness, whether these have arisen from straining the voice or from a cold or infection. They can also be extremely effective in treating thrush, mouth ulcers and gum disease. Apart from totally non-irritant and non-toxic oils such as lavender and Roman chamomile, the oils must be diluted in a carrier before gargling.

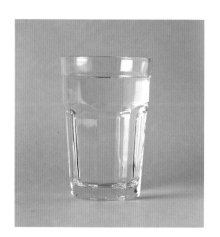

Add 2–3 drops of essential oil to 5 ml (1 tsp) strong alcohol (vodka is ideal) and add this to an eggcupful of water. A mouthwash is made by adding the same amounts of alcohol and oil to warm water.

To make up a larger amount of mixture, put 50 ml (2 fl oz/¼ cup) of vodka into a bottle and add 30–40 drops of essential oil. Add 5 ml (1 tsp) of this mixture to warm water to use as a mouthwash or gargle.

cooking

Essential oils have been used as flavourings for foods and drinks for many years. The main thing to remember is that they are very concentrated and so only 1–2 drops should be used per dish or the result will be too overpowering – and possibly toxic. The essential oil should be added to the oily part of a recipe and mixed thoroughly to ensure that it is dispersed throughout the dish.

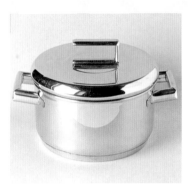

One of the simplest ways to start is to add 1–2 drops of fennel or lemon essential oil to mayonnaise as an accompaniment to fish. One or two drops of orange or neroli oil is delicious in home-made chocolates, and 1 drop of lime or spearmint oil will transform avocado soup.

perfumes

There are several essential oils that will not irritate the skin and may be worn undiluted as perfumes, including neroli, lavender, jasmine, sandalwood and rose. Simply apply a drop of the oil to the pulse points as you would any perfume. These oils may also be blended to create an individual fragrance, such as the classic combination of jasmine, rose and sandalwood, which is known as angel oil.

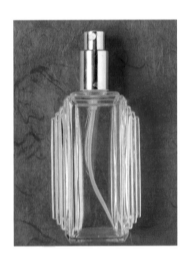

Colognes may also be created by adding a combination of essential oils to vodka as a fragrance base. Add up to 18 drops of combined essential oils to 30 ml/2 tbsp vodka and store in a glass perfume bottle.

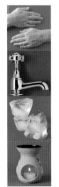

Boswellia thurifera, *syn* B. carteri

Family: Burseraceae

frankincense

Also known as: Olibanum

origin Frankincense has been in constant demand since the time of the Ancient Egyptians, who used it in skin-care preparations. It also has a tradition of use as incense in China, India and the West. Frankincense trees grow wild in North Africa, but the oil is mainly distilled from the resin in Europe.

description

Frankincense oil has a sweet, spicy, resinous odour with a fresh, slightly camphoraceous top note. It is pale yellow or greenish in colour.

therapeutic properties

Frankincense is a tonifying oil with anti-inflammatory and astringent properties. It is a wonderful rejuvenating oil to use in massage and skin lotions, though its uplifting properties are best experienced by adding it to an essential oil burner; it may also be added to the bath. Frankincense blends particularly well with citrus oils, spice oils and basil, cedarwood, myrrh, neroli, pine, sandalwood and vetiver.

The main action of frankincense is on the nervous system, where its effect is to calm and lift the spirits, while at the same time increasing energy. Its ability to assist concentration indicates its long history of use as an incense and an aid to meditation. It can also be helpful in treating anxiety and tension; a few drops of frankincense in an essential oil burner are very uplifting and beneficial if you are feeling stressed, tired or overwhelmed.

Its astringent and anti-inflammatory properties make frankincense useful in the treatment of all mucus conditions and other discharges, such as diarrhoea. It has a soothing effect on the mucous membranes and can be used for coughs, bronchitis and laryngitis – use it as a steam inhalation or in an essential oil burner. Frankincense is more cooling than cypress oil and a better expectorant when treating lung conditions, but is less effective in treating circulatory disorders.

The tonifying and rejuvenating properties of frankincense make it one of the most important oils for improving skin tone and treating ageing skin and wrinkles, as well as reducing scar tissue. It is also antiseptic and astringent and will help to close wounds and heal ulcers.

psychological profile

Frankincense is appropriate if you live at high speed and become overwhelmed by the responsibilities and material aspects of life without making time to establish a more considered and harmonious lifestyle. It is of benefit for people who have become cluttered in their atmosphere and who constantly wish they had the time for all those creative and spiritual pursuits they would like to do. Using frankincense will help you to reprioritize your life and to concentrate on those areas that will bring you greater satisfaction and happiness.

method of extraction

The bark is incised so that the tree yields an oleo-gum resin which is collected after it solidifies into amber-coloured lumps the size of a pea. This resin is then steam-distilled to produce the essential oil.

most common uses
• Meditation • Stress • Mucus conditions • Ageing skin

safety data
• Non-toxic • Non-irritant in dilution • Non-sensitizing

ylang-ylang

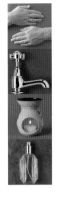

Cananga odorata

Family: Annonaceae

origin Ylang-ylang oil is produced from the flowers of a tall tree native to tropical Asia, especially Indonesia. Commercial production is mainly undertaken in Madagascar, the Comoro Islands and the island of Réunion. The name means 'flower of flowers' and the flowers have been used in folk medicine and skin creams in the Far East for thousands of years. In Indonesia they are spread on the beds of newly married couples on their wedding night. In Victorian England the essential oil was used in macassar oil, thought to stimulate hair growth. Ylang-ylang oil is a renowned base note found in many oriental and floral perfumes.

description

Ylang-ylang oil is a pale yellow, oily liquid that has a very powerful yet intensely sweet and exotic floral scent with a balsamic undertone.

therapeutic properties

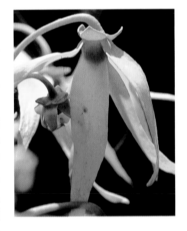

Ylang-ylang has a sedating and calming effect on the nervous system, creating a sense of relaxed well-being. It is useful for treating anxiety, depression, stress and tension, and blends well with bergamot, cedarwood, clary sage, jasmine, lemon, rose, sandalwood and vetiver. It should always be well diluted as it can be rather overpowering, causing headaches or nausea – just a drop or two of ylang-ylang in a saucerful of base oil is sufficient for massage.

This is an important oil in the treatment of high blood pressure. It will help to lower blood pressure and reduce tachycardia (abnormally rapid heart beat) and hyperpnoea (abnormally fast breathing). It has a soothing effect on palpitations associated with anxiety and panic. In treating circulatory disorders ylang-ylang may be blended with other appropriate oils and used in massage and the bath, though the best results will be obtained by visiting an aromatherapist for a therapeutic massage and advice on lifestyle.

Ylang-ylang has an excellent reputation as an aphrodisiac for both men and women, relaxing inhibitions and dispelling stress and at the same time being arousing. It can be effective as a sensual massage blend or as a room fragrancer.

Ylang-ylang adds an exotic and luxurious fragrance to many skin-care products as well as balancing the secretion of sebum. It is suitable for both dry and oily skin types and may be used in preparations to treat acne and problem skin.

psychological profile

Ylang-ylang is most appropriate if you have pushed yourself to work hard and taken on many commitments until you are no longer in control of the stress in your life. You may have forgotten how to let go and enjoy yourself, having become tense, irritable and anxious, and may easily become flushed and panicky. Using ylang-ylang will help you to relax and enable you to reprioritize your life so that you can begin to enjoy yourself again.

method of extraction

The oil is steam- or water-distilled from the freshly picked flowers of the tree. During the distillation process a number of different grades of oil are taken off. The first is known as ylang extra, and this is the most expensive and most desired by perfumers. There then follow three successive distillates known as grades I, II and III, the smell of the different grades becoming less and less complex and losing more of the subtle top notes.

most common uses
- Anxiety • Aphrodisiac • High blood pressure

safety data
- **Non-toxic** • **Non-irritant** • **Non-sensitizing**

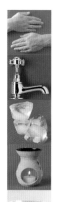

Cedrus atlantica
Family: Pinaceae

cedarwood
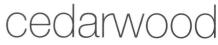
Also known as: Atlas cedar

origin Cedarwood has been valued since ancient times and the trees were used to build temples, including the temple of Solomon. The wood was prized for building because it is very hard and the natural oils present in the wood repel insects. Cedarwood essential oil was one of the earliest to be extracted, and was used by the Ancient Egyptians in cosmetics, perfumes and in the mummification process. The oil is now mainly produced in Morocco and France.

description

Cedarwood oil may be yellow or amber and is quite viscous. It has a slightly sweet, oily-woody smell that becomes more woody as it dries out.

therapeutic properties

Cedarwood is very warming as well as regenerating, tonifying, soothing and uplifting. The balancing nature of the last two properties makes it excellent in treating nervous tension, chronic anxiety, depression and tiredness; it may be added to massage and bath oil blends and steam inhalations, and it is also a pleasant room fragrancer. Cedarwood blends particularly well with bergamot, cypress, frankincense, jasmine, juniper, myrrh, neroli, rosemary, sandalwood and vetiver.

Its regenerative properties make cedarwood useful in the treatment of chronic conditions such as arthritis – blend it with other appropriate oils in a base oil and use for massage or as a compress. It is tonifying when there is weakness combined with excessive discharges, such as chronic diarrhoea or excessive urination, in which case it should be applied in a massage oil over the abdomen. Combined with sandalwood and used in the bath, or as a douche, cedarwood may also be used to treat cystitis.

This oil will help to stimulate delayed periods, and its antiseptic properties also make it a good treatment for leucorrhoea, discharges and venereal infections. Add a few drops to the bath to bring relief to pruritis. In a therapeutic compress it will prevent putrefaction in wounds, ulcers (including varicose ulcers), and any skin infection which shows signs of degenerating.

Cedarwood has a beneficial effect on the mucous membranes, especially when there is excessive catarrh, and can be used to treat coughs and bronchitis. Use as a steam inhalation or in an oil burner.

Its combination of antiseptic and astringent properties means that cedarwood is a good treatment for oily skin and hair, acne, dandruff and scalp irritation, as well as fungal infections of the skin such as athlete's foot. It is also a parasiticide and may be combined with other oils to eliminate lice and scabies.

psychological profile

Cedarwood helps to give a stronger sense of identity and encourage social interaction to those people who have problems with self-identity or are prone to daydreams and fantasies which may become morbid or perverse. These increase the inability to integrate and may even lead to mental degeneration.

other varieties

There are two other varieties of cedarwood oil: Texas (*Juniperus ashei*) and Virginian (*Juniperus virginiana*). While they share similar therapeutic properties with Atlas cedarwood, they can cause skin irritation and sensitization and are best avoided for aromatherapy.

method of extraction

The bark is incised so that the tree yields an oleo-gum resin which is collected after it solidifies into amber-coloured lumps the size of a pea. This resin is then steam-distilled to produce the essential oil.

---

most common uses
- Nervous tension and anxiety • Acne • Dandruff
- Coughs and bronchitis • Skin infections • Arthritis

---

safety data
- **Non-toxic** • **Non-irritant in dilution** • **Non-sensitizing**

cinnamon

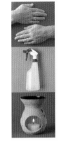

Cinnamomum zeylanicum

Family: Lauraceae

origin The cinnamon tree is a native of east India and Indonesia. The inner bark of the young twigs, sold as cinnamon sticks, has been used in cooking and as a medicine for thousands of years. In herbal medicine cinnamon is used to treat colds and flu, digestive disorders and rheumatism.

description

Cinnamon oil is a yellow or brownish-yellow liquid with a harsh, warm and spicy odour.

therapeutic properties

Cinnamon is a pungent and warming oil with stimulating and tonifying properties. It is useful for strengthening and tonifying the circulatory, respiratory and digestive systems and is restorative for weak, tired, cold people. It can irritate the skin and must be very well diluted in a base oil before application; it should not be used in dilutions stronger than 0.5 per cent and a patch test should be tried on a small area of skin before using. Because cinnamon can irritate the mucous membranes it should not be added to general bath oils and it should never be applied to the face, though it may be used in foot baths. Cinnamon blends particularly well with clove, eucalyptus, frankincense, lemon, mandarin and orange.

Cinnamon will stimulate a sluggish digestion, especially when aggravated by cold food, and will strengthen peristalsis in people prone to constipation. Its antispasmodic properties will help to relieve any kind of digestive spasm, such as colic: combine it with marjoram and orange, dilute well in a base oil and massage over the abdomen.

As a general tonifier, cinnamon may be blended into a massage oil and massaged into the lower back. This will help to strengthen the adrenal glands and general vitality as well as aiding in the cure of impotence. To treat chills and poor circulation to the extremities add a few drops of cinnamon to a teaspoon of base oil, put in a bowl of very warm water and use as a foot or hand bath.

Cinnamon can be used to treat rheumatism, especially when the pain is aggravated in cold, damp weather – try combining it with lemon and juniper in a base oil and gently massaging the area.

The strongly antiseptic properties of cinnamon make it good for treating colds and flu; it works very well in an essential oil burner or in a room spray to fumigate a room. Cinnamon is also a useful parasiticide, especially for treating lice and scabies.

For the former, combine it with oils of eucalyptus, pine, rosemary and thyme and comb through the hair; for the latter, combine with bergamot and cedarwood and apply to the skin.

psychological profile

Cinnamon is appropriate if you have become disappointed with life and feel that you will not achieve your earlier hopes. You may feel that you have become something of an outsider or even cynical and depressed. Using cinnamon will help to rekindle your interest and enthusiasm for life.

method of extraction

For aromatherapy purposes the essential oil is steam-distilled from the leaves and young twigs. An essential oil is also distilled from the bark, but this is extremely irritant and should not be used for aromatherapy.

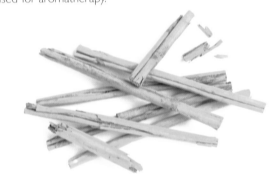

most common uses
- Sluggish digestion • Chills • Lice and scabies

safety data
- Non-toxic
- Do not use in concentrations of more than 0.5%

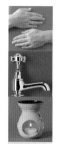

Citrus aurantium
Family: Rutaceae

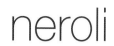

neroli

Also known as: Orange blossom, Petitgrain

origin Neroli oil is produced from the flowers of the bitter orange tree, also known as the Seville orange. The tree is native to China, but has been cultivated for hundreds of years in the countries bordering the Mediterranean. Neroli oil is one of the classic perfume and eau de cologne ingredients. Orange-flower water is a renowned skin toner for dry and mature skin.

description

A pale yellow liquid that becomes darker on ageing, neroli has an exquisite, floral, sweet smell which is powerful yet also light and refreshing.

therapeutic properties

Neroli is both calming and uplifting, although its effect in the long run is relaxing. It adds a wonderful fragrance to many massage and bath oil blends and combines particularly well with citrus oils, clary sage, jasmine, lavender and rosemary.

The main action of neroli is on the nervous system, and it is one of the most effective anti-depressant essential oils. People who feel exhausted, depressed, anxious and confused will benefit from neroli as it will aid sleep, promote relaxation and help to clear the mind and lift the spirits. It is also a useful first-aid treatment for shock and hysteria.

The relaxing action of neroli also has an effect on heart problems arising from tension, including tachycardia and palpitations. Use it to create a relaxing bath and massage oil.

Neroli has antispasmodic properties which make it a good remedy for digestive cramps, especially those arising from nervousness. It may also be useful in treating diarrhoea, especially if it is of a chronic nature or stress-related. Try combining it with geranium and massaging it over the abdomen.

Another main area of neroli's actions is on the skin. The oil has a very low toxicity and its rejuvenating properties make it useful for treating dry, mature skin, wrinkles and broken capillaries. Applied during pregnancy it will help to prevent stretch marks. It is said to stimulate the elimination of dead skin cells. It also has a deodorizing effect.

psychological profile

To benefit most from neroli you will be a somewhat private person, slightly reserved and seemingly calm and cool; you may come across as a rather aloof and sophisticated type. However, while everything appears to be under control and to your liking, this may conceal considerable anxiety, worry and stress. Using neroli will allow you to relax and become more in touch with your heart and able to express your true emotions. This will lead to feeling less remote from other people. Neroli will also help you to sleep better, relax more and participate in life more fully.

other varieties

Petitgrain essential oil is steam-distilled from the leaves and twigs of the same tree as neroli. It has a pleasant, fresh, floral and sweet smell with a herbaceous and slightly woody undertone. Like neroli, petitgrain has uplifting properties and the two can be combined. It is slightly more astringent than neroli and can be used to treat oily skin and acne.

method of extraction

Neroli oil is water-distilled from the freshly picked flowers in May and October.

most common uses
• Depression • Insomnia • Mature skin • Stretch marks

safety data
• **Non-toxic** • **Non-irritant** • **Non-sensitizing**

bergamot

Citrus bergamia
Family: Rutaceae

origin The most likely origin of the name is from Bergamo, in Lombardy, where the fruit was sold. Production of the essential oil started during the early eighteenth century in Italy, and since then it has become one of the most important perfume materials. It is the main constituent of eau de cologne as well as being used in lotions, creams, perfumes, sweets and soaps. It is bergamot oil that gives Earl Grey tea its distinctive flavour.

description

Bergamot oil is a light, yellow or pale green liquid with an extremely rich, sweet, green and fruity smell.

therapeutic properties

Bergamot is a cooling and refreshing oil. Its main action is on the nervous system, where it acts as a tonic, and is invigorating without being over-stimulating. It makes a pleasant, fragrant addition to many massage and bath oil blends, and combines particularly well with coriander, cypress, geranium, juniper, lavender, melissa, neroli, pine and rosemary.

Bergamot has a soothing effect, and is a good nerve tonic when stress makes you feel hot and sweaty. It is also useful for tension headaches. Its cooling and refreshing properties make it an oil that helps during times of stress and when you are feeling cross, irritable and overwrought.

Bergamot has carminative and antispasmodic properties which makes it useful for problems of the digestive system; especially when there is colic, painful wind and indigestion. The antiseptic properties of the oil can help in treating gastroenteritis and other gastric infections – massage it over the abdomen.

In Italy, bergamot is used for treating fevers because it is cooling. It has a special affinity for the mouth and throat and is traditionally used to treat sore throats, mouth ulcers and bad breath.

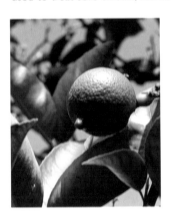

Bergamot oil alleviates genito-urinary infections when there is burning and inflammation – use in the bath or as a douche. It is also used to treat skin conditions for its antiseptic, healing and deodorizing properties and is particularly recommended in the treatment of acne, herpes, psoriasis and seborrhoea of the scalp.

Bergamot oil increases skin photosensitivity which means that the skin tans more readily. For this reason you must be careful not to apply bergamot to the skin before going out into the sun. It is possible to buy bergamot oil that has had the component bergaptene extracted, removing photosensitivity.

In first aid, bergamot is used as an antiseptic in the treatment of wounds and ulcers. It will act as a parasiticide for eliminating scabies. It also makes a deodorizing and refreshing room spray.

psychological profile

Bergamot is an appropriate oil if you are the type of person who pursues goals with a determination to succeed at any cost. It is cooling and refreshing for the cross, critical, exacting person who begins to suffer from digestive and skin problems, and whose nerves become edgy and raw.

method of extraction

For aromatherapy purposes the essential oil is steam-distilled from the leaves and young twigs. An essential oil can also be distilled from the bark, but this is extremely irritant and should not be used for aromatherapy.

most common uses
- Tonic for the nervous system • Cooling and refreshing
- Good for tension, stress and irritability • Indigestion
- Cystitis • Wounds and ulcers

safety data
- **Non-toxic • Non-sensitizing • Non-irritant**
- **Use bergaptene-free bergamot, or do not use in concentrations of more than 0.4%**

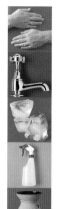

Citrus limon

Family: Rutaceae

lemon

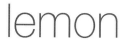

origin The lemon tree is native to India but arrived in Europe with the Crusaders as long ago as the twelfth century. The essential oil has been commercially developed for its extensive use in the perfumery and flavouring industries.

description

A transparent liquid with a fresh, sweet and green-citrus smell, reminiscent of the peel when it is ripe.

therapeutic properties

Lemon is primarily a refreshing, cleansing and tonifying oil, and is one of the most important bactericidal oils for any infection or putrefaction. It is a versatile oil to use in massage and bath oil blends, compresses, inhalations and room fragrancing. It blends well with nearly every other essential oil, and will provide a top note to 'lift' many fragrances.

Lemon is a tonic for the circulatory system and will improve a sluggish circulation and weak venous system which gives rise to chilblains or varicose veins. Its regular use is also said to reduce blood viscosity and help break down sclerotic deposits. It is also a traditional remedy for the treatment of broken capillaries visible on the skin.

This oil has a tonifying and stimulatory action on the digestive system. It can be used to treat obesity and also debility, weakness and loss of appetite. It helps to stimulate the production of pancreatic and gastric juices, and its cleansing and detoxifying properties can be of benefit to congested liver conditions and cellulite.

The moving and antiseptic properties of lemon will alleviate many respiratory conditions by combating infection and helping to eliminate mucus – use in steam inhalations or a massage blend to rub on the chest to treat colds, flu, bronchitis and asthma. Lemon also helps to stimulate the production of white blood cells, thereby strengthening the immune response. It is a good preventative during epidemics of contagious disease – use it in an essential oil burner or a plant spray in the room.

The antiseptic and astringent properties of lemon are appropriate for greasy skin and also any skin infection such as boils, acne, ulcers and eruptions. Make a compress to skin eruptions.

Lemon's astringent and tonifying properties will combat wrinkles. It is also an anti-viral oil and, applied neat, will help to eliminate warts and verrucae.

Lemon can be used against scabies and other parasitic infestations. It has insect-repelling properties and will prevent insect bites from going septic. Spray it around the house to discourage household insects such as animal fleas and ants.

lime

Lime (*Citrus aurantifolia*) shares the refreshing and uplifting properties of lemon and blends well with all the citrus fruits. Lime oil is strongly phototoxic and should not be used in concentrations of more than 0.5 per cent if going out into the sun within 12 hours of application.

psychological profile

Lemon oil is appropriate if you feel you need an astringent and cleansing treatment. You may have greasy hair and skin, a sluggish digestion, and perhaps feel generally unclean. There may have been a period in your life when you have neglected to take full care of yourself. You may have a tendency to body odour. Using lemon oil will help to tighten up your tissues, encouraging you to feel healthier and cleaner and be more self-confident.

method of extraction

Lemon oil is machine-expressed from the ripe peel of the lemon.

most common uses

- Refreshing • Cleansing • Circulatory tonic • Greasy skin
- Skin eruptions, boils • Insect repellent • Colds and flu

safety data

- Sensitization possible • Phototoxic – do not use in concentrations of more than 2% if applying to the skin within 12 hours of exposure to sunlight

grapefruit

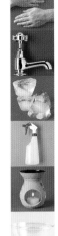

Citrus x paradisi

Family: Rutaceae

origin The grapefruit is thought to have evolved from a citrus fruit known as shaddock, which is native to the Caribbean. Cultivation now occurs in the USA, South America, the Caribbean and Israel. There are many varieties of grapefruit, including ruby or pink grapefruit, which is also available as an essential oil. Rich in Vitamin C, grapefruits are known as a cleansing and beneficial food.

description

Grapefruit has a fresh, sweet, citrus smell, similar to sweet orange. The colour may be yellow, pale green or pale orange. As with other citrus oils, grapefruit oxidizes quickly and the odour and therapeutic properties will deteriorate after 6–12 months.

therapeutic properties

Grapefruit is a cooling and slightly astringent oil. It is a mild tonic and shares refreshing and detoxifying properties with other citrus oils. It makes a pleasant, refreshing addition to many bath and shower preparations and also massage blends. Grapefruit blends particularly well with other citrus oils, clove, cypress, ginger, lavender, neroli, palmarosa and rosemary.

The main action of grapefruit oil is on the liver, where it has a cooling and detoxifying effect. It can calm symptoms of irritability, anger and overheating, and is a wonderful morning pick-me-up to use in a shower gel or bath oil following a hangover, late night or overindulgence.

Grapefruit is a mild aperient and will encourage peristalsis and thus relieve constipation. It is one of the main essential oils used in the treatment of obesity. It can help to reduce the appetite and stimulate the rate of metabolism of fats.

It has a generally detoxifying effect on the body and can help with lymphatic cleansing and reducing cellulite. Use as a massage oil, or combine with Dead Sea salts and add to the bath.

It also has a beneficial action on the respiratory system, and is good for treating colds and flu with hot, feverish symptoms. It may be combined with other appropriate oils such as eucalyptus or pine and used in a steam inhalation.

On the skin, grapefruit has cleansing, antiseptic, cooling and slightly astringent properties; it is helpful for oily skin, open pores and acne. Use in a lotion or as a facial steam. It will also help to tone and tighten loose skin, for example, after losing weight.

psychological profile

Grapefruit is appropriate if you are very self-conscious and unhappy about your appearance. You may put on weight easily, have problem skin or simply get embarrassed easily. You may also have a tendency to feel ashamed and that you are less worthy than other people. Using grapefruit will help to improve your sense of self-worth and help you to become more empowered and positive about yourself and what you can do with your life.

method of extraction

Grapefruit oil is machine-expressed from the peel of the ripe fruit.

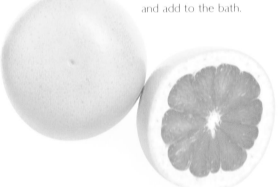

most common uses
- Detoxifying • Constipation • Cellulite • Hangovers
- Problem skin

safety data
- Non-irritant in dilution • Non-sensitizing • Slightly phototoxic • Do not use in dilutions of more than 3% if going out into the sun within 12 hours of application

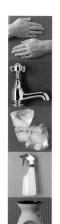

Citrus reticulata
Family: Rutaceae

mandarin

origin Originally found in China and the Far East, the mandarin orange tree was brought over to Europe at the beginning of the nineteenth century. The fruit was a traditional offering to Chinese mandarins and this is said to be the origin of the name. Mandarin oil is now mainly produced in the countries bordering the Mediterranean.

description

Mandarin oil has an extremely sweet smell with a rich, floral undertone. It is an orange or amber colour.

therapeutic properties

Mandarin oil has similar properties to those of sweet orange. It is a 'moving' oil, useful for treating conditions when stagnation and putrefaction are present. It is a pleasant addition to a wide range of massage and bath oil blends, and may also be used to fragrance a room. Mandarin blends well with citrus oils, spice oils and clary sage, geranium, juniper, lavender and neroli.

The lack of toxicity of mandarin oil makes it very suitable for children. It has a calming and soothing effect on restless children and may be used to treat hyperactivity. It can also be beneficial in the treatment of stress, nervous tension and insomnia.

The primary action of mandarin is on the digestive system, and it can be used to treat problems arising from a slow digestion such as dyspepsia and gastralgia; it will encourage peristalsis and help to relieve constipation. As a mild digestive tonic it is useful in the treatment of the elderly. It is also suitable for treating hiccoughs, indigestion or colic in children. Blend in a base oil and massage over the abdomen.

Mandarin detoxifies the body and reduces cellulite. It is also used in the treatment of water retention and obesity. It can help to tone loose skin, for example, after losing weight. The slightly astringent properties of mandarin make it good for combating oily skin and acne. It also has a role during pregnancy in preventing stretch marks – try combining it with neroli in a massage base oil.

psychological profile

Mandarin is appropriate if you have a tendency to feel sorry for yourself. Children needing mandarin may cry a lot and tend to be restless and hard to please. You may crave comfort and seek love and attention. If you do not get the affection you crave you may over-eat as compensation. Using mandarin will encourage you to be more positive about your own attributes and strengths and will help you develop a greater sense of self-worth.

other varieties

The mandarin tree was taken from Europe to the USA in the middle of the nineteenth century, where it was renamed tangerine by the Americans. Although the tree is still classified as *Citrus reticulata*, the tangerine has developed into a larger fruit than the mandarin and has a thinner and more citrus smell. Tangerine has similar therapeutic properties to those of mandarin.

method of extraction

Mandarin essential oil is machine-expressed from the peel of the ripe fruit.

most common uses
• Indigestion • Restless children • Stretch marks

safety data
• Non-toxic • Non-phototoxic • Non-irritant
• Non-sensitizing

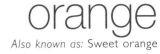

orange

Citrus sinensis, syn. C. dulcis

Family: Rutaceae

Also known as: Sweet orange

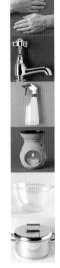

origin Orange trees are natives of the Far East, brought to Europe in the early sixteenth century and then taken on to the Americas by the Spanish and Portuguese. There are many varieties of orange tree, grown in different parts of the world. The essential oil has been produced in many countries for local use, for example in drinks. Today, most of the commercial production of orange oil is from Brazil, the USA and Cyprus.

description

Orange oil is a pale orange-yellow colour with a sweet, fresh and fruity smell.

therapeutic properties

Orange oil is very pleasant to experience and also very safe because of its low toxicity and moderate effect. It may be used for children, who generally enjoy its fresh, sweet smell. A versatile oil, it is suitable for skin conditioners, massage oils, bath oils and room fragrancing, and blends particularly well with spice oils, other citrus oils, clary sage, geranium, lavender, myrrh, neroli and rosemary. This oil has a relaxing effect but is uplifting rather than overly sedating. Its pleasant fragrance makes it beneficial when treating stress, nervous tension and related headaches, especially those connected with the digestive system. In the latter instance, combine with chamomile for the best effect.

Orange has a moving action, good for the treatment of symptoms that arise from a sluggish or obstructed system, such as flatulence and constipation. Dilute in a base oil and massage over the abdomen.

The primary function of orange is on the liver and digestive system. It is one of the main liver unblockers, helpful when there is congestion of the liver or spleen; its action is very gentle and easily tolerated. It acts as a mild aperient, helping bowel movements by encouraging peristalsis, and will also alleviate colic. Orange combines well with fennel, aniseed and peppermint for prolonged digestive conditions.

Orange oil has a general detoxifying and cleansing effect and will encourage the elimination of excess fluids and waste products from the system. Orange may be used as a massage or bath oil during a detoxifying programme and may be added to blends for the reduction of cellulite.

Due to its moderating and balancing effect, orange oil can be employed in the treatment of gastric fevers, colds and flu. Its tonifying and slightly astringent properties also indicate its appropriateness for oily skin or dull and tired skin.

psychological profile

Constitutionally, orange oil is suitable if you have trouble getting things done. You may have met many obstacles and become frustrated, eventually succumbing to laziness and finding it an effort to make any changes in your life. Bad habits of overindulgence and avoidance of exercise may develop, and you will become overweight. Using orange oil will begin to accelerate the sluggish organic processes, and the tenor of your life will also begin to change as you become more optimistic and purposeful.

method of extraction

The traditional method of obtaining orange oil was to hand-express it by rasping the peel, but most modern production is by machine expression.

most common uses

- Slow digestion • Constipation • Over-eating
- Tension headaches • Tiredness

safety data

- Non-toxic • Non-phototoxic • Non-irritant in dilution
- Sensitization rare

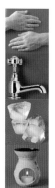

Commiphora myrrha
Family: Burseraceae

myrrh
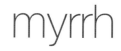

origin Myrrh is the resin of a small tree that grows in East Africa and countries bordering the Red Sea and Arabia. It has been used since ancient times in Egypt for the embalming of the dead and in China as a medicine for arthritis and skin infections. It has also been greatly valued as a sacred herb and incense ingredient. Distillation of the oil occurs mainly in Europe and the USA.

description

Myrrh oil is a sticky liquid ranging from a pale orange or amber colour to a dark red. It has a balsamic, medicinal and dry smell with an initial sweetness.

therapeutic properties

Myrrh oil is stimulating, strengthening and highly antiseptic. It may be used in massage blends, steam inhalations and room fragrancing. It blends particularly well with spice oils, cedarwood, cypress, frankincense, lemon, patchouli and sandalwood.

The main action is on the respiratory system, where its tonifying properties make it helpful in the treatment of chronic lung conditions. It is also an excellent expectorant, particularly when there is thick, white mucus. It can be used to treat coughs, colds and bronchitis, when it works particularly well in steam inhalations.

The stimulating properties of myrrh also have an effect on the digestive system, where it is appropriate for treating poor digestion, fermentation and flatulence. It can also be used to cure diarrhoea caused by a chill — combine with other appropriate oils and massage over the abdomen.

Myrrh has a very good reputation for its action on the mouth and throat. Combined with lavender and sage in a little alcohol and water it makes an excellent antiseptic mouthwash for any infection or inflammation in this area, including mouth ulcers, pyorrhoea, sore throat, bleeding gums, bad breath and thrush.

Myrrh has traditionally been regarded as a skin preserver, capable of delaying wrinkles and other signs of ageing skin. It combines well with frankincense, cypress, cedarwood and sandalwood for skin care. Its highly anti-inflammatory and antiseptic properties make it a very useful oil for the treatment of any wound that is slow to heal or is infected — apply as a lotion or compress. It has also been used to treat ulcers, gangrene and fungal infections such as ringworm.

psychological profile

Myrrh is appropriate if you are a purposeful and creative person but lack confidence in your ability to overcome difficulties and achieve what you want to. You may feel temporarily in the dark, or that you are struggling with a part of your own personality.

Using myrrh will put you back in touch with your inner sense of purpose and also help to open up the channels for the expression of love.

method of extraction

Myrrh resin is gathered by making incisions in the bark of the tree. The lumps of resin are then steam-distilled to produce the essential oil.

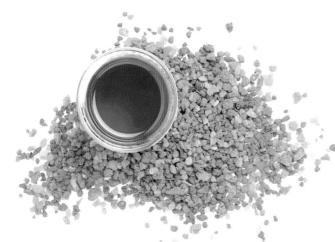

most common uses
- Mouth ulcers • Gum disease • Coughs • Ageing skin
- Skin infections

safety data
- **Non-toxic externally • Non-irritant • Non-sensitizing**

coriander

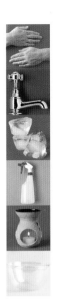

Coriandrum sativum

Family: Umbelliferae

origin Coriander seeds have been used for thousands of years and were found in the tomb of the Ancient Egyptian pharaoh Rameses II. They have been used as a remedy for digestive disorders in the West and in China. Coriander is thought to be native to the Far East but became naturalized in south-eastern Europe. It was introduced into Britain by the Romans. The leaves (herb) and the fruits (spice) are popular culinary ingredients in many parts of the world. The oil is mainly produced in Russia, Eastern Europe and North Africa.

description

Coriander oil has a fresh, aromatic and sweet-spicy smell. It is a colourless or pale yellow liquid.

therapeutic properties

Coriander is a gently stimulating and tonifying oil, mildly warming in effect. It makes a good addition to massage blends and may also be added to bath oils and room fragrancers. Coriander oil blends well with bergamot, clary sage, frankincense, jasmine, sandalwood and other spice oils.

Its gently tonifying action on the nervous system makes coriander helpful in cases of debility. It is said to improve a poor memory, and can alleviate migraine, especially if this is associated with digestive symptoms – add to a massage blend or the bath.

The main action of coriander is on the digestive system, which is why it features as an ingredient in many aperitifs and liqueurs. It is an excellent digestive tonic, encouraging better assimilation, and is an important oil in the treatment of anorexia nervosa, helping to stimulate the appetite, improve an undermined digestion and strengthen the nervous system. Other digestive disorders that coriander oil can treat include colic, diarrhoea, dyspepsia, flatulence and nausea. To relieve digestive discomfort, blend coriander into a base oil with other appropriate essential oils and massage over the abdomen.

Coriander is also known to have aphrodisiac properties. It is particularly appropriate when the libido is low as a result of tiredness and debility. Add to a massage or bath oil blend with other aphrodisiac oils or use to fragrance the room.

Coriander has an analgesic and warming effect, making it a helpful addition to blends treating rheumatic pains, muscular stiffness, sprains, strains and neuralgia. It is also an effective deodorant in that it both masks unpleasant smells and prevents the growth of bacteria that cause body odour. Blend it into lotions and flower waters to use as deodorants, colognes and body splashes.

psychological profile

Coriander is appropriate if you present a misleading appearance; you may seem confident, independent and even arrogant, but underneath you are a rather needy and clingy person who does not actually like yourself. You probably feel that your parents had high expectations of you and that you now have similarly high expectations of yourself, but are having difficulty living up to them. This split between how you feel and what you show to the world may lead to depression, eating disorders and feelings of desperation. Using coriander oil will bring a feeling of comfort and inner strength that will help you to come to terms with who you really are and begin to express your vulnerable side.

method of extraction

The fruits are crushed and the oil is then steam-distilled.

---

most common uses
- Anorexia • Poor digestion • Rheumatism • Deodorant

---

safety data
- **Non-toxic • Non-irritant in dilution • Non-sensitizing**

Cupressus sempervirens
Family: Cupressaceae

cypress

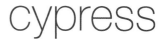

origin Cypress trees are native to the countries bordering the Mediterranean. It has been used as an astringent herbal medicine since ancient times and is valued greatly in Tibet as an incense ingredient. Cultivation and distillation occur mainly in France and Morocco, and the oil is used as a fragrance in aftershaves and colognes.

description

Cypress oil is pale yellow or green in colour and has a sweet, resinous, fresh odour reminiscent of a pine forest.

therapeutic properties

Cypress's main characteristic is its astringent properties and its main action is on the circulatory system. Cypress may be used in massage and bath oil blends, in steam inhalations and room fragrancing. It blends particularly well with cedarwood, clary sage, frankincense, juniper, lavender, mandarin, marjoram and orange.

Cypress refreshes and tones the nervous system. It may be used to treat nervous debility, nervous strain and weariness brought about by stress.

Cypress is very useful in the treatment of varicose veins or broken capillaries – dilute in a base oil and massage over the affected area. It is the main oil for treating haemorrhoids – try adding a couple of drops to the bath. Cypress combines well with ginger and may be massaged on to the hands or feet or used in a footbath to treat poor circulation and chilblains.

The astringent properties of cypress make it effective in treating excessive discharges – it can be used for hot and burning diarrhoea, frequent urination and most forms of haemorrhage. To stop a nosebleed, put a couple of drops of cypress oil on a tissue and hold under the nose for a few moments.

Cypress has a tonifying effect on uterine and pelvic tissue and can relieve heavy and prolonged menstrual bleeding. It can be helpful during the menopause and will relieve hot flushes; use in the bath and as a massage oil.

Cypress can help to relieve muscular aches and pains. It may be used as a compress or massage oil to relieve rheumatism. It will reduce swelling and oedema of the joints.

This oil has a detoxifying effect on the system. It helps to prevent the build-up of excess fluid and toxins within the tissues and may be used in the treatment of water retention, obesity and cellulite. Use in massage and bath oils.

Cypress is suitable for oily skin and also for areas of loose skin, for example, after losing weight. It may be used as a facial steam or in a massage oil or lotion. It will also help to check excessive perspiration and is a natural deodorant – foot baths with cypress and lavender oil are an effective way to deal with foot odour.

Cypress also has antispasmodic properties and can be used in steam inhalations to relieve spasmodic and loose coughs, hayfever, bronchitis and asthma.

psychological profile

Cypress works best for those people who tend towards excess and over-indulgence. Such people may be lazy and overweight, and perhaps of an easy-going and chatty nature. If appropriate, cypress will help to focus and increase energy.

method of extraction

The oil is extracted by steam distillation of the needles and twigs.

most common uses
• Varicose veins and haemorrhoids • Poor circulation
• Heavy periods • Profuse perspiration
• Spasmodic coughs

safety data
• **Non-toxic** • **Non-irritant** • **Non-sensitizing**

Cymbopogon citratus, C. flexuosus
Family: Gramineae

lemongrass

origin There are two main types of lemongrass: West Indian (*Cymbopogon citratus*) and East Indian (*Cymbopogon flexuosus*). Both varieties are native to India, although the former is now mainly cultivated in the Caribbean. Lemongrass is a fast-growing, aromatic perennial grass that grows up to 1.5 m (5 ft) tall. It is used in India to treat fevers and infectious illnesses and appears as a culinary herb throughout Asia.

description

Lemongrass essential oil has a fresh, intensely sweet, lemony and herbaceous smell and is a pale yellow or amber liquid.

therapeutic properties

Lemongrass has the refreshing and antiseptic properties of lemon but is more warming. It should be well diluted (do not use in concentrations of more than 2 per cent) and may be used in massage oils, insect-repellent preparations and room fragrancing. Lemongrass blends particularly well with coriander, eucalyptus, lavender, peppermint, rosemary, thyme and vetiver.

The main actions of lemongrass are on the digestive system and skin. It is also a mild antidepressant and will relieve stress and nervous exhaustion.

Lemongrass will help to stimulate the appetite and tone a sluggish digestive system. It has been used to treat colitis and, because of its antiseptic properties, it is helpful for enteritis and other gastric infections. Combine with geranium in a base oil and massage over the abdomen.

The tonifying properties of lemongrass are beneficial for poor muscle tone and slack tissues. It is an excellent component for any sports oil blend, both for a pre-sport massage and to treat aching muscles or muscle strain after sports. Combine with rosemary and vetiver in a base oil and massage into muscles before and after sport.

Lemongrass has a tonifying, deodorizing and astringent effect on the skin. It can be used to treat open or blocked pores and acne. It may also be added to a facial steam in order to deep-cleanse the skin.

This oil is widely used as an insect repellent for mosquitoes and fleas. It is also a parasiticide, eliminating lice, scabies and ticks.

psychological profile

Lemongrass is appropriate if you feel you have been a victim of circumstances or other people's behaviour during your life. You may be someone who is easily used and taken for granted by other people and you find it difficult to assert yourself, or to free yourself from restrictions. Using lemongrass will help you to become aware that there may be other ways of responding to your situation, and then new possibilities will begin to open up for you.

method of extraction

Lemongrass essential oil is produced by steam distillation of the chopped grass. After distillation the exhausted grass is used as cattle feed.

most common uses

- Enteritis • Acne • Sports preparation
- Insect repellent • Parasiticide

safety data

- **Non-toxic • Avoid use on hypersensitive or damaged skin**
- **Do not use in more than 2% concentration**

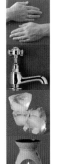

Cymbopogon martinii
Family: Gramineae

palmarosa

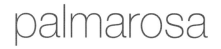

origin Palmarosa is a grassy-leaved herbaceous plant of the same family as lemongrass and citronella. It is native to India but is now also cultivated – and the oil produced – in Indonesia, the Comoros Islands, East Africa and Brazil. The essential oil is used in perfumery, particularly in soap, and was frequently employed in the past to adulterate the more expensive rose oil.

description

Palmarosa oil is a pale yellow or pale green liquid with a sweet, rosy, floral smell.

therapeutic properties

Palmarosa is a cooling and tonifying oil with healing and regenerative properties similar to those of lavender, and is also a balancing oil, being both calming and uplifting. It is a pleasant oil to use and may be added to massage blends, bath oils and room fragrancers. Palmarosa oil combines well with rose, bergamot, cedarwood, geranium, mandarin, sandalwood and ylang-ylang.

This oil has a soothing and mildly strengthening effect on the nervous system and is useful in the treatment of stress, anxiety and nervous tension. It has a mild aphrodisiac effect and is helpful when stress and tension are getting in the way of sexual fulfilment.

The action of palmarosa on the digestive system is as a gentle tonic and aid to digestion and assimilation. It will help to improve the appetite and may be used in the treatment of anorexia nervosa. Palmarosa is an effective antiseptic in the treatment of diarrhoea, gastroenteritis and dysentery; try combining it with bergamot and geranium. It will help to rebalance the intestinal flora after an intestinal infection or a course of antibiotics – use as a massage oil and massage over the abdomen, or add to a bath oil blend.

Palmarosa is best known for its skin care properties. It has a balancing action on the skin and can help to hydrate dry skin and balance the sebum secretions of oily skin. It will reduce scar tissue and its antiseptic properties are helpful for acne and minor skin infections. Palmarosa stimulates cellular regeneration and will reduce wrinkles and improve the appearance of tired or ageing skin; it may also be used to help prevent stretch marks. Apply to the skin in massage oils, compresses, creams and lotions and use as a facial steam.

psychological profile

Palmarosa is most appropriate if you tend to live in the past and do not feel optimistic about the future. You may feel that your life has not worked out how you wanted it to and you are disappointed and depressed. You may also fear the ageing process. It may be that you have experienced a particular crisis, such as losing your job or your partner, or there may be a more gradual feeling that life never fulfilled the expectations of your younger days. Using palmarosa will help you to feel more optimistic about your present life and to get more in touch with your inner sense of worth.

method of extraction

The essential oil is steam- or water-distilled from the fresh or dried grass. Palmarosa oil is frequently adulterated by the similar but inferior oil of gingergrass (*Cymbopogon martinii var. sofia*).

---

most common uses
• Stress • Diarrhoea • Skin care

---

safety data
• Non-toxic • Non-irritant • Non-sensitizing

cardamom

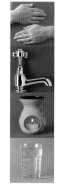

Elettaria cardamomum

Family: Zingiberaceae

origin The seeds and pods of cardamom have been used for centuries as a culinary spice in India, its native country. Cardamom has been employed in traditional Chinese medicine and in Indian Ayurvedic medicine for over 3,000 years, primarily for the treatment of respiratory diseases, fevers and digestive complaints. The essential oil also has a long history of use and has been produced since the sixteenth century. Cardamom oil is a perfume ingredient, especially in oriental-type fragrances. The oil is now produced mainly in India, Europe and the USA.

description

The oil is colourless to pale yellow and has a sweet-spicy, aromatic smell with a woody and almost floral undertone.

therapeutic properties

Cardamom is a warming and restorative oil which has a tonifying and calming action on the nervous system. It is pleasant to use in massage blends and combines particularly well with bergamot, cedarwood, clove, frankincense, orange, sandalwood and ylang-ylang.

The restorative properties of cardamom make it useful in the treatment of mental fatigue – try combining it with rosemary and burning it in the room. It will also relieve nervous tension. Cardamom has aphrodisiac properties, useful when feelings of stress and tension are getting in the way of sexual enjoyment. It is particularly helpful in the treatment of impotence. Combine with other appropriate oils such as jasmine or sandalwood and use in massage or burn in the room.

The main action of cardamom is on the digestive system: it is antispasmodic and carminative and will alleviate nausea, flatulence, indigestion, colic and heartburn. It may be diluted in a base oil and massaged over the abdomen, or the seed may be chewed to release the essential oil. It can be used as a general tonic for a sluggish digestive system and help to encourage better assimilation of food. It is also used in the treatment of anorexia. Cardamom is an important oil in the treatment of headaches related to digestive disorders.

The antiseptic properties of cardamom make it a good addition to mouthwashes for the treatment of bad breath.

Try combining it with myrrh and lavender and diluting in alcohol and water for use as a mouthwash.

psychological profile

Cardamom is appropriate if you have become a dry and melancholic type of person. You probably have a sedentary job and tend to have an intellectual approach to life, disliking excessive displays of emotion. You tend to be a rather fearful person and are anxious about your health. Other people may find you over-critical and rather unapproachable. Using cardamom will help you to get back in touch with the feeling of joy and encourage you to express greater warmth and friendliness with others.

method of extraction

Cardamom essential oil is steam-distilled from the dried seeds.

---

most common uses

• Digestive tonic • Nausea • Heartburn • Bad breath
• Poor assimilation

---

safety data

• **Non-toxic** • **Non-irritant** • **Non-sensitizing**

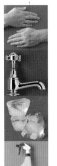

Eucalyptus globulus
Family: Myrtaceae

eucalyptus
Also known as: Blue gum

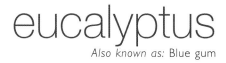

origin The eucalyptus tree is indigenous to Australia and was used as a medicinal herb by the Aborigines. In the nineteenth century a German botanist, von Muller, introduced the tree and its essential oil to the rest of the world. It is now cultivated in North Africa, Spain, California and India, as well as Australia.

description

A clear or pale yellow liquid, eucalyptus has a strong medicinal-camphoraceous smell and a faint woody undertone.

therapeutic properties

Eucalyptus is a warming and drying oil with excellent antiseptic properties. It may be used in massage blends and bath oils and excels as a steam inhalation. It blends very well with cedarwood, cypress, lavender, lemon, marjoram, pine, tea tree and thyme.

Eucalyptus has a refreshing effect on the nervous system and may be used to treat tiredness, poor concentration, headaches and debility. Use in inhalations or burn in the room.

The Australian Aborigines used eucalyptus in the treatment of all kinds of fever, including malaria. The essential oil is especially good for infections of the respiratory tract such as colds, flu, sinusitis, bronchitis and pneumonia. Because it is a warming oil it works especially well if you are feeling chilled. It is also a decongestant and makes an excellent inhalation to relieve over-production of mucus. It can be combined with aniseed to treat a cough or with cypress to treat catarrh.

Eucalyptus is an important remedy for the treatment of rheumatism and arthritis, especially when there is a lot of stiffness and loss of mobility, and the symptoms are worse when it is cold and damp. Try combining it with lavender and pine and using as a compress or massage lotion.

As an antibiotic oil eucalyptus can be used to treat infections of the urinary tract, especially if there is pus in the urine. Try it when cystitis is brought on by a chill. It is also good for genital infections such as leucorrhoeal – dilute it well and use it in a sitz bath. The anti-biotic properties of eucalyptus make it helpful in the treatment of skin infections and wounds, herpes and ulcers. It may be dabbed directly on to the skin to relieve the pain or itching of insect bites and stings. It is also anti-fungal, helping to alleviate infections such as athlete's foot.

Eucalyptus oil makes an excellent antiseptic room spray to fumigate a sickroom. It is also an effective insect repellent, especially if combined with cypress and lemon.

psychological profile

Eucalyptus is indicated if you recognize that it is time for a change in your life, but feel bogged down. You will feel restless, but have become trapped by fear of change and a lack of direction. This in turn leads to a state of confusion. Eucalyptus will allow you to gain clarity and move forward in your life.

other varieties

Eucalyptus citriodora is also highly antiseptic but is more cooling in its action than *E. globulus*. It has a pleasant lemony smell. Use this variety for respiratory infections when the mucus secretions are yellow, indicating there is heat in the system. *E. citriodora* is also useful for rheumatism when the joints are hot and red.

method of extraction

The oil is extracted by steam distillation of the leaves and twigs.

---

most common uses
- Colds and flu • Bronchitis • Mucus congestion/sinusitis
- Rheumatism • Cystitis • Infectious diseases

---

safety data
- Non-toxic externally • Toxic internally • Non-irritant
- Non-sensitizing

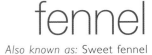
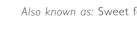

fennel

Foeniculum vulgare var. dulce

Family: Umbelliferae

Also known as: Sweet fennel

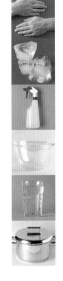

origin There are many cultivated varieties of fennel, all of them related to wild fennel, which is native to the countries bordering the Mediterranean. The variety used in aromatherapy is sweet fennel, which is cultivated in France, Italy and Greece. Fennel has been used as a sacred and medicinal herb for thousands of years. It was believed to ward off evil spirits and impart longevity, courage and strength.

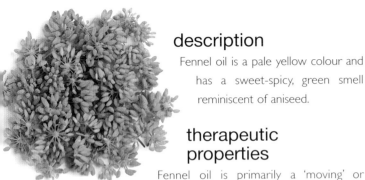

description

Fennel oil is a pale yellow colour and has a sweet-spicy, green smell reminiscent of aniseed.

therapeutic properties

Fennel oil is primarily a 'moving' or unblocking oil and its main action is on the digestive system. It may be used in massage blends and inhalations, but not at concentrations of more than 1.5 per cent as there may be some toxicity in concentrated doses. It blends particularly well with geranium, lavender, marjoram and rose.

A carminative and digestive stimulant, fennel will relieve flatulence and digestive spasms. When food is not properly carried through the digestive system, putrefaction occurs and gas will form; fennel is one of the main oils to encourage food to be digested properly and to help expel gas. It may be combined with a tiny amount of cinnamon and massaged over the abdomen to stimulate and strengthen the digestion.

Fennel is similar in action and smell to aniseed, but aniseed works more on the upper digestive tract and stomach while the action of fennel is more on the lower digestive processes and bowel. Fennel can be used to relieve constipation – dilute in a carrier oil and massage over the abdomen. It is also useful in the treatment of nervous indigestion such as is brought on by hurrying or after an emotional upset. It is the main oil for treating a swollen or distended abdomen and will relieve bloating after a rich or large meal.

Fennel oil also has an important action on the lungs. It is a mild expectorant and will help to relieve a phlegmy cough. Combine with other appropriate oils in a base oil and use in a chest rub, or burn in the room.

Fennel is a diuretic and increases the loss of fluids from the body. It can be used in a massage blend to detoxify the body,

for example, when treating cellulite. It has an oestrogenic action on the body and can help to increase milk production in nursing mothers. It may also help to relieve engorged or painful breasts; use as a compress.

Fennel oil has been shown to be effective in eliminating lactobacillus, which is thought to be the main bacterium that causes tooth decay. This indicates the usefulness of fennel in dental preparations, such as toothpastes and mouthwashes. Fennel will also help to mask unpleasant odours.

psychological profile

Fennel will be of most benefit to you if you are the type of person who holds back from expressing yourself. This may be as a result of a repressive childhood and inadequate opportunity to communicate deep emotions. This can result in a lack of enthusiasm, a fear of communicating and little opportunity to experience and learn. The habit of withholding expression on the emotional level can lead to flatulence and constipation physically. If appropriate, fennel can help you to relax and be more open to the experience of life.

method of extraction

The essential oil is steam-distilled from crushed fennel seeds.

---

most common uses

- Flatulence • Constipation • Nervous indigestion
- Bloatedness • Phlegmy coughs

---

safety data

- Sensitization possible
- **Do not use in concentrations of more than 1.5%**

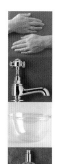

Helichrysum angustifolium,
H. italicum *subsp.* serotinum
Family: Asteraceae

helichrysum

Also known as: Everlasting flower, Immortelle

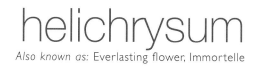

origin An aromatic herb, native to the Mediterranean, with yellow, daisy-like flowers. The flowers do not wither and are popular with florists, hence their name Everlasting flowers, or the French *Immortelle*. The essential oil is costly and highly valued in perfumery as well as aromatherapy.

description

It is a yellow liquid, sometimes with a tinge of red. The smell is heady and honey-like, with a warm and spicy undertone.

therapeutic properties

Helichrysum is a cooling and moving oil with profoundly regenerative and anti-inflammatory properties. Its main actions are on the nervous system and the skin. It is similar to chamomile in that it has an anti-allergenic effect, helping the individual to become less sensitive to allergens. Helichrysum blends very well with chamomile, geranium, lavender, rose and citrus oils. It works better in blends than on its own, and can make a wonderful addition to massage oils, skin lotions and bath oils.

Helichrysum has a profound action on the nervous system, where it has a soothing yet strengthening action. It will help to sweeten the temperament and lift the spirits, and may be used to treat depression, nervousness, exhaustion and any stress related conditions. Combine it with geranium to make a superbly balancing blend, with lavender for a relaxing blend, and for children blend with mandarin to treat symptoms of nervousness and anxiety. It will work best in bath or massage oils.

Helichrysum has vasodilatory and antispasmodic actions which make it useful in the treatment of certain circulatory disorders including high blood pressure, varicose veins, acne rosacea and phlebitis.

The antispasmodic action also makes helichrysum useful for treating some respiratory disorders such as asthma and whooping cough. It has decongestant properties making it helpful in treating some types of sinusitis and catarrh, especially those that are allergy- or stress-related. In this case it will work best blended with chamomile and used as a chest rub or inhalation.

With regard to the skin, helichrysum has excellent anti-inflammatory and regenerative properties. Its action on the skin is similar to lavender, and it can be combined with lavender to treat the effects of blows, bruising or operations. Combine it with frankincense, lavender or rose in a base of comfrey macerated oil to reduce scarring. Blended with chamomile it is one of the most important oils to treat allergic skin conditions, eczema and even psoriasis. Its action is gentle enough that it can be used to treat children's skin conditions, especially if blended with Roman chamomile.

psychological profile

If you need helichrysum you are probably a person who appears rather shy and self-conscious, although underneath you will have a stubborn streak. You are actually quite ambitious, although rarely put yourself forward for a new and challenging situation because of a fear of failure or showing yourself up. This lack of confidence can lead to feelings of frustration, lack of fulfilment and being taken advantage of.

Using helichrysum will help to boost your confidence, make you less concerned about appearances and more independent. It will encourage the realisation that you can achieve that which you most desire if you commit yourself to it fully and are prepared to work calmly through any obstacles.

method of extraction

Steam distillation of the fresh flowering tops.

---

most common uses
- Stress • Nervous exhaustion • Depression
- Allergies • Eczema

---

safety data
- **Non-toxic • Non-irritant • Non-sensitizing**

jasmine

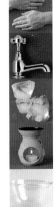

Jasminum officinale

Family: Oleaceae

Also known as: Common white jasmine

origin A native of north-west India, jasmine has been highly valued for the scent of its flowers for thousands of years and is known as the 'king of perfumes' because of its importance to the fragrance industry; indeed, a whole industry grew up around it in the Grasse region of France. Because the flowers are too delicate to be steam-distilled, jasmine used to be extracted by a labour-intensive method known as enfleurage, but today the usual method is by solvent extraction (see below). Jasmine absolute is produced mainly in France, Morocco and India.

description

Jasmine has an intensely rich, warm, heady, floral scent. It is a viscous, dark orange-brown liquid.

therapeutic properties

Jasmine is the most uplifting of all the oils. Its main effect is on the emotions, where it promotes a state of relaxed awareness; wearing jasmine helps to increase self-confidence and is anti-depressant. It is at once refreshing, soothing and calming, most effective when there is a clear and direct link between psychological stress and physical discomfort. Its relaxing properties make jasmine a useful oil when there are symptoms of contraction, tension and blockage, for example, a tight chest or tense muscles. Jasmine blends well with bergamot, clary sage, orange, rose, sandalwood and ylang-ylang.

The relaxing yet uplifting properties of jasmine suggest its use as one of the classic aphrodisiac oils, its exotic smell creating an atmosphere of relaxation and enjoyment. It can be beneficial in the treatment of both impotence and frigidity. Use as a sensual massage oil.

Jasmine will help ease menstrual discomfort and cramps, and also relieve labour pains if used either to perfume the room or diluted in a base oil and massaged into the lower back between contractions.

In skin care, jasmine is beneficial for treating hot, dry and inflamed skin, especially if this is worse during times of emotional stress. It may be applied undiluted to the skin as a perfume.

psychological profile

Jasmine is most suitable when you are going through a time of trauma and grief. It is also appropriate if you have become trapped by lingering feelings of sadness or grief. The use of jasmine can help to encourage an acceptance of all the experiences of life and promote enjoyment and relaxation.

method of extraction

Jasmine for aromatherapy use is not strictly speaking an essential oil but an absolute. First, a concrète is produced from jasmine flowers by a process of solvent extraction. Then the solvent is removed and the absolute is obtained from the concrète by separation with alcohol. Jasmine absolute is a very costly substance because of the large volume of flowers required to produce a small amount of it.

---

most common uses
• Uplifting • Aphrodisiac • Labour pains • Dry skin

---

safety data
• **Non-toxic** • **Non-irritating** • **Non-sensitizing**

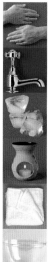

Juniperus communis
Family: Cupressaceae

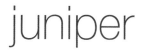

juniper

origin Juniper is an evergreen shrub or tree which produces small black berries. It is widespread throughout the northern hemisphere. Juniper has a long history of use as a herbal medicine in the treatment of urinary disorders, gout and rheumatism, and respiratory problems. Gin is flavoured by the berries.

description

Juniper oil has a piercing, fresh, warm, woody-herbaceous smell. The oil from the berries is slightly sweeter and less harsh than that from the wood, needles and twigs. It is a colourless or pale yellow liquid.

therapeutic properties

Juniper is a warming, stimulating and tonifying oil. It makes an excellent refreshing and detoxifying addition to many bath oils and massage oils, and may also be used in inhalations and room freshening. It blends particularly well with cedarwood, cypress, ginger, lavender, pine, rosemary and all the citrus oils.

The main action of juniper is on the kidneys and urinary system. It can be appropriate for both excessive and diminished urination and is one of the most important oils in the treatment of cystitis, especially when this is worsened by cold weather.

Juniper will encourage the elimination of uric acid and other toxins that a cold, sluggish system may fail to excrete efficiently. For this reason it is known as a blood purifier. It combines well with cypress to treat fluid retention, obesity and cellulite, and can also be used in the treatment of urinary stones (as compresses over the lower back) and gout (in footbaths or compresses).

Juniper is an important oil in the treatment of rheumatism and arthritis, especially in cases that are worse in cold weather. Combine it with a rubbing oil and massage the affected parts or use it in a compress.

This is a good oil for tonifying the glandular system, particularly the adrenals and pancreas – use it in baths and massage blends. It has also been used to treat leucorrhoea, and absent, painful or scanty periods. It was thought that juniper oil should be avoided by pregnant women, because juniper berries taken internally can cause miscarriage, but in fact juniper oil used externally is not abortifacient and is safe to use at normal dilutions during pregnancy.

The stimulating, astringent and detoxifying properties of juniper make it a good oil to treat clogged, oily and unhealthy skin. It will help the body to remove impurities and will improve skin that is prone to blackheads and acne. A few drops of juniper oil make an excellent, deep-cleansing steam facial. It can also be used to treat weeping eczema and dermatitis.

psychological profile

Juniper is appropriate if you were misunderstood and lonely in childhood. You may have appeared shy and, from fear of rejection, kept to yourself. In later life this may have developed into aloofness and a lack of the ability to give and receive warmth and affection. The lack of emotional care as a child may also develop into a neglect in looking after yourself physically. The use of juniper will promote a more optimistic outlook and encourage a warmer and friendlier state of being.

method of extraction

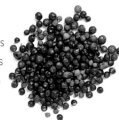

Juniper oil is steam-distilled from the berries alone or from the berries, needles and twigs of the shrub. Distillation occurs mainly in France and eastern Europe.

most common uses

- Cystitis • Water retention • Cellulite • Rheumatism
- Oily skin • Acne

safety data

- **Non-toxic • Non-irritant in dilution • Non-sensitizing**

lavender

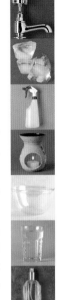

Lavandula angustifolia,
syn. L. officinalis, L. vera

Family: Lamiaceae (*formerly* Labiatae)

origin An aromatic shrub native to the Mediterranean, lavender has a long history of use as a medicine, fragrance and insect repellent. The essential oil production is long-established in the Provence region of France and also occurs in many other countries.

description

A colourless or pale yellow liquid, lavender oil has a very familiar, fresh, floral, slightly harsh and sweet smell.

therapeutic properties

This is the most versatile and well-used of all the essential oils. It may be used in massage blends, bath oils, room fragrancing, compresses, douches and steam inhalations, and is one of the few essential oils that may be applied to the skin without dilution.

Lavender is a balancing or regulating oil. In the long run it does tend towards calming, although initially it has a reviving effect – a footbath with a few drops of lavender has superb restorative effects. Like jasmine, it can be used to treat any physical symptoms that are the result of stress or nervous tension.

Lavender is relaxing as it calms cerebro-spinal activity. It may be used to treat irritability, depression, insomnia, hysteria, shock and nervous tension. It also has mild analgesic properties, which make it an important oil in the treatment of headaches and migraine, and good for all forms of neuralgia, shingles, sciatica, muscular pains and rheumatism. It will relieve earache in children; massage a few drops around the ear.

Its restorative and calming effect on the heart means that it helps high blood pressure and palpitations – use lavender in massage and bath preparations, and as an inhalant to relieve fainting and shock. The antispasmodic properties of lavender make it efficacious in the treatment of any kind of spasmodic cough. The excellent antiseptic properties are effective in treating flu, bronchitis and pneumonia.

Lavender may be used to treat colic and flatulence. It is of most benefit when treating digestive problems with a nervous origin, including diarrhoea, indigestion, nausea and so on. Dilute in a base oil and massage into the abdomen.

The anti-bacterial and anti-inflammatory properties of lavender have a pronounced effect on the urinary system and genitals – use in the bath. It is excellent for treating cystitis, leucorrhoea, thrush and other genital infections. The antispasmodic properties can soothe menstrual cramps.

Lavender is extremely useful in a variety of skin conditions, including wounds, ulcers and sores of all kinds. As a first-aid remedy it can be used neat on abrasions, wounds, burns, insect bites and stings. Other skin conditions that lavender may help are dermatitis, eczema, acne, acne rosaceae, psoriasis and scarring. Combined with lemon and used as a compress, it will treat boils.

Lavender may be combined with other oils to eliminate lice and scabies and to repel mosquitoes. Its deodorizing properties make it a useful room spray and antiseptic.

psychological profile

If you are a sensitive person who is easily embarrassed and inhibited you need lavender. You may have learned to conceal your shyness by appearing to be efficient, practical and organized, yet behind this you are aware of your sensitivity and vulnerability to other people. Using lavender will help you to accept your sensitivity and make the most of new situations that so often leave you feeling frustrated and unable to express yourself.

method of extraction

The oil is steam-distilled from the fresh flowering tops of the plant.

---

most common uses

- Stress • Insomnia • Headaches • Neuralgia • Thrush
- First aid: wounds, burns, shock • Insect repellent

---

safety data

- Non-toxic • Non-irritant • Non-sensitizing

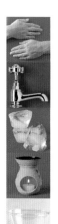

Matricaria recutita, *syn.* Chamomilla recutita
Family: Asteraceae (*formerly* Compositae)

chamomile

Also known as: Blue chamomile, German chamomile

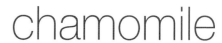

origin Chamomile is a flowering herb that has been used medicinally for thousands of years. The flowers are taken as an infusion for digestive disorders and to treat nervous tension and insomnia. Chamomile is cultivated in central and northern Europe.

description

A deep ink-blue viscous liquid that becomes brown with age, chamomile oil has an intensely heavy, sweet and herbaceous smell with a fruity undertone.

therapeutic properties

Chamomile is a profoundly soothing and calming oil, especially on the nervous and digestive systems. It is widely used in massage blends, skin care creams and bath oils, and blends very well with clary sage, lavender, lemon, marjoram and rose.

Chamomile is suitable for treating any digestive complaint arising from a nervous origin, including diarrhoea, colic, indigestion and peptic ulcers. Because of its low toxicity it is also suitable for treating children's digestive upsets.

The pain-relieving properties of chamomile make it excellent for treating teething pains in infants, especially when combined with fretfulness or earache. Chamomile also stimulates the production of white blood cells and is useful when treating any kind of virus or infection, especially in children.

Its antispasmodic properties make it a good treatment for menstrual cramp, and it is a mild emmenagogue, bringing on a menstrual period delayed due to cold or emotional upset. It is very soothing for genital irritation, particularly vaginal pruritis. Chamomile compresses can be excellent in relieving the pain and inflammation of mastitis, especially when combined with lavender or rose. It can be helpful during the menopause for menstrual irregularities, especially when associated with irritability or nervous complaints. Try blending it with rose and using for massage and in the bath.

Chamomile has a very calming and sedative effect on the nervous system, helping to relieve insomnia, irritability and nervousness. Combined with lavender or geranium and massaged over the site, it will help to relieve the pain of neuralgia or sciatica. It soothes inflamed joints and aching muscles.

One of the most important uses of chamomile is in treating skin inflammation; its soothing properties make it particularly appropriate for allergic skin conditions. It may also be used to treat eczema, herpes, wounds, dryness and any stress-related skin condition. Use it in the bath, in a lotion or as a compress.

psychological profile

Children needing chamomile are nervous and sensitive; adults requiring it feel misunderstood because they tend to hide their inner sensitivity under a layer of defensive behaviour, irritability and emotional over-reaction. Using chamomile oil will help to soothe reactions and calm any nervousness, enabling free expression of sensitivity.

other varieties

Roman chamomile, distilled from *Chamaemelum nobile*, is pale yellow and has a milder, sweeter smell than blue chamomile, which comes through in its effect. It is particularly suitable for treating infants or people with weak constitutions.

method of extraction

The oil is produced by steam distillation of the flowers.

---

most common uses

- Colic • Menstrual cramps • Neuralgia • Inflammation
- Eczema and allergies

---

safety data
- **Non-toxic** • **Non-irritant** • **Non-sensitizing**

tea tree

Also known as: Ti tree

Melaleuca alternifolia
Family: Myrtaceae

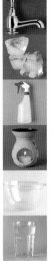

origin This species of the *Melaleuca* family is native to Australia. Tea tree has been used medicinally for thousands of years by the Australian Aborigines. During the Second World War it was included in first-aid kits to treat infections.

description
A colourless or pale yellow liquid, tea tree oil has a strong, spicy, fresh camphoraceous smell.

therapeutic properties
Tea tree is a stimulating and tonifying oil used primarily for its germicidal properties. It is highly antiseptic and can combat many different kinds of bacterial infection, including streptococcal and staphylococcal types, and has also been shown to have significant anti-viral and anti-fungal properties. It also stimulates the immune response. It blends particularly well with other strongly antiseptic oils, such as clove, eucalyptus, lavender, lemon, pine, rosemary and thyme.

Tea tree oil is used to treat many kinds of respiratory tract infections. It is extremely useful in helping to throw off colds and flu, and works particularly well in a steam inhalation.

Another important area of action for tea tree oil is the genito-urinary tract. It is effective for both acute and chronic cystitis and has become one of the main treatments for many genital infections, including thrush, non-specific urethritis (NSU), genital herpes, genital warts, pruritis and trichomonas. Due to its low toxicity, it can safely be used in high concentration in baths and can be applied in pessaries.

As an excellent anti-fungal, tea tree can be applied locally to treat such conditions as athlete's foot and ringworm. It is widely used in lotions to treat acne as well as combating infection in ailments such as corns, calluses, whitlows, boils, wounds, cuts and burns. To disinfect a cut or soothe insect stings and bites, apply tea tree neat – it will not even sting.

Tea tree can be used as a mouthwash to treat bad breath, mouth ulcers and gum infections. Many cases of warts and verrucae have been eliminated by the use of tea tree oil – dab it on neat on a daily basis. Tea tree is also effective in the treatment of cold sores and other types of herpes.

psychological profile
Although tea tree will work effectively for a wide range of first-aid and acute ailments, it is most appropriate if you are prone to complaints that are lingering and slow to heal. You may also have the feeling that you are never quite reaching your full potential, and that you are somehow disadvantaged and held back by circumstances beyond your control. Using tea tree will help you to realize that you can have an effect on your life and that you can take at least the next step towards a more fulfilling, happy and purposeful existence.

other varieties
There are two other types of *Melaleuca* that share the strongly antiseptic and stimulating properties of tea tree. Niaouli (*M. viridiflora*), also native to Australia, is primarily used in the treatment of skin complaints and respiratory illnesses. Cajuput (*M. cajuputi*) is native to Indonesia and the Philippines and is used mainly in the treatment of respiratory conditions.

method of extraction
The oil is steam- or water-distilled from the leaves and twigs.

---

most common uses
- Colds and flu • Cystitis • Thrush • Herpes • First aid
- Skin infections

---

safety data
- **Non-toxic externally • Non-irritant**
- **Skin sensitization rare but possible**

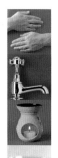

Melissa officinalis
Family: Lamiaceae (*formerly* Labiatae)

melissa
Also known as: Lemon balm

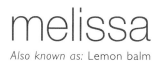

origin Melissa is an aromatic herb native to central and southern Europe. It has been used as a medicinal herb in the treatment of melancholy and heart problems for thousands of years. Commercial production of the oil is carried out mainly in France.

description

Melissa oil is a pale yellow liquid with a pleasant lemony, fresh and sweet-herbaceous smell.

therapeutic properties

This is a sweet, calming oil. Its main action is on the nervous system and it is useful for treating many symptoms with a nervous origin. It may be used in massage blends or bath oils and, although it is expensive, just one or two drops can transform an essential oil blend. Melissa combines particularly well with citrus oils, chamomile, geranium, lavender, marjoram and rose.

Melissa's calming yet uplifting effect is very useful in the treatment of stress headaches and migraines. It is especially appropriate when the headache is associated with tension in the neck and shoulders. Melissa combines well with chamomile to treat neuralgia and any nerve pains in the body. It can be combined with rosemary or bergamot to relieve brain fatigue from over-concentration and is also good for treating depression, hysteria and anxiety.

The antispasmodic properties of melissa have a calming effect on the heart. It reduces palpitations and panic attacks and is appropriate when overwork and overstimulation have weakened the heart and caused high blood pressure. Combine it with marjoram and use in the bath and for massage. The anti-spasmodic properties are also helpful for painful periods.

Melissa has an important action on the digestive system. It is a carminative to relieve flatulence, colic, dyspepsia and so on, and can also help to relieve nausea.

The cooling effect of melissa relieves fevers, especially when restlessness and distress are marked. Melissa can also help respiratory problems that are anxiety-related, such as asthma. To treat respiratory problems, either dilute melissa in a base oil and massage on to the chest or use in a vaporizer or oil burner.

Melissa's anti-inflammatory properties are helpful for inflamed skin and allergic skin conditions. It may be used for ulceration and also for eczema, especially when stress-related. Keep it on hand as a first-aid remedy for bee or wasp stings.

psychological profile

Melissa is most appropriate if you are the type of person who appears sweet, open and extremely considerate, but do not show the darker side of your nature for fear of not being liked. You may have developed an over-concern and anxiety for the welfare of others. Although you may appear charming and cheerful, underneath there is a growing tension and frustration at not being able to express your whole self. Symptoms such as nervousness, headaches, insomnia and even heart symptoms will develop as the body suffers from these hidden tensions. Melissa will encourage you to find ways to express the whole of your personality and will enable you to relax and enjoy life to the full.

method of extraction

Melissa oil is steam-distilled from the herb. Because the yield of oil is extremely small, melissa has the reputation of being one of the most frequently adulterated essential oils. True melissa oil is very expensive.

---

most common uses
- Depression • Insomnia • Headaches • Palpitations
- Colic • Inflamed skin conditions

---

safety data
- Non-toxic • Sensitization possible
- Do not use in concentrations of more than 2%

peppermint

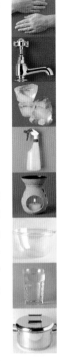

Mentha x piperita

Family: Lamiaceae (*formerly* Labiatae)

origin Peppermint is a perennial herb that is a cultivated hybrid of other types of mint. Mint is naturalized in Europe and North America and is also cultivated throughout the world; it has been used as a medicinal herb for thousands of years. The essential oil comes primarily from the USA. The majority is used in the flavouring and toothpaste industries.

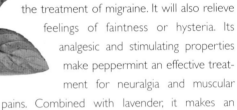

description

Peppermint oil has a fresh, strong, minty smell with a sweet undertone. It is a pale yellow or pale green liquid.

therapeutic properties

Peppermint is cooling, refreshing, warming and stimulating. The reason for this paradox is that the body increases circulation and warms up in response to the cooling action of peppermint applied to the skin. Peppermint adds a stimulating note to many massage and bath oil blends, but use only one or two drops or the smell will overpower any other oils used. It blends particularly well with eucalyptus, lavender, lemon, pine and rosemary.

The primary action of peppermint is on the digestive system, in particular the stomach. It encourages the easy absorption of food, and can be used for any symptom of a sluggish digestion, such as indigestion and flatulence. It also helps to stop regurgitation, sour risings, belching and hiccups.

Peppermint is a digestive antiseptic and can be used to treat gastric fevers, diarrhoea and food poisoning. It is also antispasmodic, and will relieve gastric spasm and colic. For digestive problems, peppermint combines well with oils of fennel and orange, and may be diluted in a base oil and massaged over the abdomen.

This oil can be used to treat nausea from any cause, including morning sickness and travel sickness. Peppermint aids the digestion of fats by encouraging the flow of bile, and has a detoxifying effect on the liver.

The secondary action of peppermint is on the respiratory system. It can be used for its antispasmodic and decongestant properties in the treatment of spasmodic coughs, asthma, bronchitis and sinusitis, and can relieve flu and head colds. Use in an essential oil burner.

Peppermint is refreshing and a general tonic of the nervous system. It will relieve nervous fatigue, and is an important oil in the treatment of migraine. It will also relieve feelings of faintness or hysteria. Its analgesic and stimulating properties make peppermint an effective treatment for neuralgia and muscular pains. Combined with lavender, it makes an excellent foot bath for tired or aching feet.

psychological profile

Peppermint is appropriate for times of transition, when one phase of life is completed and a new one about to begin, such as when changing schools or adapting to a new lifestyle. You may know that you need to leave a job or a relationship or move house, but do not yet know which direction to take. Using peppermint will help you to make a break with the past and strengthen your resolve and courage to take the next step.

other varieties

Spearmint oil (*M. spicata*) is milder and sweeter than peppermint but shares similar properties.

method of extraction

The essential oil is steam-distilled from the flowering herb.

---

most common uses

- Indigestion • Nausea • Muscle pains • Coughs and colds
- Deodorant

---

safety data

- Non-toxic externally
- Do not use in cases of cardiac fibrillation
- Do not use in concentrations of more than 3%

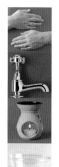

Ocimum basilicum

Family: Lamiaceae (*formerly* Labiatae)

basil

origin There are many varieties of the herb basil growing throughout the world, and all have a long tradition of use in cooking and as a herbal medicine. Essential oil production mainly occurs in France, Egypt, eastern Europe and the USA.

description

The oil has a sweet, spicy, green and slightly balsamic odour and is colourless or a pale yellow colour.

therapeutic properties

Basil is a very useful essential oil but there is concern about possible toxicity when using it for prolonged periods of time, so use it in moderation and only for relatively short periods, such as three weeks. It may be used in steam inhalations, and in small amounts in massage and bath oil blends. It combines particularly well with bergamot, chamomile, clary sage, geranium, lavender, lemongrass, marjoram and rose.

The main action of basil oil is on the nervous system; it is an excellent nerve tonic and has a balancing, reviving and strengthening effect. It can be used to relieve brain fatigue, nervousness, anxiety, depression, tension headaches and nervous insomnia.

When sexual problems are the result of tension, debility and overwork, the tonifying and restorative action of basil can be of help. Basil can be used to treat absent or very scanty periods, especially when this is due to debility and stress. The antispasmodic properties of basil make it useful to treat menstrual cramp; dilute the oil and massage over the abdomen.

Basil also has a beneficial action on the digestive system, particularly the small intestine. It will relieve flatulence and is especially good when digestive disorders are the result of nervous tension, such as nervous indigestion. Dilute in a base oil and massage in over the abdomen.

Basil can be used to treat spasmodic respiratory conditions such as coughs. It is also said to help restore the sense of smell – use in a steam inhalation. Basil oil is useful for debility following a prolonged fever or for lingering colds and catarrh.

Basil may be used to treat muscular weakness and muscular aches and pains. Use as a rubbing oil or compress. Basil may also be used to treat gout and rheumatism.

In first-aid treatment basil may be used to relieve wasp stings and insect bites. It also acts as a successful insect repellent.

psychological profile

Basil is appropriate if you have worn yourself out by overwork, particularly by mental effort or in a high-stress working environment. People who need basil have pushed themselves to the point where they are exhausted and their nervous system is overwrought. Basil will have a calming and strengthening effect.

other varieties

Of the many varieties of basil, only two chemotypes are generally used to produce essential oil – French basil and exotic basil. Of these, French basil is preferable for use in aromatherapy as it is less toxic and less likely to cause sensitization and irritation than the exotic type.

method of extraction

Basil essential oil is produced by steam distillation of the flowering herb.

---

most common uses
- Nervous debility • Mental fatigue • Catarrh
- Loss of sense of smell

---

safety data
- Non-irritant in dilution • Possible carcinogenic components – use in moderation• Do not use in concentrations of more than 2% • Avoid in therapeutic doses during pregnancy

marjoram

Origanum majorana

Family: Lamiaceae (*formerly* Labiatae)

Also known as: Sweet marjoram

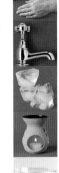

origin This well-known culinary herb originated in the eastern Mediterranean and is now cultivated in central and southern Europe and North Africa. It has been used as a medicinal herb for thousands of years, and was a particular favourite of the Ancient Greeks. In herbal medicine marjoram is valued for its restorative, warming and relaxing properties.

description

Marjoram oil is a pale yellow or pale amber liquid with a warm and spicy, slightly camphoraceous smell.

therapeutic properties

A warming and relaxing oil, marjoram makes an excellent addition to any massage blend or bath oil when a relaxing and calming effect is desired. It blends particularly well with bergamot, cypress, eucalyptus, geranium, lavender, orange and rosemary.

Marjoram tonifies the circulatory system, having a general vaso-dilatory effect. It can be used in the treatment of high blood pressure and narrowing of the arteries.

The sedative properties of marjoram make it effective for treating anxiety, insomnia and nervous debility. It is said to be an anaphrodisiac – that is, it reduces the sexual impulse. It also has analgesic properties useful for headaches and migraines, especially those caused by stress. Its analgesic and warming properties suggest its use in the treatment of sinus pains and head colds and make it a good addition to an oil blend for the treatment of muscle pains, sprains, strains, rheumatism, arthritis, over-exertion and so on. Try combining it with eucalyptus or rosemary and use as a bath or massage oil, or compress.

Marjoram is very effective at relieving painful periods, working best if massaged into the abdomen. It is also an important oil in the treatment of PMT, especially with feelings of anxiety, weariness and irritability. Sweet marjoram is safe to use externally at normal dilutions during pregnancy.

Marjoram is an antispasmodic and can help to alleviate colic, flatulence and dyspepsia. It also acts as a mild laxative by both stimulating and strengthening intestinal peristalsis.

psychological profile

Marjoram will be most appropriate if you have become exhausted and stressed as a result of overwork. You may suffer from insomnia and find it difficult to relax, and you may have thrown yourself into work as a compensation for unexpressed creative outlets or sexual activity. Eventually, enjoying life and relaxing becomes difficult. Using marjoram will allow you to relax and will open up the possibilities of a more fulfilling and enjoyable life.

other varieties

There are many different varieties of marjoram and its close relative oregano, and there is much confusion between them. Spanish marjoram (*Thymus mastichina*) has similar properties to sweet marjoram, though it has a harsher smell and slightly stronger action.

method of extraction

The oil is steam-distilled from the dried flowering herb.

---

most common uses

- High blood pressure • Stress • Insomnia • Period pains
- Headaches and migraines • Muscle pains
- Rheumatism

---

safety data

- **Non-toxic externally • Non-irritant • Non-sensitizing**

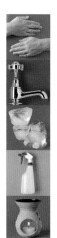

Pelargonium graveolens
Family: Geraniaceae

geranium

Also known as: Rose geranium, geranium Bourbon, Pelargonium

origin A native of South Africa, *Pelargonium graveolens* was exported to Europe in the late seventeenth century. There the pelargoniums were hybridized, and later re-exported during the nineteenth century to the French and British colonies. The essential oil was first distilled in France in the early nineteenth century; today it is produced mainly in Réunion, China and Egypt. Geranium is one of the most important perfumery oils.

description

The oil has a powerful, sweet, green, floral smell with a fruity-minty undertone. It is a pale green to olive-green liquid.

therapeutic properties

Geranium is a cooling and moistening oil, good where heat and dryness are present. It is calming but not necessarily sedating, as it also has an uplifting and strengthening effect; it is a balancing oil. Geranium oil is quite versatile, making a fragrant addition to many blends for massage and the bath; complementary oils are bergamot, lavender, lemon, marjoram, neroli, orange, palmarosa, rose and sandalwood.

Geranium calms and cools the nervous system, which makes it useful for treating restlessness and anxiety. It is one of the most important oils for treating menopausal symptoms, including hot flushes and vaginal dryness. Add it to baths and massage oils.

Its calming effect makes geranium helpful in treating palpitations and panic attacks; it is particularly appropriate for people who wake at night with these symptoms.

The cooling properties of geranium can help to relieve symptoms arising from heat in the abdomen. These may include either constipation with dryness, or burning, yellow diarrhoea. Geranium is an effective treatment for dysentery or gastro-enteritis. In the treatment of diarrhoea it should be diluted in a base oil and massaged into the abdomen, or used as a compress over the abdomen. Its anti-inflammatory properties can help treat gastritis or peptic ulcers. It is also appropriate for cystitis with burning urination; add a few drops to the bath.

The analgesic properties of geranium can help to relieve the pain of neuralgia and shingles. Use it in a massage blend or bath oil or as a compress.

Geranium has an excellent reputation in skin care and is a popular ingredient in many creams and lotions. It has a regulating effect on the secretion of sebum, making it suitable for dry or oily skin types, and it is a useful antiseptic and anti-inflammatory in the treatment of acne. Its soothing properties make it appropriate for dry, inflamed skin; combine with chamomile or melissa in the treatment of dry eczema. Geranium may be applied to the skin as a lotion or compress or used in a facial steam.

psychological profile

Geranium is appropriate if you are finding it difficult to let go of your past achievements and have become congested and 'stuck', fearful to continue to the next stage of your life. You may have lost confidence in the natural flow of life and become fearful, irritable and defensive. Geranium will help to relieve these feelings and will refresh and relax you, enabling you to move on and enjoy life again.

method of extraction

The bark is incised so that the tree yields an oleo-gum resin which is collected after it solidifies into amber-coloured lumps the size of a pea. This resin is then steam-distilled to produce the essential oil.

---

most common uses

• Anxiety • Hot flushes • Palpitations • Diarrhoea • Acne
• Dry, inflamed skin

---

safety data

• Non-toxic • Non-irritant in dilution
• Sensitization rare but possible

pine

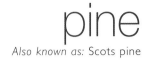

Pinus sylvestris *(and other varieties)*
Family: Pinaceae

Also known as: Scots pine

origin Scots pine is native to Eurasia and is also cultivated in the USA, Europe and Scandinavia. The needles have been used medicinally for hundreds of years. Pine has one of the largest productions of any essential oil. It is used extensively in disinfectants, detergents, insecticides and paint manufacture, in the paper industry and in perfumery.

description
Pine oil has a fresh, sweet, balsamic smell. It is a colourless or pale amber liquid.

therapeutic properties
Pine has a refreshing and 'opening' effect. Of medium temperature, it can be used for either hot or cold conditions. It may be added to massage and bath oils and also is excellent in steam inhalations. Pine combines particularly well with cedarwood, eucalyptus, juniper, lavender, lemon, marjoram and tea tree. Pine has a reviving effect on the nervous system and can be used to treat nervous exhaustion and poor concentration.

The main action of pine is on the respiratory tract – it is a powerful respiratory antiseptic and is also a decongestant. It has a strengthening effect on the lungs and can be used to treat bronchial infections, such as bronchitis, asthma, flu, coughs and colds. It will clear mucus from the chest and throat and catarrh from the sinuses. Combine with cypress to relieve the symptoms of hayfever.

The antiseptic properties of pine also have a beneficial effect on the urinary system, especially when used in the bath. It is a useful oil for treating urinary infections, such as urethritis, cystitis, pyelitis and prostatitis. Combine with eucalyptus or thyme to treat both urinary infections and venereal infections, such as non-specific urethritis (NSU).

This is a pleasant oil to add to the bath to ease aches and pains after a tiring day. It may also be used in compresses or massage oils to treat rheumatism, arthritis, sprains and strains.

Pine is a parasiticide against scabies and lice. It is also a good deodorant – try using it in a footbath to treat smelly feet.

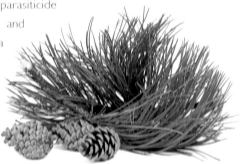

psychological profile
Pine is appropriate if you have a strong tendency to feel guilty. You may have been repressed as a child and punished for having a rebellious spirit or non-conformist attitudes. This type of early experience will tend to make you fearful of enjoyment and to negate inner feelings that may cause conflict. This can produce a tendency to rigidity and self-punishment, and on the physical level induce tension and a tight chest. Using pine will help to break through all types of rigidity and will enable you to reconnect with your own sensitivity, affording you greater enjoyment and happiness in life.

other varieties
Other varieties of pine that are available as an essential oil include dwarf pine (*Pinus pumilio* or *P. mugo*) and also longleaf pine (*P. palustris*). Dwarf pine should not be used in aromatherapy as it is a skin irritant and common sensitizer. Longleaf pine is frequently used in the USA. It has very similar therapeutic properties to Scots pine.

method of extraction
Pine oil for aromatherapy use is steam-distilled from the needles. Distillation occurs mainly in the USA and Eastern Europe.

most common uses
- Decongestant • Bronchitis • Hayfever
- Urinary infections • Rheumatism

safety data
- Non-toxic • Do not use in dilutions of more than 3%
- Sensitization possible

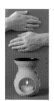

Piper nigrum
Family: Piperaceae

black pepper

origin The pepper plant is a trailing, vine-like shrub native to India. Black pepper, one of the most important and oldest known spices, is the dried whole fruit. It has been used in India and China for over 4000 years as a medicine and culinary spice and became a key part of the spice trade from Asia to the West. In traditional Chinese medicine it is regarded as a treatment for malaria and a wide range of digestive disorders. The main areas of cultivation are India and Indonesia.

description

Black pepper oil has a fresh, warm, spicy, dry-woody smell. It is a colourless or slightly green liquid.

therapeutic properties

Black pepper is a hot and drying oil and is suitable where there is coldness, weakness and depleted energy as it has tonifying, strengthening and stimulating properties. It may be used in massage and rubbing oils and in steam inhalations. It will irritate the skin in strong concentrations and must be very well diluted before application; do not use in concentrations of more than 0.5 per cent. It combines very well with cedarwood, frankincense, juniper, lemon, marjoram, palmarosa and sandalwood.

As a stimulant to the digestive system, black pepper alleviates constipation, indigestion, flatulence, dyspepsia and a sluggish digestion. Combine with cardamom and fennel in a base oil and massage over the abdomen.

Its profoundly warming properties suggest black pepper's usefulness in treating respiratory conditions, especially if you are chilly and producing copious amounts of white mucus. It can be used in a steam inhalation to relieve head colds with these symptoms. The strongly anti-microbial properties of black pepper suggest its use in the treatment of flu and many other infections and viruses.

As a stimulant to the circulatory system, black pepper can be used in blends to treat poor circulation and cold hands and feet; combine with cedarwood and ginger and use as a massage oil or foot bath. It may also be used to treat chilblains.

Black pepper oil will stimulate the eliminative processes and can be used in detoxifying blends, for example, combined with juniper or rosemary. It is good in massage blends for the treatment of cellulite.

Black pepper can also be blended into an excellent rubbing oil to relieve rheumatism, aches, sprains and pains. Because it has a very stimulating effect on muscles it should be considered for conditions involving muscular palsy, wasting and paralysis.

psychological profile

Black pepper oil is appropriate for chilly, weak and debilitated people, who are weary and suffer from feelings of hopelessness. The martial quality of black pepper suggests that these people may once have been fiery and energetic, but have suppressed their emotions (anger, in particular) and become frustrated, introverted and weak. The use of black pepper oil will help to strengthen such people and develop their physical and creative energy.

method of extraction

The oil is steam-distilled from dried, crushed peppercorns.

---

most common uses

• Sluggish digestion • Colds and flu • Cellulite
• Aches and pains • Poor circulation

---

safety data

• Non-toxic • Non-sensitizing
• Do not use in dilutions of more than 0.5%

patchouli

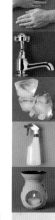

Pogostemon cablin

Family: Lamiaceae (*formerly* Labiatae)

origin A large-leaved herb of up to 1 m (3 ft) high, patchouli is native to tropical Asia. It has been used for centuries as an incense and also for its disinfectant and insect-repellent properties. It was traditionally incorporated into carpets and woven fabrics to give them fragrance. The distinctive and tenacious smell of patchouli has made it a popular ingredient for the perfumery industry. Distillation of the oil occurs in Asia, Europe and the USA.

description

Patchouli oil has a dry, aromatic, woody, almost musky smell. It is a thick liquid that varies in colour from amber to dark reddish-brown.

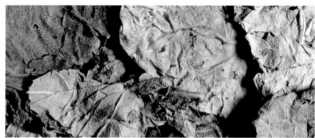

therapeutic properties

Patchouli is a stimulating and strengthening oil with astringent properties. It may be added to massage and bath oils and a little goes a long way. It may also be used to fragrance a room and is an effective deodorant. Patchouli combines well with cedarwood, geranium, neroli, orange, rose and sandalwood.

This oil has a pronounced effect on the nervous system and is an anti-depressant, but its smell is not to everyone's taste and it will only be of benefit to those who enjoy using it. It has a traditional role as an aphrodisiac and as a remedy for frigidity. Patchouli can also be used to treat nervous exhaustion, stress and anxiety.

The astringent and tonifying properties of patchouli make it a good treatment for diarrhoea – try combining it with geranium and massaging over the abdomen. Its stimulating properties can also help to relieve constipation when this is due to sluggish peristalsis and lack of muscle tone.

Patchouli shares many properties with myrrh, and can be used in steam inhalations when too much mucus is produced. It is anti-bacterial and anti-viral and may be combined with other essential oils in the treatment of many infections or viruses.

The astringent and antiseptic properties of patchouli indicate its use in the treatment of acne, oily skin, weeping sores and impetigo. It can help healthy skin tissue to regenerate and can be used to improve scars and stretch marks. Patchouli is an important oil in the treatment of ageing skin and it can help to reduce wrinkles. In skin care patchouli combines especially well with rose. It is also anti-fungal and can be used in cases of athlete's foot and other fungal infections.

psychological profile

The smell of patchouli is strongly associated with the 1960s, when it was used to evoke a mood of warmth, sexuality and a relaxed style of living. To benefit most from patchouli, you will be a person lacking in energy and drive. You may be somewhat weak, easily influenced and over-sensitive, finding it difficult to concentrate and focus on the requirements of everyday life. Using patchouli will impart a warmth and energy that will stimulate you to direct your attention, and feel more 'earthed' in your surroundings.

method of extraction

The leaves are first lightly fermented or scalded to break the cell walls and then subjected to steam distillation to produce the essential oil.

most common uses

- Anti-depressant • Aphrodisiac • Diarrhoea
- Acne • Scars

safety data

- **Non-toxic • Non-irritant • Non-sensitizing**

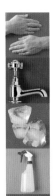

Ravensara aromatica
Family: Lauraceae

ravensara

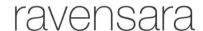

origin Ravensara is a tall forest evergreen tree native to Madagascar and cultivated on the island of Réunion. All parts of the tree are aromatic and the fruits are used as a spice – Madagascar nutmeg or clove nut. The leaves have been used by Malagasies for digestive and respiratory problems, and also made into a healing ointment. In fact, the name ravensara is derived from two local words meaning 'good leaf'.

description

A colourless liquid with a fresh, warm camphoraceous smell.

therapeutic properties

Ravensara is a warming and stimulating oil with excellent anti-microbial and immuno-enhancing properties. It may be used in massage blends and bath oils, and is especially good in chest rubs or inhalations. It blends particularly well with cinnamon, clove, cypress, eucalyptus, lavender, rosemary and thyme.

Ravensara has a reviving action on the nervous system and is an excellent tonic for nervous exhaustion, and for people who have been living under great stress. Its refreshing action can help lift depression. Ravensara also acts as a tonic for the endocrine system and is useful in the treatment of such ailments as glandular fever. Use in a bath or massage oil, or as a steam inhalation.

Ravensara is one of the most effective essential oils in the treatment of viral infections, such as colds or flu. If used at the first sign of a chill, cold or flu it can help to prevent the symptoms from developing. For the treatment of viral infections use in inhalations, chest salves or a rubbing oil and consider combining it with eucalyptus or tea tree.

Ravensara is an excellent treatment for both chronic and acute ailments of the respiratory tract, including coughs, bronchitis and also rhinitis and sinusitis. Use in inhalations or chest salves.

The anti-viral properties of ravensara make it a useful remedy for the treatment of all kinds of herpes. For genital herpes or cold sores around the mouth blend it with tea tree. Ravensara is also an excellent treatment for shingles – combine it with lavender in a base of St John's wort macerated oil for best results.

Ravensara is a digestive tonic and helps to stimulate digestive secretions. It is also a useful antiseptic for

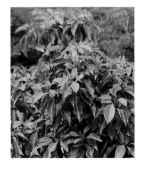

treating gastroenteritis and food poisoning. Use as a massage oil and apply to the abdomen.

It has a relaxing and pain-relieving action on the muscles and joints and may be used for relieving sprains and strains, rheumatism and arthritis. Use in compresses or as a rubbing oil.

psychological profile

Ravensara can be used by anyone who is going through a time of transition, or when the process of change has become stuck in some way and illness has resulted. If you have been through a period of your life which has called for great adaptability and willingness to change, but that has caused feelings of stress, weariness or defensiveness, then ravensara is highly appropriate. Its use will encourage enthusiasm for the new, and will promote the capacity to learn from experience and then move on.

other varieties

Bay laurel (*Laurus nobilis*) is another member of the *Lauraceae* family and shares the anti-microbial and stimulating properties of ravensara. Bay laurel is an excellent nerve tonic. It is useful for treating colds, coughs and flu, particularly when the symptoms drag on for a long time, or recur.

method of extraction

Steam distillation of the young, leafy twigs.

---

most common uses
• Colds and flu • Coughs • Viral infections • Herpes

---

safety data
• **Non-toxic** • **Non-irritant** • **Non-sensitising**

rose

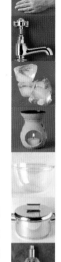

Rosa centifolia, R. damascena

Family: Rosaceae

origin Roses have been used as a medicinal plant since antiquity; *Rosa centifolia* (the cabbage rose or Provence rose) is believed to have originated in Persia and is now cultivated for extraction mainly in Morocco and France. *Rosa damascena* (the damask rose), probably a native of China, has been primarily cultivated in Bulgaria for the perfumery industry. While both varieties share similar therapeutic properties, *Rosa centifolia* is the most commonly available for aromatherapy.

description

Rose essential oil is a pale yellow liquid, while the absolute is orange-red and viscous. Both have a deep, rich and sweet rosy-floral smell.

therapeutic properties

Rose oil is cooling, relaxing and tonifying. It is similar to bergamot, geranium and jasmine in that it decreases sympathetic nervous system activity, while at the same time strengthening the parasympathetic nervous system. This means it increases feelings of vitality and creates a sense of relaxed well-being. Rose is useful for treating a wide range of stress-related conditions in adults and hyperactivity in children. It has a low toxicity and is delightful in the bath or as a massage blend; it blends well with bergamot, chamomile, clary sage, geranium, jasmine, lavender and patchouli.

Rose oil is a great anti-depressant, helping people feel more attractive and confident. It is an excellent massage oil for scarring, and has been useful in the treatment of anorexia.

Its primary action is on reproduction and sexuality. It has a cleansing and tonifying effect on the uterus and is helpful for menopausal women or those who are prone to heavy, clotted and painful periods. It is one of the most important oils in the treatment of PMT. As well as being a renowned treatment for infertility and frigidity in women, using rose oil increases the sperm count in men.

Rose has a tonifying effect on the vascular system and may be added to skin creams and oils to treat broken capillaries. It is particularly appropriate when symptoms of heart disease are related to stress.

On the digestive system, rose has a strengthening and detoxifying effect. Its antiseptic and anti-inflammatory properties can be used to treat gastroenteritis and gastric ulcers. It can also relieve feelings of nausea and help to regenerate damaged intestinal walls, as well as being a mild aperient useful in the treatment of chronic constipation. It has a soothing effect on the liver and gall bladder. Rose has a rejuvenating and healing effect on the skin and also has profound anti-inflammatory properties which can be used to treat dryness, inflammation, heat and itching of the skin.

Cabbage rose

(Rosa centifolia)

psychological profile

Rose is appropriate if you have grown up with a romantic picture of love far removed from reality. You may have had the capacity for expressing yourself in a very loving way, but because reality didn't live up to your expectations you became bitter and resentful. Using rose will help to remove feelings of frustration and disappointment and will enable you to love in a way that is more understanding and tolerant of human nature.

method of extraction

In recent years, the most common form of rose extract has been the absolute obtained by solvent extraction on the rose flowers, the oil being less available and expensive, but both are suitable for aromatherapy.

---

most common uses
- Anti-depressant • Aphrodisiac • PMT • Infertility
- Anti-inflammatory

---

safety data
- **Non-toxic • Non-irritant • Non-sensitizing**

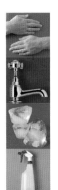

Rosmarinus officinalis
Family: Lamiaceae (*formerly* Labiatae)

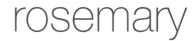
rosemary

origin A native of the Mediterranean countries, rosemary has been used as a medicine and a sacred herb for thousands of years. It is also one of the classic culinary herbs.

description
Rosemary oil is an almost colourless or pale yellow liquid with a strong, fresh, camphoraceous and herbaceous smell.

therapeutic properties
Rosemary is a very versatile stimulating, warming and tonifying oil. It may be used in massage blends and compresses, steam inhalations, in the bath and for room fragrancing. Rosemary combines well with many oils, especially basil, lavender, lemongrass, olibanum, orange, peppermint, petitgrain and pine.

The primary action of rosemary is on the circulatory system; it stimulates a weak heart and is useful for treating low blood pressure and cold extremities.

Rosemary increases the circulation of blood to the brain and nervous system and can help to improve memory, concentration and mental alertness, so it is a very good oil to use in a burner in any room where people are trying to concentrate. It is an important remedy in the treatment of headaches and is helpful for many people who suffer with migraines.

The moving qualities of rosemary make it a good digestive tonic, promoting the flow of bile, helping to unblock an obstructed gall bladder and clearing gallstones. It is also used to treat hepatitis and jaundice.

Rosemary is an antiseptic and antispasmodic oil which can be employed to treat gastro-intestinal infection, painful digestion, flatulence and colic. It will alleviate diarrhoea and colitis, particularly in weak, nervous people.

Rosemary is a mild emmenagogue, and will help to relieve painful periods. Dilute in a base oil and massage over the abdomen, or add a few drops to a warm bath.

Rosemary is a beneficial oil for people prone to chronic lung conditions.

It is antiseptic and tonifying and can be used to treat colds, flu and coughs. It is also one of the main detoxifying oils; combine with lavender and juniper as a massage oil to detoxify the lymphatic system.

The warming, moving qualities of rosemary make it helpful in the treatment of arthritis and rheumatism, especially when symptoms are worse in cold weather. Rosemary will also bring relief to sprains and strains, making it a classic ingredient of sports blends. Dilute the oil and rub into painful areas.

Traditionally, rosemary has been an important treatment for problems of the hair and scalp. It stimulates the circulation to the latter and can be used to treat alopecia and dandruff. It is a parasiticide and can be used to remove lice and scabies.

psychological profile
Rosemary is an energizing oil suitable if you are cold, debilitated, weak and nervous. This may be the result of prolonged grief or of a past emotional shock that was never fully resolved, inhibiting you from freely expressing love. Using rosemary will help you to regain contact with your body and unblock your emotions, enabling you to feel stronger, more 'in your body', and better able to form close emotional relationships again.

method of extraction
Rosemary is steam-distilled from the flowers and leaves of the herb. The bulk of the production occurs in France, Spain, Croatia, Tunisia and Morocco.

---

most common uses
• Poor circulation • Headaches • Aids concentration
• Sprains and strains • Lymphatic drainage

---

safety data
• Non-toxic • Non irritant in dilution • Non-sensitizing

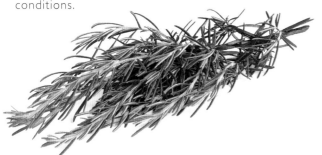

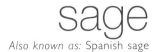

sage

Salvia lavandulifolia

Family: Lamiaceae (*formerly* Labiatae)

Also known as: Spanish sage

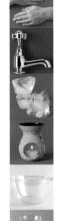

origin Sage is native to the countries bordering the Mediterranean, but is now cultivated throughout the world. Like all forms of sage, Spanish sage has been used as a medicinal herb for thousands of years.

description

A pale yellow liquid, Spanish sage oil has a fresh, herbaceous and camphoraceous smell.

therapeutic properties

Sage is a powerful stimulant and tonifier of the nervous system, appropriate for people who are exhausted and particularly for those who have been under stress. It can also help to build up the stamina of anaemic people, aid convalescence and relieve prolonged nervous depression. For all these conditions sage must be well diluted before use and discontinued when progress is established because of its strongly stimulating properties.

Sage oil can alleviate chronic lung conditions, helping to strengthen lung tissue, and is particularly good for long-drawn-out respiratory conditions such as chronic bronchitis. It is beneficial for people who are prone to recurrent colds and flu as it will help to strengthen immunity and vitality.

In very small doses sage is antispasmodic and can be used to treat indigestion and dyspepsia in weak, debilitated people. It will help to improve a sluggish digestive system and stimulate the appetite. It can be used to relieve diarrhoea.

Sage has an important action on the female reproductive system and can regulate menstrual periods. Its antispasmodic properties will help to relieve painful periods if it is very well diluted. It also has a regulatory effect on hormonal problems during the menopause, and is particularly useful in relieving hot flushes and excessive perspiration; use in the bath or in a massage blend. Sage oil should never be used during pregnancy as it can stimulate uterine contractions, nor when breastfeeding because it will tend to reduce the flow of milk.

The stimulating properties of sage can be used to relieve muscular aches and pains, rheumatism and arthritis. Use in a massage blend or a compress.

Sage is an important remedy in the treatment of glandular disorders. It has a stimulating effect on the lymphatic system and can be helpful in cases of glandular fever and post-viral syndrome.

This oil makes an excellent mouth wash for gingivitis, receding or bleeding gums and mouth ulcers. Sage's astringent properties can be used to treat oily skin and hair, and it is an effective treatment for dandruff.

psychological profile

Sage is suitable if you have an undermined constitution resulting from a prolonged period of overwork or of living in an overstressed situation. In the past you may have been a high achiever and had plenty of energy, but you have become 'burnt out'. You will feel constantly tired and depressed. Using sage will help to strengthen your vitality so that you regain your energy and enjoyment in life.

other varieties

Common sage (*Salvia officinalis*) is also available as an essential oil, but it is high in thujone which can cause epilepsy and muscular spasm, so should be avoided.

method of extraction

The oil is steam-distilled from the wild herb.

most common uses
- Debility • Recurrent colds and flu • Hot flushes
- Excessive perspiration • Gum disease
- Oily skin and hair

safety data
- **Non-irritant in dilution • Non-sensitizing • Do not use in pregnancy • Not to be used by people with epilepsy**

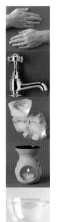

Salvia sclarea
Family: Lamiaceae (*formerly* Labiatae)

clary sage

origin This distinctive variety of sage originated in the countries bordering the Mediterranean. It is an impressive plant, growing 60–90 cm (2–3 ft) high, with tall flower spikes rising above hairy leaves. Clary sage has been used for hundreds of years in the treatment of eye problems and digestive disorders. It is also used to flavour muscatel wine in Germany and vermouth in France. It is a classic ingredient of fine perfumes and colognes.

description
Clary sage has a rich, bitter-sweet and herbaceous smell that is very tenacious. It is a colourless, pale yellow or pale green liquid.

therapeutic properties
Clary sage has a tonifying, warming and sedating effect – used in small amounts it can create feelings of well-being and calmness. At the same time it will gently stimulate and strengthen the body's vitality, which makes it an excellent oil to use during convalescence and to treat depression, weakness and debility.

This oil must be well-diluted and used in moderation because it can cause drowsiness. It should be avoided when drinking alcohol as it can exaggerate the feeling of intoxication. It is excellent in massage and bath oil blends and is also pleasant to use in an essential oil burner. It combines particularly well with cardamom, coriander, geranium, jasmine, lavender, lemon, rose and sandalwood.

A renowned anti-depressant, clary sage lifts the spirits and is excellent for treating nervous tension, post-natal depression and many stress-related diseases. It can be used during the recuperative period following a break-down and acts as an aphrodisiac when frigidity or impotence are clearly connected to stress and tension. The benefits of clary sage in treating nervous system disorders can be greatly enhanced by blending it with other appropriate oils, such as jasmine, sandalwood and geranium.

Clary sage has a tonifying effect on the female reproductive system and can strengthen a weak uterus. It will help with absent, scant and painful periods. During labour, it may be massaged over the lower back or burnt in the room to ease labour pains and strengthen contractions. It can help ease feelings of stress and nervous tension during the menopause, and will also relieve excessive perspiration associated with hot flushes.

Clary sage is an effective muscle relaxant and will relieve painful muscles and muscle strain. It has hypotensive properties and can be used to treat high blood pressure, especially when this is caused by stress. It is also antispasmodic and can be used to treat asthma (especially when this is stress-related) and coughs.

psychological profile
Clary sage is appropriate if you are a nervous, fearful person who has become run down and debilitated and may lack the will to carry on. A family history of depression and hardship is likely, and as a child you may have been subjected to a lot of negativity and pessimism. Using clary sage will encourage energy and optimism for life.

method of extraction
The flowering tops of the herb are steam-distilled.

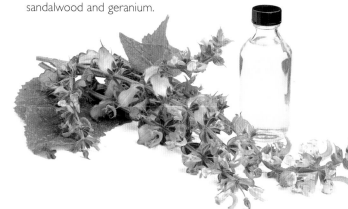

most common uses
- Anti-depressant • Convalesence
- Stress and nervous tension • Painful periods

safety data
• Non-toxic • Non-irritant in dilution • Non-sensitizing

sandalwood

Santalum album

Family: Santalaceae

Also known as: East Indian sandalwood

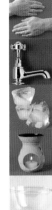

origin Sandalwood trees are found throughout India, though the main cultivation occurs in the southern states. The sandalwood tree is a root parasite, drawing mineral nutrients from its host. Sandalwood has been used for thousands of years to make carved objects, and as a fragrant incense. It is an important remedy in Ayurvedic and traditional Chinese medicine. In perfumery, it is an excellent fixative. The essential oil is produced by the heartwood of mature trees.

description

Sandalwood oil has a long-lasting soft, deep, sweet and woody smell. It is a yellow or brownish viscous liquid.

therapeutic properties

Sandalwood combines relaxing and restorative properties and is a cooling oil that has a pronounced effect on both physical and emotional problems. Because of its calming effect on the brain it was traditionally used as an aid to meditation; it will also help to quieten a restless body and soothe the nervous system. Sandalwood combines well with rose to calm anxiety; other oils it blends well with include bergamot, cedarwood, jasmine, palmarosa, vetiver and ylang-ylang.

This oil is one of the most renowned aphrodisiac oils, particularly for men. In Chinese medicine it is said to strengthen the yang. A massage with sandalwood in a base oil will enhance feelings of physical enjoyment.

Sandalwood is one of the main oils for treating genito-urinary tract infections, including cystitis, leucorrhoea, non-specific urethritis (NSU) and other venereal infections. It is antiseptic and encourages the body to clear out infective organisms. It may be used in the bath to cure any thick, sticky discharge.

The cooling properties of sandalwood are effective for soothing inflamed mucous membranes and lung tissue, while its decongestant and antiseptic properties are beneficial in the treatment of bronchitis, laryngitis and any chronic respiratory tract infection. It may be used as a rubbing oil or as an inhalation. Sandalwood is also appropriate for any hot and painful digestive symptoms, including diarrhoea and dysentery. It will help to soothe an inflamed gall bladder.

In cosmetics and skin care, sandalwood has been in use for centuries. It has emollient and anti-inflammatory properties that are extremely soothing for dry, itching and inflamed skin. It is also mildly astringent and may be used on oily skin. It may be used in a cream or lotion or as a compress.

psychological profile

Sandalwood is appropriate if you feel stuck in your life, or constantly experience repeating patterns. You may approach life in a rational, intellectual way without this being balanced by the intuitive, feeling side of your nature. Your mind may go over the same episodes in your life until eventually you become confused and further from any solutions. Using sandalwood enables you to come up with fresh solutions and actions. It helps to create a wider vision of life.

method of extraction

Sandalwood oil is steam-distilled from the heartwood of the tree. There are four grades, the finest used in perfumery being Mysore sandalwood. The majority of sandalwood oil is known as Agmarked Sandalwood Oil, which is guaranteed to conform to Indian government standard.

most common uses
- Aphrodisiac • Meditation • Cystitis • Venereal infections
- Chronic coughs • Dry skin • Weeping eczema

safety data
- **Non-toxic** • **Non-irritant** • **Non-sensitizing**

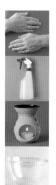

Syzygium aromaticum,
syn. Eugenia caryophyllata
Family: Myrtaceae

clove

origin Clove trees originated in Asia and have been cultivated for at least 2000 years. The flower buds are dried to produce the spice we know as cloves, an important part of the spice trade since the sixteenth century. Today, the main centres of cultivation are Zanzibar, Madagascar and Indonesia. Preparations of clove have been used medicinally for thousands of years to treat skin infections and infestations, digestive disorders and toothache.

description

Clove oil is a pale yellow or straw-coloured liquid. The smell is strong, spicy and woody with a fruity, fresh top note.

therapeutic properties

Clove is a warming and stimulating oil. It is a powerful antiseptic and highly appropriate for use in infectious diseases and the treatment of septic wounds and ulcers. It also aids the formation of scar tissue. When using clove oil on the skin it must be very well diluted or it may be an irritant; do not use in dilutions stronger than 2 per cent and do a patch test on a small area of skin first. It is a useful addition to a room spray for fumigating a room – combine it with other strongly antiseptic oils such as bergamot, eucalyptus, lavender and thyme.

Cloves also have anti-neuralgic properties, hence the oil's well-known use for soothing the pain of toothache or abscesses. To relieve toothache, half-fill an egg cup with warm water, mix in two drops of clove oil, soak a small piece of cotton wool in the dilution and then place against the painful tooth.

Clove has anti-rheumatic and pain-relieving properties beneficial in the treatment of rheumatism, arthritis and muscular sprains and strains. Dilute well and use in a rubbing oil.

Its stimulating action makes clove an appropriate addition to oils such as rosemary for stimulating the memory and concentration. Use in an essential oil burner. Its warming and stimulating properties also make it an aphrodisiac. Clove has antispasmodic and carminative properties and can be of use in relieving flatulence, dyspepsia and diarrhoea from a chill. Dilute well in a base oil and massage over the abdomen. Its warming and antiseptic action means it is a good treatment for colds, flu and chills. It will also help to strengthen the immune system.

Clove is a useful insect repellent and parasiticide. It is of particular use against scabies – combine with cedarwood, cinnamon and lemon in a base oil and apply to the skin. To eliminate fleas and moths, combine with eucalyptus, lavender and lemon and use in a plant spray.

psychological profile

Clove is appropriate if you are generally a cheerful, outgoing and optimistic person but have been brought down by an illness, infection or trauma. You may have been suffering with a recurrent or painful condition for some time and are now becoming increasingly despondent and fed up. Using clove will help to impart a sense of warmth and cheerfulness and restore your sense of optimism and enjoyment of life.

method of extraction

Clove essential oil is water-distilled from the clove buds. Essential oils are also distilled from the leaves and stems but these are more toxic than the oil from the buds and should not be used for aromatherapy.

---

most common uses
- Infectious diseases • Toothache • Parasiticide
- Insect repellent

---

safety data
- Non-toxic externally
- Do not use in concentrations of more than 2%

thyme

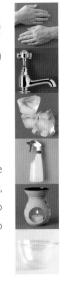

Thymus vulgaris

Family: Lamiaceae (*formerly* Labiatae)

Also known as: Common thyme, Red thyme (oil), White thyme (oil)

origin Thyme is native to the Mediterranean and is widely grown as a culinary herb. It has also been used as a medicinal herb for thousands of years.

description

Red thyme oil is a reddish-brown liquid with a powerful, warm, spicy-herbaceous smell. White thyme oil has a fresh, herbaceous, green smell, sweeter and slightly milder than red thyme, and is colourless or pale yellow.

therapeutic properties

Thyme oil is hot, pungent and stimulating. It can act as a general nerve tonic, making it useful for any exhausted or debilitated condition. It is also a powerful germicide, effective against many types of bacteria, viruses and fungi. It may be used in massage blends but can be an irritant, so do not use in concentrations of more than 3 per cent. Thyme may also be added to the bath, but it can irritate mucous membranes so should not be used in concentrations of more than 1 per cent in bath oils. Add it to other strongly antiseptic oils such as clove, eucalyptus, lavender, lemon and pine and use in a room spray or burner to fumigate.

The primary action of thyme is on the genito-urinary tract. It is one of the most important oils in the treatment of venereal infections and has been used effectively in the treatment of non-specific urethritis (NSU), leucorrhoea and trichomonas. It is also effective against many types of urinary infections including cystitis and pyelitis.

Thyme oil is a very effective pulmonary antiseptic, so it is useful in treating respiratory infections, including colds, flu, coughs and especially bronchitis. It may be used in steam inhalations, as a chest rub or in an essential oil burner. It is particularly beneficial where there is debility associated with the respiratory infection. It is similar to eucalyptus in its expectorant properties and is also an antispasmodic, helpful for spasmodic coughs and asthma.

Similarly to tea tree, thyme has been shown to be effective in combating infection and strengthening the immune response by stimulating the production of white blood cells. It is one of the main essential oils used in the treatment of HIV-related diseases.

Thyme has a warming and tonifying effect on the digestive system. Its antiseptic properties make it useful in treating dysentery and gastroenteritis. Combine with rosemary or geranium and massage into the abdomen.

As a warming and stimulating oil, thyme can be used in massage blends and baths to ease muscle stiffness, aches, pains, rheumatism and arthritis. Well diluted, thyme can be applied to the skin to heal infections, acne, boils and sores. It will also eliminate head and body lice and scabies.

psychological profile

Thyme is appropriate if you tend to neglect or abuse your body. Over time you may have become weak, debilitated and prone to lingering infections and viruses. Using thyme will help to build up your immune system and clear out the ill effects of past habits.

other varieties

Wild thyme (*Thymus serpyllum*) has similar properties to common thyme (*T. vulgaris*). Thyme 'linalol' is milder and less toxic than common thyme and is therefore more suitable for children or those people with a weakened constitution.

method of extraction

Thyme oil is steam- and water-distilled from the flowering tops and leaves. Two types of thyme oil are produced from the plant: red thyme is the crude distillate, while white thyme is further redistilled or rectified.

---

most common uses

- Cystitis • Bronchitis • Infectious illnesses • Rheumatism
- Gastroenteritis • Skin infections

---

safety data

- **Do not use on hypersensitive or damaged skin**
- **Do not use on infants under 2 years old**
- **Dilute well before use**

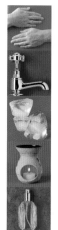

Vetiveria zizanioides,
syn. Andropogon muricatus
Family: Gramineae

vetiver

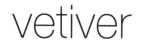

origin Vetiver is a tall perennial grass related botanically to citronella, lemongrass and palmarosa. A native of India, it is cultivated for essential oil production in southern India, Indonesia, the Caribbean and South America. The grass has a practical agricultural use as the dense lacework of rootlets helps to prevent soil erosion on steep slopes during torrential tropical rains. The roots have been used in Asia for centuries for their fragrance, and are woven into aromatic matting and screens. Vetiver oil has always been in great demand by perfumers as a base note in many oriental, woody and chypre fragrances. Distillation occurs either near the area of cultivation, or the grass is exported for distillation in the USA and Europe.

description

Vetiver oil is an amber, olive or dark brown viscous liquid which has a sweet, heavy smell with a woody, earthy undertone and a lemony top note.

therapeutic properties

The main action of vetiver is on the nervous system and it is both sedating and strengthening in effect. It is excellent in the treatment of depression, nervous tension, debility, insomnia and many stress-related diseases, and acts as an aphrodisiac where there is a clear connection between impotence or frigidity and stress. Vetiver may be used in massage blends and the bath; it has a rather powerful smell but is very pleasant when diluted. It blends well with other anti-depressant oils, such as clary sage, jasmine, lavender, patchouli, rose, sandalwood and ylang-ylang.

Vetiver stimulates the circulatory system and makes a useful massage oil for elderly or debilitated people with poor circulation. It also helps to stimulate the production of red blood cells and is thus beneficial for anaemia.

Vetiver makes a useful warming and pain-relieving rubbing oil, suitable for deep massage of muscular aches and pains, sprains, stiffness, rheumatism and arthritis. It may be added to sports oil blends and massaged into muscles before and after sports.

In skin care, vetiver helps to regulate the secretion of sebum. It is also a useful antiseptic and is slightly astringent. Use it in lotions, compresses and baths to treat oily skin, acne and weeping sores.

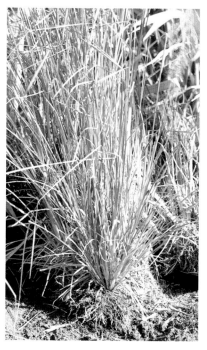

psychological profile

Vetiver is most appropriate when you are feeling emotionally overwhelmed. You may be weepy, feeling under pressure and uncertain which direction to take. It may be that you have been dominated by a particular situation or person and need to learn to make decisions for yourself. You may be leaving an institution, or relationship, or entering a different phase of your life. Using vetiver will enable you to keep calm and deal with the stress of change so that you can begin to see new opportunities and directions.

method of extraction

The oil is steam-distilled from the rootlets, which are washed, dried, cut and chopped, then usually soaked again in water prior to distillation.

most common uses
• Anti-depressant • Aphrodisiac • Oily skin
• Muscular aches and pains

safety data
• Non-toxic • Non-irritant • Non-sensitizing

ginger

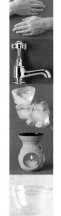

Zingiber officinale
Family: Zingiberaceae

origin The ginger plant is native to coastal regions of India. It is a perennial herb with a tuberous rhizome root that has been used as a culinary and medicinal spice for several thousand years. The essential oil is used to add warmth and depth to fragrances, and also as a flavouring for food and drinks.

description

The essential oil has a familiar hot, sweet, pungent and spicy odour. It is pale yellow or light amber in colour.

therapeutic properties

Ginger is a hot, moving and tonifying oil for use in cold and weak conditions. It makes an excellent warming massage or rubbing oil. It may also be used in footbaths, but as it may irritate sensitive mucous membranes it is best avoided in general bath oils. Ginger blends particularly well with cedarwood, coriander, frankincense, juniper, palmarosa, sandalwood, vetiver and all citrus oils.

One of the main areas ginger acts on is the lungs. Its tonifying qualities help chronic cold conditions in people who have a tendency to keep catching colds and flu. Ginger encourages the body to produce heat and sweat and throw off fevers, and acts as an expectorant. The moving effects of ginger help to relieve headaches caused by congestion and blocked sinuses.

The stimulating properties of ginger make it a very important oil for strengthening the immune system – use it in foot baths or inhalations at the beginning of winter to encourage immunity against colds and flu. It stimulates and strengthens the adrenal cortex and may be blended into a massage oil and massaged over the kidney area to improve vitality if you are cold and weak.

Ginger is an excellent oil for treating circulatory problems. It will combine well with cypress to treat chilblains, or can be used alone in a footbath to improve chronically cold feet.

One of ginger's most important uses is in treating ailments of the digestive system. It is most beneficial if you have a slow and weak digestion; it will relieve flatulence and help to improve assimilation and tone the digestive process. It will also bring relief to diarrhoea brought on by a chill.

Ginger can be used to treat arthritis and rheumatism when the symptoms are worse in cold and damp weather. It will work well if combined with peppermint and juniper in a base oil and massaged into the joints. Ginger may also be used to relieve muscle fatigue or aches and pains after over-exertion, as well as help with sprains and strains.

The strengthening and tonifying properties of ginger indicate its use as an aphrodisiac. It will work best if added to a base oil and massaged in over the kidney area.

As a first-aid remedy, ginger can help to relieve travel sickness, morning sickness and nausea. Place a couple of drops on a tissue and inhale the vapours at frequent intervals.

psychological profile

Ginger is useful if you are the type of person who is easily swayed by circumstances and frequently side-tracked. Everything has become an effort and all courses of action seem to have too many difficulties to work out well. You may feel flat, apathetic and indecisive. Using ginger oil will create a sense of determination and confidence, so that you can work through difficulties with a greater sense of your own inner power.

method of extraction

The oil is steam-distilled from the dried rhizomes.

---

most common uses

- Colds and flu • General debility • Poor circulation
- Weak digestion • Rheumatism • Nausea

---

safety data

Non-toxic • Non-sensitizing • Non-irritant in dilution

essential oils and their properties

This table provides a quick reference to the properties of the different essential oils, and how they may be used therapeutically.

	acne	allergies	anxiety	apathy	blisters	bronchitis	bruises	burns	candida	colds	concentration	confusion	coughs	cramp	cuts	depression	eczema	exhaustion	fear	flu	headache
basil			✓		✓						✓					✓		✓			
bergamot			✓	✓							✓			✓	✓						✓
cardamom												✓									✓
cedarwood	✓				✓					✓	✓										
chamomile	✓	✓	✓		✓			✓								✓		✓			✓
cinnamon				✓						✓							✓			✓	
clary sage			✓									✓				✓		✓			
clove																					
coriander			✓						✓	✓			✓				✓			✓	✓
cypress							✓					✓	✓								
eucalyptus					✓				✓	✓			✓							✓	✓
fennel					✓	✓							✓	✓							
frankincense			✓		✓					✓						✓		✓			
geranium	✓		✓								✓					✓					
ginger			✓	✓					✓			✓					✓			✓	
grapefruit	✓		✓	✓					✓	✓	✓									✓	✓
helichrysum		✓	✓				✓				✓				✓	✓	✓				
jasmine			✓									✓							✓		
juniper	✓											✓									
lavender	✓	✓	✓		✓		✓	✓	✓					✓	✓	✓	✓	✓			✓
lemon	✓		✓							✓	✓										
lemongrass	✓																				
mandarin			✓		✓											✓					
marjoram			✓						✓				✓	✓	✓			✓			✓
melissa		✓	✓										✓		✓	✓					✓
myrrh	✓				✓			✓		✓			✓				✓	✓			
neroli											✓										✓
orange			✓													✓					
palmarosa	✓		✓													✓					
patchouli	✓								✓												
pepper			✓	✓					✓					✓			✓		✓		
peppermint			✓						✓											✓	✓
pine					✓				✓	✓	✓		✓						✓	✓	✓
ravensara					✓				✓	✓	✓		✓			✓		✓	✓		
rose			✓										✓			✓			✓		
rosemary				✓						✓	✓		✓				✓			✓	✓
sage					✓								✓				✓			✓	✓
sandalwood			✓		✓								✓					✓			
tea tree	✓				✓	✓	✓	✓	✓	✓					✓					✓	
thyme	✓	✓			✓			✓	✓	✓			✓	✓			✓			✓	✓
vetiver	✓														✓	✓		✓			
ylang-ylang																✓					

	hyperactivity	insect bites	insect repellent	insomnia	irritability	jet lag	laryngitis	mood swings	muscle aches	panic attacks	period pains	PMT	rheumatism	shock	sprains	stress	sunburn	toothache	upset stomach	warts	worry
basil		✔	✔	✔					✔	✔	✔					✔					
bergamot				✔	✔											✔					
cardamom																			✔		
cedarwood																					
chamomile	✔	✔		✔						✔	✔	✔						✔	✔	✔	
cinnamon			✔									✔									
clary sage	✔			✔				✔				✔				✔					✔
clove			✔															✔			
coriander						✔			✔	✔			✔	✔							
cypress					✔		✔		✔				✔								
eucalyptus			✔						✔												
fennel													✔								
frankincense										✔											✔
geranium					✔		✔					✔				✔					
ginger									✔				✔		✔	✔			✔		
grapefruit									✔												
helichrysum	✔			✔												✔					✔
jasmine								✔								✔					
juniper									✔				✔								
lavender	✔	✔	✔	✔	✔	✔	✔	✔	✔	✔	✔		✔	✔	✔	✔	✔		✔		✔
lemon			✔				✔						✔							✔	
lemongrass			✔																		
mandarin	✔			✔												✔					✔
marjoram				✔	✔				✔	✔	✔	✔	✔		✔	✔					
melissa	✔	✔	✔	✔	✔					✔	✔	✔		✔		✔			✔		✔
myrrh			✔				✔														
neroli				✔										✔		✔					
orange																✔					
palmarosa																✔					
patchouli																					
pepper									✔				✔		✔						
peppermint			✔			✔												✔	✔		
pine									✔				✔		✔						
ravensara							✔		✔				✔		✔	✔			✔		
rose								✔			✔	✔				✔	✔				
rosemary						✔			✔				✔		✔						
sage							✔		✔		✔		✔			✔					
sandalwood				✔				✔													✔
tea tree		✔												✔	✔					✔	
thyme			✔										✔		✔	✔					
vetiver							✔		✔						✔	✔					
ylang-ylang				✔	✔					✔			✔								

essential oils for perfumery

This table gives guidance and suggestions for making your own fragrances to suit your general mood. It can also be used for self-help aromatherapy; check the far-right column for the overall therapeutic effect you wish to achieve.

TOP NOTES			
ESSENTIAL OIL	**BLENDS WELL WITH**	**THERAPEUTIC USE**	**EFFECT**
basil	bergamot, chamomile, clary sage, geranium, lavender, lemongrass, marjoram, rose	nerve tonic, balancing, reviving, strengthening	relaxing, uplifting
bergamot	lavender, melissa, rosemary	nerve tonic	uplifting
cardamom	bergamot, cedarwood, clove, frankincense, orange, sandalwood, ylang-ylang	digestive tonic, anti-spasmodic, carminative	tonifying, calming
clary sage	cardamom, coriander, geranium, jasmine, lavender, lemon, rose, sandalwood	strengthens nervous system, stress, anxiety	soothing, sedating
coriander	bergamot, clary sage, frankincense, jasmine	digestive, mildly warming, tonifying	aphrodisiac
eucalyptus	cedarwood, cypress, lavender, lemon, marjoram, pine	antiseptic, decongestant	warming, refreshing
grapefruit	citrus oils, clove, cypress	detoxifying, astringent	refreshing, uplifting
juniper	citrus oils, cedarwood, cypress, ginger, lavender, pine, rosemary	stimulates elimination of toxic fluids	cleansing
lavender	geranium, rosemary	stress, jet lag, insomnia	relaxing, balancing
lemon	any	antiseptic, astringent	stimulating
mandarin	citrus oils, spicy oils, clary sage, geranium, lavender, neroli	digestive, peristalsis	refreshing, uplifting
neroli	citrus oils, clary sage, jasmine, lavender, rosemary	anxiety, depression, insomnia	relaxing, calming, uplifting
orange	citrus oils, spice oils, clary sage, geranium, lavender, myrrh, neroli, rosemary	sluggish digestion, liver detoxifier	relaxing, uplifting
peppermint	fennel, orange	digestive, antiseptic	warming, stimulating
petitgrain	citrus oils, clary sage, jasmine, lavender, rosemary	nerve tonic	uplifting, anti-depressant
pine	cedarwood, eucalyptus, juniper, lavender, lemon, marjoram, tea tree	decongestant, urinary infection, rheumatism	refreshing, reviving
tea tree	clove, eucalyptus, lavender, lemon, pine, rosemary, thyme	anti-viral, anti-fungal, antiseptic	stimulating, tonifying
thyme	clove, eucalyptus, lavender, lemon, pine	strongly anti-microbial, strengthens immune system	warming, stimulating

MIDDLE NOTES

ESSENTIAL OIL	BLENDS WELL WITH	THERAPEUTIC USE	EFFECT
cedarwood	bergamot, cypress, frankincense, jasmine, juniper, myrrh, neroli, rosemary, sandalwood, vetiver	warming, regenerating, tonifying, soothing	balancing
cinnamon	lavender, melissa, rosemary, frankincense, lemon, mandarin, orange	warming, stimulating	restorative
clove	bergamot, eucalyptus, lavender, thyme	warming, stimulating, antiseptic	stimulating, pain-relieving
geranium	bergamot, lavender, lemon, marjoram, neroli, orange, palmarosa, rose, sandalwood	calming, cooling	calming, uplifting
jasmine	bergamot, clary sage, orange, rose, sandalwood, ylang-ylang	increases self-confidence, anti-depressant	uplifting, relaxing
marjoram	bergamot, cypress, eucalyptus, geranium, lavender, orange, rosemary	relieves aching muscles, period pain	warming, relaxing
olibanum	citrus oils, spice oils, basil, cedarwood, myrrh, neroli, pine, sandalwood, vetiver	tonifying, astringent, anti-inflammatory	aids meditation
palmarosa	bergamot, cedarwood, geranium, mandarin, rose, sandalwood, ylang-ylang	healing, regenerative	calming, uplifting, digestive tonic
Roman chamomile	clary sage, lavender, lemon, rose	anti-inflammatory	sedative
rose	bergamot, chamomile, clary sage, geranium, jasmine, lavender, patchouli	cooling, relaxing, tonifying	anti-depressant, aphrodisiac
ylang-ylang	bergamot, cedarwood, clary sage, jasmine, lemon, rose, sandalwood, vetiver	treats anxiety, depression, stress, tension	sedating, calming

BASE NOTES

ESSENTIAL OIL	BLENDS WELL WITH	THERAPEUTIC USE	EFFECT
benzoin	coriander, cypress, frankincense, jasmine, juniper, lemon, myrrh, rose, sandalwood, spice oils	skin irritation, poor circulation	anti-inflammatory, carminative, astringent
patchouli	cedarwood, geranium, neroli	anti-depressant, antibacterial, anti-viral	stimulating, astringent
sandalwood	bergamot, cedarwood, jasmine, palmarosa, vetiver, ylang-ylang	calming, soothing	relaxing, aphrodisiac, cooling
tonka	bergamot, citronella, clary sage, helichrysum, lavender	tonic, insecticidal	tonic, narcotic
vanilla	benzoin, sandalwood, spice oils, vetiver	balsamic	soothing
vetiver	clary sage, jasmine, lavender, patchouli, rose, sandalwood, ylang-ylang	anti-depressant, aphrodisiac	sedating, strengthening

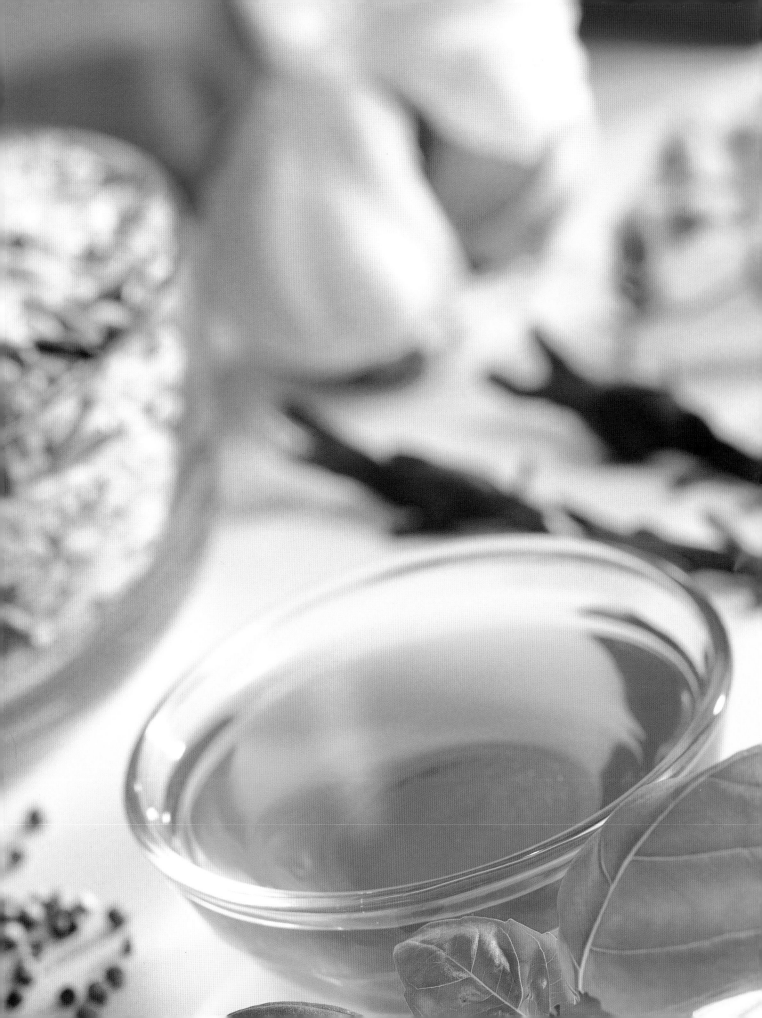

glossaries of natural ingredients, technical terms and therapies

glossary of natural ingredients

Following is a description of many of the natural ingredients, including herbs and essential oils, used in the recipes in this book. Use this information as a guide to choosing appropriate ingredients when making cosmetics for your hair and skin. More detailed information on essential oils is given in the profiles on pages 164–205.

Achillea millefolium (yarrow) This herb has astringent, tonic, vulnerary, diaphoretic and diuretic properties. A very good all-round tonic, yarrow aids poor circulation and helps to relieve menstrual problems, such as delayed periods, but it should be avoided internally during pregnancy. Yarrow is also excellent for oily or problem skin.

Agnus-castus see *Vitex agnus-castus.*

Allium cepa (onion) The bulb of this plant has antiseptic properties for the skin.

Allium sativum (garlic) The bulb of this member of the onion family is an antibiotic and anti-catarrhal, which is used to treat colds, flu, sinusitis, catarrh and any similar infections.

Almond see *Prunus dulcis.*

Aloe vera (syn. *A. barbadensis*) A mucilage, known as aloe vera juice, is extracted from this plant. It is used externally for its soothing, cooling and anti-irritant properties. It is excellent for treating burns, insect bites and so on. Aloe is an easy plant to grow and you can simply break off a leaf and use the juice that is produced. It is often referred to as a gel, but aloe vera juice has more of the consistency of a liquid.

Althaea officinalis (marsh mallow)

Althaea officinalis (marsh mallow) The herb is a demulcent and healer and is used externally as a poultice combined with slippery elm (*Ulmus rubra*) to draw boils and heal ulcers and slow-healing wounds. The same properties can be derived from the root as they can from the herb. Marshmallow tincture is an extract of the herb, produced using alcohol and, as such, has the same properties. See also *Ulmus rubra.*

Angelica archangelica (angelica) The leaves can be used in an infusion and will help to tone the whole system, particularly the digestive system and the lungs. The root can also be used as a circulatory stimulant. It is also a diuretic and an antiseptic (internally and externally).

Anise see *Illicium anisatum.*

Annatto see *Bixa orellana.*

Apium graveolens (celery) Celery seeds are good for itchy and irritated skin.

Apple see *Malus domestica.*

Apple cider vinegar This can be used as an astringent and pH adjuster for both skin and hair – it is a traditional hair rinse when diluted with water. It also contains malic acid which aids in the removal of dead skin cells. See also *Malus domestica.*

Apricot see *Prunus armeniaca.*

Arctium lappa (burdock) Both the root and leaves of the plant are used. Burdock is an excellent blood purifier for skin disease – taken internally and externally as a wash. As it is antiscorbutic, it may also be used to treat boils and skin infections.

Arnica tincture The tincture of the herb *Arnica montana* is produced using water and alcohol. It is renowned for its ability to heal bruised skin and ease aching muscles, making it an excellent remedy for sports injuries.

Arrowroot This is derived from the rhizomes of a plant of the Marantaceae family. It is used to thicken liquids and for its demulcent properties.

Astragalus gummifer A white or reddish gum called tragacanth is derived from this plant. The gum is used as a thickener in cosmetics and sensitization is possible.

Avena sativa (oats) The cereal nourishes, softens and cleanses the skin. It is excellent to use in facial scrubs and exfoliant preparations, and is mild enough to be used on sensitive skins.

Avocado pear see *Persea americana*.

Balm see *Melissa officinalis*.

Balsam of tolu see *Myroxylon balsamum*.

Banana see *Musa acuminata*.

Basil see *Ocimum basilicum*.

Bay see *Laurus nobilis*.

Calendula officinalis (marigold)

Beeswax Wax produced by the honeybee (*Apis mellifera*) which contains a mixture of fatty acids and esters. It is used in a range of cosmetics and toiletries as a thickener and emulsifier.

Bergamot see *Citrus bergamia*.

Bilberry see *Vaccinum myrtillus*.

Bixa orellana (annatto) The colouring agent from this tree, annatto, contains bixin and several orange-red pigments. It is used as a natural colourant for food and cosmetics.

Black pepper essential oil see *Piper nigrum*.

Blackcurrant see *Ribes nigrum*.

Bladderwrack see *Fucus vesiculosus*.

Boswellia thurifera (Frankincense, olibanum) Frankincense essential oil is distilled from the resin of this tree, which is native to mountainous areas of southern Arabia and India. It has been used for thousands of years as incense, and a few drops placed on an essential oil burner will be uplifting and aid concentration. Its tonifying and rejuvenating properties are of benefit to mature skins.

Bran The fibrous coating of wheat kernels that is used as an exfoliating agent.

Brassica napus (rape, colza) Rape seed oil is expressed from the seeds of this crop. It is used as a lubricant in soft soaps. It is non-toxic but sensitization is possible.

Brassica nigra (black mustard) Mustard powder, which is made from the ground seeds of this plant, is a stimulant and rubifacient. It increases circulation to a localized area of skin.

Burdock see *Arctium lappa*.

Cajuput see *Melaleuca cajuputi*.

Calendula officinalis (common marigold) This herb is spasmolytic, anti-haemorrhagic, emmenagogic, vulnerary, styptic and antiseptic, making it a very useful first-aid remedy. Used externally as a wash or cream it is good to heal burns and sores, while the crushed fresh leaf will prevent bleeding and is itself antiseptic. The remedy may also be used externally for varicose veins, ulcers and haemorrhoids, and applied as an eye lotion to treat conjunctivitis. Calendula ointment is used as a soothing and healing treatment for irritated or inflamed skin, for rashes and for eczema. Calendula tincture is an extract of the herb, produced using alcohol, that is antiviral, antibacterial and antifungal. Like the ointment, the tincture can be used to soothe irritated and inflamed skin, and it is an excellent antiseptic healer, which helps to prevent scarring from cuts, burns and boils.

Camellia sinensis (tea) The dried leaf of this familiar shrub is used in cosmetics as a dye and to darken hair colour.

Cananga odorata Ylang-ylang essential oil is distilled from the fresh flowers of this tree, which grows in India, Indonesia and the Philippines. The essential oil has a powerful, exotic, floral smell, which has a relaxing effect on the nervous system. It is traditionally used in perfumery and as an aphrodisiac.

Canarium luzonicum Elemi essential oil is distilled from the resin of this tree, which is found in the Philippines. Elemi has a citrusy, spicy aroma. It is strongly antiseptic and also has a tonifying and tightening effect. Used on the skin it has a similar action to myrrh, being cooling and drying. In hair preparations, it balances the secretion of sebum of the scalp.

Candelilla wax This is obtained from species of the family Euphorbiaceae and is used in conditioners and lipsticks for its emollient effect.

Capsella bursa-pastoris (shepherd's purse) This is an antihaemorrhagic, urinary, antiseptic, astringent plant, which is useful in the treatment of internal and external bleeding.

Capsicum (pepper) The dried ripe fruit of various species of this shrubby plant is used in external applications in ointments for the treatment of rheumatism. Cayenne pepper, the purest of herbal stimulants, is derived from *C. frutescens*. Used externally as a counter-irritant, it is useful in the treatment of rheumatism, arthritis and sciatica. Great care must be taken with the dosage, because this is a very hot remedy indeed.

Cardamom see *Elettaria cardamomum*.

Carrageen A hydrocolloid extracted from an edible seaweed called Irish moss (*Chondrus crispus*) found on rocky shores of the Atlantic in North America and northern Europe. It is used as a thickener in toiletries and food products, and has skin-soothing properties.

Carrot see *Daucus carota*.

Castor oil see *Ricinus communis*.

Cayenne pepper see *Capsicum*.

Cedarwood see *Cedrus atlantica*.

Cedrus atlantica Cedarwood essential oil is derived from the tree *C. atlantica* (Atlas cedar). It has a pleasant, mild, balsamic, woody odour, and it is one of the oldest oils to be produced, having been employed by the ancient Egyptians in the embalming of the dead. It can be used to treat oily skin, oily hair and dandruff.

Celery see *Apium graveolens*.

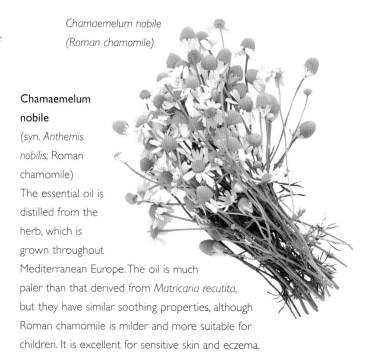

Chamaemelum nobile
(Roman chamomile)

Chamaemelum nobile (syn. *Anthemis nobilis;* Roman chamomile) The essential oil is distilled from the herb, which is grown throughout Mediterranean Europe. The oil is much paler than that derived from *Matricaria recutita,* but they have similar soothing properties, although Roman chamomile is milder and more suitable for children. It is excellent for sensitive skin and eczema.

Chamomile see *Chamaemelum nobile* and *Matricaria recutita*.

Chaste tree see *Vitex agnus-castus*.

Chickweed see *Stellaria media*.

Cider vinegar see *Apple cider vinegar*.

Cinnamomum camphora (camphor tree) Ho leaf oil is steam-distilled from the leaves of the tree. It has a clean, sweet and floral-woody smell. It is a balancing and calming oil, useful during times of stress. Ho wood oil is toxic and should not be used.

Cinnamomum zeylanicum (cinnamon) The inner bark of this Asian tree is used as a culinary spice and medicinal herb. It is a stimulant and increases the blood flow to a localized area. Cinnamon essential oil is distilled from the inner bark and leaves of the tree. The oil has a powerful, warm, sweet-spicy odour, but it must be well diluted before use because it can be an irritant.

Cinnamon see *Cinnamomum zeylanicum*.

Citronella see *Cymbopogon nardus*.

Citrus aurantifolia (lime) The essential oil is expressed from the unripe peel of the fruit. It has a sharp, fresh smell and astringent and refreshing properties. This oil should not be applied before going into the sun because it may photosensitize the skin — increasing the risk of sunburn.

Citrus aurantium (bitter orange tree) The blossom of the tree is distilled to make neroli essential oil. Neroli has a delightfully refreshing, powerfully floral smell, and is a classic ingredient of high-quality perfumes. It is a relaxing and uplifting oil, of benefit in treating anxiety, depression and insomnia. In skin care it is useful for dry, mature skin.

Citrus bergamia (bergamot, bergamot orange) Bergamot essential oil is expressed from the peel of the fruit of the tree *C. bergamia*, which is native to Sicily. The oil has an uplifting, sweet, fruity odour. It can be used to make a pleasant, cooling and refreshing massage or bath oil. The oil may photosensitize the skin to the sun, causing sunburn, unless the bergaptene has been removed.

Citrus limon (lemon) The fruit of the tree is an astringent and toner, and it decreases the production of sebum. It contains high amounts of vitamin C, and it can be used on the hair to enhance blonde highlights. Lemon essential oil is expressed from the peel of ripe lemons. It has a fresh, sweet smell, truly reminiscent of ripe lemons. It is highly antiseptic and has an astringent effect on the skin. It may be used to treat boils, broken capillaries, greasy skin, herpes and insect bites.

Citrus x paradisi (grapefruit) This refreshing and cooling citrus fruit is high in vitamin C and AHAs. The essential oil is expressed from the peel of the fruit. It has a fresh, sweet, citrus odour and is detoxifying and astringent.

Citrus reticulata (mandarin) The essential oil is expressed from the ripe peel of the fruit. The smell is extremely sweet, and it is a pleasant, safe and refreshing oil to use for adults and children.

Citrus sinensis (syn. *C. dulcis*; orange, sweet orange) Orange essential oil is expressed from the peel of this orange. It is a sweet, refreshing, pleasant oil, with detoxifying properties. Orange flower water, traditionally a by-product of the distillation of orange essential oil, has recently been manufactured by combining neroli oil with water, using a dispersing agent. It is specific for mature and dry skin types.

Clary sage see *Salvia sclarea*.

Clove see *Syzygium aromaticum*.

Clover see *Trifolium pratense*.

Cocoa butter see *Theobroma cacao*.

Coconut see *Cocos nucifera*.

Cocos nucifera (coconut tree) The oil obtained from the pressing of coconuts, the fruit of this palm tree, is used extensively in the production of soaps. It is also an excellent ingredient in skin and hair-care products, when it has an emollient effect. Powdered coconut milk is soothing, softening and moisturizing for the skin. The aroma is more pleasant than that of powdered cow's milk.

Coffea (coffee) Ground coffee is a soothing anti-inflammatory. As a hair rinse, coffee enhances dark highlights.

Coffee see *Coffea*.

Coltsfoot see *Tussilago farfara*.

Comfrey see *Symphytum officinale*.

Commiphora myrrha (myrrh) Myrrh essential oil is distilled from a resin that occurs naturally in the trunks of this small tree, which is native to countries bordering the Red Sea. The oil is an amber-coloured, sticky liquid. It has preserving and antiseptic properties, and it is used to treat infections of the gums, mouth and throat.

Coriander see *Coriandrum sativum*.

Coriandrum sativum (coriander) The essential oil is distilled from the crushed, ripe seeds of this small herb, which is native to southeast Europe. The oil has a fresh, spicy scent. It is a natural deodorant and aphrodisiac.

Coriandrum sativum (coriander)

Corn see *Zea mays.*

Cucumber see *Cucumis sativus.*

Cucumis sativus (cucumber) This salad vegetable has soothing, cooling, refreshing and toning properties. It calms skin irritation.

Cupressus sempervirens (cypress) The essential oil is distilled from the needles and twigs of this evergreen conifer. The smell has a freshness reminiscent of walking through a pine forest. It is an astringent oil that tonifies the venous system and is useful for treating varicose veins, haemorrhoids and broken capillaries.

Cydonia oblonga (quince) The seed of this small tree is used as a mucilage to thicken cosmetics and as a suspending agent. It can also be used to make a hair gel.

Cymbopogon citratus (lemongrass) Lemongrass essential oil is obtained by distillation from this grass. It has a strong, fresh-grass and lemony scent. Lemongrass is a strong anti-bacterial oil, useful for treating problem skin, open pores and acne. It is also an effective insect repellent.

Cymbopogon martinii (palmarosa) Palmarosa essential oil is distilled from this grass, which grows wild in India. It has a pleasant, sweet, rose-like scent and a mildly stimulating effect. It has a regenerative action on the skin.

Cymbopogon nardus (citronella) Citronella essential oil, which has a powerful lemony scent, is distilled from this grass. Its main use is as an effective insect repellent.

Cypress see *Cupressus sempervirens.*

Dandelion see *Taraxacum officinale.*

Daucus carota (carrot) Carrots contain beta-carotene (provitamin A), an antioxidant that protects the skin from free radical damage. Topical application promotes the production of new cells. Eating excess amounts may temporarily discolour the skin. Carrot oil,

which is also naturally rich in beta-carotene, is excellent for dry and mature skin.

Echinacea angustifolia (echinacea, coneflower) The plant is a blood cleanser, making it useful whenever there is blood poisoning, carbuncles, boils or insect bites. It helps to cleanse morbid matter from the digestive system and encourages lymphatic elimination, so helping to expel poisons, toxins and pus from the body. It may be of benefit in treating fevers and is useful in the treatment of skin conditions.

Echinacea angustifolia (echinacea)

Elder see *Sambucus nigra.*

Elemi see *Canarium luzonicum.*

Elettaria cardamomum (cardamom) The essential oil that is distilled from this tree, which grows abundantly in India and Sri Lanka, has a warm, spicy, aromatic smell. It has been used in Eastern medicine for more than 3,000 years.

Equisetum arvense (horsetail) The herb contains silica and is useful for strengthening hair and nails.

Eucalyptus citriodora (lemon-scented gum) This species of eucalyptus has a fresh, sweet, lemony aroma. It is more cooling and refreshing than ordinary eucalyptus, although it shares its antiseptic properties.

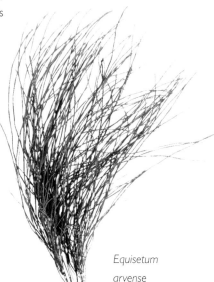

Equisetum arvense (horsetail)

Eucalyptus globulus (eucalyptus, blue gum) Eucalyptus essential oil is distilled from the leaves of this Australian tree. It is a warming and antiseptic oil, with a strongly camphoraceous and medicinal smell. It is an effective treatment for skin infections and irritation resulting from insect bites.

Euphrasia officinalis (eyebright) As the common name suggests, this makes a very good eyewash if used as a cool, sterile infusion. It also helps to relieve hayfever when it affects the eyes.

Evening primrose see *Oenothera biennis*.

Eyebright see *Euphrasia officinalis*.

Fennel see *Foeniculum vulgare*.

Foeniculum vulgare (fennel) Sweet fennel essential oil is steam-distilled from the crushed seeds of *F. vulgare var. dulce*, a plant cultivated in Mediterranean Europe. It has a very sweet, fresh smell, which is reminiscent of aniseed. Chewing fennel seeds will freshen the breath. An infusion can also be made to use as an eyewash for conjunctivitis.

Foeniculum vulgare (fennel)

Fragaria vesca (strawberry) This fruit is said to be able to whiten stained teeth, and it can be added to face masks for its cleansing, cooling and astringent properties.

Frankincense see *Boswellia thurifera*.

Fucus vesiculosus (bladderwrack) Like many seaweeds, this plant contains many nutritious trace elements, which are often deficient in the modern diet. It is particularly rich in iodine, so it may help those who suffer from an under-active thyroid.

Garlic see *Allium sativum*.

Geranium see *Pelargonium graveolens*.

Ginger see *Zingiber officinale*.

Glycine max (soya bean) Soya oil is expressed or extracted from soya beans. The oil consists mainly of triglycerides or linoleic and oleic acids. Soya oil is a pale yellow, odourless oil, which is useful for massage or as a base to which essential oils can be added. Sensitization is possible.

Golden rod see *Solidago virgaurea*.

Golden seal see *Hydrastis canadensis*.

Grapefruit see *Citrus × paradisi*.

Grapeseed see *Vitis vinifera*.

Gum A true plant gum is the dried exudate from various plants, obtained when the bark is cut or another injury is sustained. Plant gums are soluble in water and produce very viscous colloidal solutions, sometimes called mucilages, used to thicken liquids.

Gum arabic This fine yellow or white powder, soluble in water, is obtained from some species of Acacia. It is also known as gum acacia. It is used as an emulsifying and suspending agent and for the formation of gels. Sensitization is possible.

Hamamelis virginiana (witch hazel) Witch hazel leaves have astringent, anti-inflammatory and cooling properties. The name witch hazel also refers to a lotion made from an extract of the leaves in alcohol and water. The lotion is used as a cooling and astringent skin toner and to treat bruised, inflamed or itchy skin; it is useful in first aid for the treatment of injury and insect bites. It is also an excellent cosmetic ingredient for oily or problem skin.

Henna see *Lawsonia inermis*.

Hibiscus The flowers of some species are high in vitamin C and are the source of a strong, deep-red dye.

Ho leaf see *Cinnamomum camphora*.

Honey The sweet syrup made by bees is an excellent humectant for moisturizing the skin, and also has antiseptic properties.

Horsetail see *Equisetum arvense*.

Hydrastis canadensis (golden seal) The sacred herb of the Comanche Native Americans. Once called the King of Tonics, it is certainly a wonderful healer for inflammation of the mucous membranes. Externally, it is useful in skin diseases and infections.

Hypericum perforatum (St John's wort) This herb makes a marvellous remedy for spinal and nervous problems such as neuralgia, sciatica and fibrositis. It is antibacterial and can be used for healing when applied locally to burns, wounds or contusions. St John's wort tincture is an extract of the herb, produced using alcohol. It is antibacterial, astringent and healing. St John's wort oil is a macerated oil that is obtained by infusing the herb in vegetable oil – traditionally olive oil. It is excellent for treating neuralgia, sciatica and any nerve pains, as well as burns, rashes and shingles. It should not be applied before exposure to the sun since it may cause skin photosensitivity.

*Hypericum perforatum
(St John's wort)*

Illicium anisatum (anise) The essential oil is distilled from the dried and crushed seeds of the tree, which originated in the Near East. The essential has a fresh, sweet smell, and it can be used for cramping, digestive problems and for spasmodic coughs. It has a relatively high toxicity and is best used for only short periods of time.

Iris pallida The rhizome of the iris, known as orris root, has been used for many years as a fixative for fragrances, including in pot pourris.

Jasmine see *Jasminum officinale.*

Jasminum officinale (common jasmine) Jasmine absolute is the most uplifting of all the oils. It has an intensely rich and exotic smell, produced from the delicate flowers of the plant. The essential oil can be worn as a perfume, creating a sense of relaxation and enjoyment.

Jojoba see *Simmondsia chinensis.*

Juglans nigra (black walnut) The leaves of the tree can be used to darken the hair.

Juniper see *Juniperus communis.*

Juniperus communis (juniper) The essential oil is distilled from the berries of the juniper tree. It is used in skin preparations to aid oily skin, blocked pores and acne. Juniper oil added to the bath is refreshing and will stimulate the elimination of toxic fluids.

Karite butter see Shea-nut butter.

Laurus nobilis (bay, bay laurel) The leaves of this small tree are frequently used in cooking. The medicinal properties involve stimulating and cleansing. The essential oil is used mainly for treating sprains and strains.

Lavandula angustifolia (syn. *L. officinalis;* lavender) This herb is soothing, calming and healing for delicate and sensitive skins. Lavender essential oil, with its familiar, sweet fragrance, is one of the most widely used of all essential oils. It has a balancing effect on the nervous system and will relieve headaches and help prevent insomnia. It is very pleasant to use in a massage and in baths. The oil is an excellent antiseptic and aid to healing, useful for burns, wounds, bites, dermatitis and any inflammation of the skin.

Lavender see *Lavandula angustifolia.*

Lawsonia inermis (henna) The powdered leaf of the shrub is traditionally used to dye the skin and hair red.

Lemon see *Citrus limon.*

Lemon balm see *Melissa officinalis.*

Lemongrass see *Cymbopogon citratus.*

Lime see *Citrus aurantifolia* and *Tilia* x *europaea.*

Malus domestica (apple) Apples are a good source of vitamins A and C as well as containing trace elements of potassium, calcium and magnesium. They also contain malic acid, a 'protein digester', which aids in the removal of dead skin cells. Organic apple juice can be used neat on the skin as an effective toner to remove excess surface oil.

Mandarin see *Citrus reticulata.*

Marigold see *Calendula officinalis* and *Tagetes minuta.*

Marjoram see *Origanum majorana*.

Marsh mallow see *Althaea officinalis*.

Matricaria recutita (syn. *Chamomilla recutita*; German chamomile) This herb grows throughout Europe and west Asia and makes a very effective remedy, not to mention a poultice that can be used externally for ulcers. The active, yet volatile, oils are best extracted by infusion, but care must be taken not to allow the steam to escape. It may be given with complete safety to nervous children (or adults, for that matter) or to those who suffer from insomnia; it is also good for children's teething problems. Used externally as a wash or steam bath, it will help clear the skin and can be a useful eyewash. Chamomile flower water is traditionally a by-product from the distillation of chamomile essential oil, but it is now produced commercially by combining chamomile essential oil with water using a dispersing agent. The flower water is excellent for dry and sensitive skin. Blue chamomile oil, the essential oil that is distilled from the herb, has remarkable anti-inflammatory properties and a considerable range of uses, including the treatmer allergies, stomach cramps, period pains, insomnia and all kinds of skin irritation and inflammation. See also *Chamaemelum nobile*.

Melaleuca alternifolia (tea tree) Tea tree essential oil is obtained from the leaves of this tree, which is native to Australia. Its excellent germicidal and antifungal properties give it a wide range of uses, including the treatment of colds, flu, herpes, thrush, athlete's foot, warts and other skin infections.

Melaleuca cajuputi (cajuput) An essential oil is distilled from this tree, which grows abundantly in the Philippines and Malaysia. Like that of eucalyptus, the odour is strongly camphoraceous and medicinal. Cajuput essential oil is mainly used in inhalations for respiratory infections, and is especially suitable for relieving symptoms of colds, coughs, sinus infections and sore throats.

Melissa officinalis (lemon balm) This fragrant herb produces one of the most refreshing herbal tisanes. It can often lift the spirits and is

a good tonic for the heart, circulation and nervous systems. It is an aid to digestion and helps to relieve tension. The essential oil has a sweet, lemony smell, popular with both children and adults. Melissa essential oil is very uplifting and calming, and it is useful for treating inflamed skin conditions.

Mentha x piperita (peppermint) Peppermint essential oil is distilled from this herb. Peppermint is known for its decongestant, stimulating and refreshing properties. Menthol, which is usually obtained from peppermint, has decongestant and cooling properties.

Mentha x piperita (peppermint)

Mentha spicata (spearmint) Spearmint makes a refreshing and fragrant infusion, which is cooling for the skin.

Menthol see *Mentha x piperita*.

Mullein see *Verbascum thapsus*.

Musa acuminata (banana) The fruit contains high levels of vitamins and minerals, especially potassium. It is humectant and moisturizing.

Mustard see *Brassica nigra*.

Myroxylon balsamum (tolu balsam tree) The aromatic resin, known as balsam of tolu, of this South American tree is a dark brown fluid that darkens and hardens on ageing. It is used as a conditioner, although some people may have allergic reactions to it.

Myrrh see *Commiphora myrrha*.

Neroli see *Citrus aurantium*.

Nettle see *Urtica dioica*.

Oats see *Avena sativa*.

Ocimum basilicum (basil) The sweet, spicy, fresh essential oil that is distilled from the herb basil has a calming yet uplifting effect. The oil may irritate sensitive skin if it is not well diluted before use, and it should not be used for prolonged periods.

Oenothera biennis (evening primrose) Pressed oil from the flowers of this plant contains high concentrations of the essential fatty acid, gamma linolenic acids (GLAs), which the human body is unable to make and which must, therefore, be provided in the diet. It is beneficial externally for dry skin and some kinds of eczema.

Olea europaea (common olive) A fixed oil is expressed from the fruit of the tree. Olive oil comprises triglycerides or oleic, linoleic and palmitic acids, and it is used as an emollient and as a soap base. Externally it is soothing, nourishing and lubricating.

Olibanum see *Boswellia thurifera*.

Olive see *Olea europaea*.

Onion see *Allium cepa*.

Orange see *Citrus sinensis*.

Origanum majorana (marjoram, sweet marjoram) The essential oil is steam-distilled form the dried leaves and flowering tops of this well-known herb. It is a warming and relaxing oil, useful for treating stress, anxiety and insomnia. It is also used to relieve aching muscles, rheumatism, strains and period pains.

Orris root see *Iris pallida*.

Oryza sativa (rice) The grain of this plant is composed essentially of starch. Ground rice can be added to creams and face masks to act as an exfoliant. Rice bran oil is extracted from the endosperm of the grain. It is suitable for use in cosmetics and toiletries when low in free fatty acids and all the lipase has been deactivated.

Palm Palm oil is obtained from the seed of the palm tree, cultivated since ancient times. It is used in soaps and as a cosmetic ingredient for its lubricant properties. It has no known toxicity. Palm kernel oil is an edible fat obtained from palm kernels to make soap. It is also used as an ingredient in cosmetics for its emollient properties. It also has no known toxicity.

Palmarosa see *Cymbopogon martinii*.

Parsley see *Petroselinum crispum*.

Patchouli see *Pogostemon cablin*.

Pelargonium graveolens (geranium, rose geranium) Geranium essential oil is produced from the leaves of this species. It is a cooling and calming oil, useful for treating anxiety and tension. It also has a balancing effect on the skin, making it suitable for dry, oily or problem skin. Pleasant to use in the bath or as a massage oil.

Peppermint see *Mentha × piperita*.

Persea americana (avocado pear) The fruit of the tree is naturally rich in unsaturated oils, which hydrate, nourish and moisturize the skin. Avocado oil, which is expressed from the flesh of the avocado pear, is dark green. It is an excellent emollient and natural colourant, containing oleic, linoleic and palmitic acids.

Petroselinum crispum (parsley) This popular culinary herb also soothes, cleanses and heals the skin, and it is used when the skin is irritated and inflamed. It contains high levels of vitamins A and C.

Pine see *Pinus sylvestris*.

Pinus sylvestris (pine, scots pine) Pine essential oil is distilled from the needles and wood chippings of this tree. It has a refreshing, sweet, woody smell, and is an effective antiseptic and deodorant.

Piper nigrum (black pepper) The essential oil is produced by steam distillation of the dried, crushed fruits of this climbing plant, which is grown mainly in Indonesia and India. It is a hot, dry, spicy oil, with a deeply warming effect, and it is useful for relieving muscular aches and pains and for its detoxifying properties. Black pepper oil must be well diluted before it is applied to the skin.

Pogostemon cablin (patchouli) Patchouli essential oil is distilled from the dried leaves of this small plant. It has a persistent, dry-wood smell and is used in perfumery for its fixative properties. Patchouli is claimed to be an aphrodisiac, and it can be used to reduce scarring and to treat oily and problem skin.

Potato see *Solanum tuberosum*.

Prunus armeniaca (apricot) Apricot kernel oil, also known as peach kernel oil, is the oil expressed from the kernels of the fruit of this tree. It has very similar properties to *P. dulcis* oil.

Prunus dulcis (almond, sweet almond) Sweet almond oil is expressed from the kernels of varieties of *P. dulcis*. It is a light, odourless oil, with soothing, nourishing and skin-conditioning properties. It is a popular massage base oil and is also used as an emollient in many skin-care creams and lotions; sensitization is possible. Almond meal, the residue that is left after almond oil has been expressed, is an excellent exfoliant. Ground almonds also make a good exfoliant.

Quassia amara (syn. *Simaba cedron*; quassia) Quassia chips are derived from the bark of this tree and from *Picrasma excelsa*, which are native to South America. The chips have an extremely bitter taste, but a hair rinse made from quassia chips can be used as an effective treatment for head lice.

Quillaja saponaria (soap-bark tree) The inner dried bark of this tree is known as soap bark, quillaja or quillay. Extracts are used as a natural detergent and natural foaming agent. Quillaja is a saponin, and it is used in shampoos, shower gels and creams and also as a foam stabilizer in soft drinks. It is non-toxic to mammals but is toxic to crustaceans, and its use is, therefore, of environmental concern.

Quince see *Cydonia oblonga*.

Rape see *Brassica napus*.

Raspberry see *Rubus idaeus*.

Rheum x hybridum (rhubarb) This edible garden plant is used medicinally as an astringent and purgative. Externally, it may be used to lighten the hair. The leaves should not be eaten.

Ribes nigrum (blackcurrant)

Rhubarb see *Rheum x hybridum*.

Ribes nigrum (blackcurrant) The leaves of the shrub are used as an astringent to decrease the production of sweat and to reduce pore size.

Rice see *Oryza sativa*.

Ricinus communis (castor oil plant) The thick, colourless oil that is extracted from the plant provides a protective, waterproof coating to both the skin and hair.

Rosa (rose)

Rosa spp. (rose) Pink and red rose buds may be used medicinally for their cooling and soothing action. They may be used as an infusion for itchy, inflamed or sunburned skin. Hips, the fruits or berries from wild rose bushes, notably R. canina (dog rose) and R. gallica (French rose), which contain high concentrations of vitamin C, make a pleasant infusion for drinking on their own or combined with hibiscus. Rose-hip oil, which is extracted from the hips of R. canina, is claimed to be of use in treating scar tissue. Rose water was traditionally a by-product of the steam-distillation of rose essential oil, but it is now manufactured commercially by combining rose absolute with water, using a dispersing agent. A cooling, anti-inflammatory lotion for itchy, inflamed or reddened skin, it also helps to maintain the skin's natural water balance. It is a good skin toner with a pleasant fragrance and is suitable for any skin type. Rose essential oil is an exquisite oil produced from R. centifolia (Provence rose, cabbage rose) and R. damascena (damask rose). It is a cooling and soothing oil, which is excellent for treating stress-related conditions and menstrual problems, including PMT. It is beneficial for dry, inflamed and mature skins. Rose absolute is produced by solvent extraction, while the very costly true rose oil is steam-distilled.

Rose see *Rosa* spp.

Rosemary see *Rosmarinus officinalis*.

Rosmarinus officinalis (rosemary) The herb is found growing wild throughout the Mediterranean countries, and it has been used for centuries as a culinary and medicinal herb. The volatile oils have strong antiseptic properties. It makes an excellent rinse for the hair. Rosemary essential oil is refreshing and stimulating. It is excellent for hair and scalp problems, including hair loss and dandruff.

Rubus idaeus (raspberry) The leaves of this shrub are anti-spasmodic, astringent and stimulant. It is effective in treating sore throats and bleeding gums, and other oral infections.

Sage see *Salvia lavandulifolia*.

St John's wort see *Hypericum perforatum*.

Salvia lavandulifolia (Spanish sage) This herb, native to north Mediterranean countries, is a natural antibiotic. It is an antiseptic to the skin and darkens the hair. It is also useful in the treatment of dandruff. Sage relieves excessive sweating, but it should not be taken during pregnancy. Sage essential oil is distilled from the wild herb. It has a fresh, herbaceous and camphoraceous smell. It is a strongly simulating oil, which will relieve muscular aches and pains, reduce excessive sweating and is traditionally used in mouthwashes and gargles for oral infections, including sore throats.

Salvia sclarea (clary sage) The essential oil derived from this herb has a bitter-sweet, herby odour. It has a soothing and sedating effect, while at the same time strengthening the nervous system. It is useful for treating stress, anxiety and depression and for hastening convalescence.

Sambucus nigra (elder) Its somewhat astringent property has made elderflower water a favourite wash for greasy or problem skin. A steam facial will do much to clear blackheads.

Sandalwood see *Santalum album*.

Rubus idaeus (raspberry)

Sambucus nigra (elder)

Santalum album (sandalwood) Sandalwood essential oil is distilled from the wood of the tree. It has long been regarded as having aphrodisiac properties, and it makes a popular massage oil. Sandalwood is particularly beneficial for dry skin.

Saponaria officinalis (soapwort) Infusions of soapwort have been used as a cleanser for the hair and skin for centuries.

Seaweed A number of different seaweeds, most notably bladderwrack (*Fucus vesiculosus*), carrageen (*Chondrus crispus*) and kelp, have a use in cosmetics and toiletries. Seaweed is a rich natural source of many minerals, vitamins and trace elements, and they have a long history of use in external applications as cleansing, detoxifying, toning and conditioning agents. See also Carrageen.

Shea-nut butter (also known as karite butter) A natural fat obtained from the fruit of the tree *Butyrospermum parkii*. It has no known toxicity.

Shepherd's purse see *Capsella bursa-pastoris*.

Simmondsia chinensis (jojoba) Jojoba oil is a semi-liquid, oil-like wax obtained from the leaves of this shrub. It has excellent emollient properties.

Slippery elm see *Ulmus rubra*.

Soap bark see *Quillaja saponaria*.

Soapwort see *Saponaria officinalis*.

Solanum tuberosum (potato) Potatoes are high in vitamin C. They will reduce puffiness around the eyes if sliced and placed on the eyes.

Solidago virgaurea (golden rod) This herb has astringent and toning properties.

Soya see *Glycine max.*

Spearmint see *Mentha spicata.*

Stellaria media (chickweed) This common garden weed has a cooling action on the body tissues and is useful for external inflammation – as a poultice for boils, for example, or in an ointment for itching, eczema and skin rashes.

Strawberry see *Fragaria vesca.*

Symphytum officinale (comfrey) The old country name, 'knitbone', tells of the great healing potential of this herb. Used externally as a compress, it helps fractured bones to mend and cuts, ulcers and bruises to heal with minimal scar formation. It is very nutritious. Comfrey tincture is an alcoholic extraction that provides the same properties as the herb.

Syzygium aromaticum (syn. *Eugenia caryophyllata;* clove) Clove essential oil is obtained by distillation of the flowerbuds of the evergreen clove tree, which originated in the Moluccas. It has a strongly stimulating effect and also has pain-relieving properties, which are especially valuable for relieving toothache. It is a very antiseptic oil and is useful as a room fumigant. Clove oil may irritate the skin and must be well diluted before use.

Tagetes minuta (syn. *T. glandulifera*) The essential oil is distilled from a species of marigold. It is a bright orange-green colour and has a sweet, herbaceous smell. It is useful for treating foot problems, such as corns and verrucas. Tagetes oil should not be applied before exposure to the sun as it may cause skin photosensitivity.

Taraxacum officinale (dandelion) This plant has superb medicinal qualities. The leaves are strongly diuretic and rich in potassium, which means that no potassium supplement is required. It is, therefore, very useful in any condition in which there is fluid retention. It is also a blood purifier and spring tonic. Its cleansing properties make it a useful herb for treating many skin problems, such as acne.

Tea see *Camellia sinensis.*

Thymus vulgaris (thyme)

Tea tree see *Melaleuca alternifolia.*

Theobroma cacao (cacao, chocolate-nut tree) Cocoa butter is the fat that is obtained from the roasted seeds of the cocoa bean, the fruit of this tree. The butter contains stearic, palmitic and oleic acids, and it is used as an emollient and conditioning agent.

Thuja occidentalis (thuja) Thuja tincture is a strong anti-viral remedy derived from this tree. Apply sparingly to warts and verrucas.

Thyme see *Thymus vulgaris.*

Thymus vulgaris (thyme) An infusion of the herb is fragrant as well as being antiviral, antifungal and antibacterial. It is traditionally used to add shine and strength to dark hair. Thyme essential oil is distilled from the herb. It is a warming and stimulating oil that will relieve muscular pain. It is used to treat many kinds of infections – for example, skin, respiratory and urinary – because it is strongly antimicrobial and also strengthens the immune response. The oil must be well diluted before use because it may irritate sensitive skin.

Tilia x europaea (lime) A very soothing remedy is made from the flowers of the tree, which may be used both internally and externally.

Tolu balsam see *Myroxylon balsamum.*

Tragacanth see *Astragalus gummifer.*

Trifolium pratense (red clover) Taken internally, the flowers purify the blood and can aid many skin conditions. It is rich in minerals.

Tussilago farfara (coltsfoot) This plant's generic name comes from the Latin word meaning 'to cough'. It is one of nature's great pulmonary remedies, useful in all chest complaints. Both flowers and leaves are used, and the plant is rich in magnesium, so it may also help in skin complaints.

Ulmus rubra (syn. *U. fulva;* slippery elm) This tree provides one of nature's most useful remedies. Slippery elm is nutritious, demulcent and healing, with a very gentle action. Applied externally as a poultice, it is wonderfully soothing and drawing for injured or inflamed parts. It helps to speed healing, when it may be combined with comfrey (*Symphytum officinale*), marsh mallow (*Althea officinalis*) and marigold (*Calendula officinalis*).

Urtica dioica (stinging nettle) Rich in minerals, this is one of nature's finest spring tonics (especially the new green shoots). It is excellent for anaemia and will slough off the clogging foods of winter, reviving the system. It can be eaten as food either in soups or as a vegetable. It also makes a useful external wash for a dry, flaking scalp.

Vaccinum myrtillus (bilberry, whortleberry) The fruits of this shrub contain fruit acids that can be used to whiten the teeth.

Valerian see *Valeriana officinalis*.

Valeriana officinalis (valerian) This herb is an effective sedative, used to treat nervous tension, anxiety and insomnia.

Verbascum thapsus (mullein) The oil is a macerated oil made using the herb mullein and vegetable oil. It is used to treat earache and blocked ears.

Verbena officinalis (vervain) An antispasmodic and relaxing nervine herb, used to relieve symptoms of depression, stress and tension.

Urtica dioica
(nettle)

Vervain see *Verbena officinalis*.

Vetiver see *Vetiveria zizanioides*.

Vetiveria zizanioides (syn. *Andropogon muricatus*; vetiver) Vetiver essential oil is distilled from the roots of this scented grass, which grows mainly in India and Indonesia. It has a sweet, woody and earthy smell and astringent properties. It may be used to treat oily skin, acne and weeping skin conditions.

Vitex agnus-castus (chaste tree, agnus-castus) The berries are used to produce agnus-castus, which has a reputation as a normalizer of pituitary functions. It is useful in cases of PMT, menstrual irregularity and whenever male or female hormonal imbalance is involved.

Vitis vinifera (grape) Grapeseed oil, which comes from the vine, is quickly and deeply absorbed by the skin, making it suitable for light massage of delicate or oily skin. It is odourless and almost colourless, and is, therefore, an ideal base to which essential oils can be added.

Walnut see *Juglans nigra*.

Wheatgerm oil This heavy, rich oil is a natural source of vitamin E. Used alone, it is rather a heavy oil with a distinctive odour; for massage, it can be combined with a lighter oil, such as almond oil, or it can be used to help avoid stretch marks during pregnancy.

Whortleberry see *Vaccinum myrtillus*.

Witch hazel see *Hamamelis virginiana*.

Yarrow see *Achillea millefolium*.

Ylang-ylang see *Cananga odorata*.

Yoghurt Produced by the action of bacteria on milk, yoghurt cleanses and conditions the skin and is readily absorbed. It contains lactic acid, which is thought to stimulate cell production. It is a useful treatment for thrush (*Candida albicans*) when applied locally.

Zea mays (maize, sweet corn) Cornstarch (cornflour) is the milled powder derived from maize. The size of the particles makes it an excellent exfoliant, although sensitization is possible. Corn oil, which is also obtained from maize, is used as an emollient and naturally contains tocopherols and lecithin, which are excellent for moisturizing; again, sensitization is possible. Corn silk, which is obtained from the cobs of maize, is a soothing demulcent for the urinary system and is especially useful for the burning pains of cystitis and other infections of the urinary tract.

Zingiber officinale (ginger) The root of this plant, a native to the tropical coastal regions of India, is a very good circulatory stimulant. The essential oil is deeply warming, helping to encourage good circulation of the blood. It may be used to treat rheumatism, sprains and strains.

glossary of technical terms

Increasingly, manufacturers of cosmetics are obliged to list all the ingredients they use on their product packaging. This glossary includes explanations of many of the chemical ingredients of commercially prepared cosmetics as well as definitions of many chemical terms to help you interpret this information.

Absolute An aromatic, volatile substance obtained by solvent extraction from a single botanical species, such as rose absolute and jasmine absolute. None of the solvent should remain after the process is complete, when absolutes may be used like essential oils.

Acetamide MEA A synthetic raw material used as a hair conditioner and solvent. It has low toxicity to the skin and eyes.

Acetic acid An acid in vinegar and used as a preservative in foods and a solvent for gums and volatile oils.

Acetone A solvent used mainly in nail varnishes and nail polish removers. It is an irritant, however, and its use in cosmetics has been banned or restricted in many countries.

Acid colours Synthetic dyes used to colour food, cosmetics and toiletries. The list of allowable acid colours has been reduced dramatically in recent years because they are highly irritant.

Acids Substances that, when added to water, liberate hydrogen as an ion. They also react with bases to form salts. Acids have a low pH value (pH7 being neutral). Note that strong acids can be highly irritant, if not corrosive, but weak acids are beneficial to the skin, which is naturally slightly acidic.

Acne Although this is the commonest skin complaint, affecting an estimated 80 per cent of teenagers at any one time, its causes are still not fully understood. It affects both females and males in the same numbers, although the condition is usually more severe in young males.

Active ingredients The ingredients contained in any formula that give the desired physiological effect — for example, the component in a moisturizing cream that improves the moisture content of the skin.

Alkalis Substances with a pH above 7 that are often used as neutralizers in cosmetics and toiletries. Strongly alkaline substances are corrosive — for example, caustic soda.

Alkaloids Plant substances with an organic nitrogen base that often have pharmacological properties. For example, valerianine is an alkaloid present in the herb valerian.

Alkyloamides A common family of ingredients, including Cocamide DEA, MEA, MIPA or PEG, used in shampoos, bubble baths and liquid hand and body cleansers. They are employed for thickening, gelling, emulsifying and solubilizing. The major drawback with alkyloamides is that they can be contaminated with nitrosamines during manufacture of the product. Nitrosamines are suspected animal carcinogens. Correct formulation and the use of a reputable supplier will help eliminate the risk.

Allantoin A product that is synthetically produced by the oxidation of uric acid and found naturally in comfrey root and uva ursi. Used as a humectant, conditioner and detoxicant, it has soothing and anti-irritant properties.

Allergy A hypersensitive reaction to specific substances that develops in some people. It is characterized by an irritation, such as redness or itching.

Aluminosilicates Silicates containing aluminium, which are a major compound found in many clays, such as kaolin or bentonite.

Amber A synthetic substitute for ambergris.

Ambergris A waxy substance, secreted by sperm whales. It was traditionally used as a fixative in perfumery, although nowadays it has been replaced by synthetic fixatives. See also Amber.

Amino acids Group of compounds containing both the carboxyl (COOH) and the amino (NH2) groups. They are the building blocks of proteins and are crucial to the maintenance of the body. Essential amino acids — for example, histidine, leucine and lysine — cannot be manufactured by the body and must be supplied in the diet. However, non-essential amino acids arginine, cystine and taurine, for example – are manufactured by the body.

Ammonium laureth sulphate A synthetic detergent that is used extensively as the primary surfactant in shampoos as a foaming and cleansing agent. Some problems can arise from the ethoxylated detergents. See also Ethoxylate.

Ammonium lauryl sulphate The ammonium salt of sulphated lauryl alcohol, which is used as a foaming and cleansing agent. The absence of any ethoxylation makes it slightly less mild than ammonium laureth sulphate but excludes the problems associated with ethoxylation. See also Ethoxylate.

Ammonium pareth-25 sulphate An anionic surfactant used for its foaming and cleansing properties. It is an inexpensive detergent that, if used in high concentrates, can cause eye and skin irritation.

Amphoteric surfactant see Surfactant.

Amygdalin A glucoside found in the kernels of most fruit belonging to the Rosaceae family, particularly bitter almonds. It is used widely as a flavouring material in the form of essence of bitter almonds. Although harmless in small doses in its natural form, it becomes toxic when distilled, hence the toxicity of bitter almond oil.

Anionic surfactant see Surfactant.

Antibacterial Any agent or process that inhibits the growth and reproduction of bacteria. Preservatives have antibacterial properties, and are used to protect products from degradation. Many essential oils are antibacterial.

Antioxidants Substances that prevent the formation of free radicals, which can cause the oxidative deterioration that causes rancidity in oils or fats and also premature ageing. Examples of natural antioxidants include vitamins A, C and E. See also Free radicals.

Antiperspirants Substances that inhibit perspiration and cause blocking of the skin's pores. They are generally based on either aluminium zirconin or zinc salts.

Arachidonic acid An essential fatty acid that is found in beeswax and some natural oils.

Astringents Products that cause a tightening and contraction of the skin tissues, generally used to tone skin and close pores.

Azulene An anti-inflammatory component found in chamomile flowers. Chamazulene is the blue component that gives chamomile oil its distinctive colour.

Barrier cream A cream that provides a barrier when applied to the skin and produces a protective coating. Generally, barrier creams are quite oily products or contain lanolin. A simple barrier cream for the nappy area for babies is zinc and castor oil.

Bentonite A form of clay that swells in the presence of water to give a gel. It is used as a thickening agent, for example, in face masks, and is considered non-toxic.

Benzaldehyde The major component of bitter almond oil. It is often synthesized for its almond fragrance and is used in cosmetics and toiletries. It can produce allergic reactions in sensitive individuals.

Benzalkonium chloride A cationic surfactant used in conditioners and shampoos for conditioning the hair and as an anti-dandruff ingredient. It has bactericidal activity and is also used in mouthwashes and aftershave preparations. It can be a severe irritant to the eyes and skin if used in high concentrations.

Benzene A petrochemical used as a solvent and manufacturing agent in lacquers, varnishes and cosmetics. Highly toxic in even minute proportions, it has known carcinogenic activity.

Benzoic acid A white powder that is used as an anti-microbial agent both in food products and in toiletries. It is slightly toxic and can cause skin irritations.

Benzoin A resin obtained from various Styrax species, which has a warming odour. It is used as a fixative, preservative and antioxidant and for its skin-healing properties. In its natural state it is solid, so it is dissolved in a solvent for ease of use. It is good for dry, cracked or chapped skin and also has antiseptic properties. It should not be taken internally.

Benzophenones These are used as fixatives in perfumes. Benzophenone-3 absorbs ultra-violet light and is therefore used as a sunscreen agent, especially for UVA protection. Allergic reactions can occur.

Benzyl alcohol A colourless liquid that is used as a bactericide and solvent. It has an anaesthetizing action, and high concentrations can cause irritation.

Betaines Derivatives of trimethyl glydine that occur chiefly in plants. Surfactants, such as coco betaine, are formed by linking them to a fatty acid chain. They are used in shampoo products, for example, to decrease the irritancy potential of some anionic surfactants, such as sodium laureth sulphate. They have no known toxicity.

Bha (butylated hydroxanisole) A synthetic white, waxy solid used as an antioxidant to prevent oxidative deterioration of oils and fats.

Bht (butylated hydroxytoluene) A synthetic antioxidant, which can cause sensitization.

Borax (sodium borate) A mild alkali that is used in cosmetics and toiletries as a water softener, preservative and texturizer. When making simple creams and lotions it may be safely used in combination with beeswax as an emulsifier. Not toxic externally, but there is some toxicity internally and it should not be applied to broken skin. Keep out of reach of children.

Botanical extract A general term for an extract of herbs and plants. The extracting solvent can be water, oil, alcohol or any synthetic solvent such as propylene glycol.

2-bromo-2 nitropropane 1-3 diol An antimicrobial agent used in toiletries, active against bacteria and fungi. It can react with secondary amines and form nitrosamines, which are known carcinogens. Used at high levels it can cause irritation.

Butyl paraben Butyl p-hydroxybenzoate. See Parabens.

Calamine A pink powder made of zinc oxide with a small amount of ferric oxide. It is a traditional mixture used for relieving itchy skin and rashes. It is not generally considered to be toxic.

Calcium carbonate Commonly known as chalk, a naturally occurring calcium salt found in limestone, coral and marble. It is used as an abrasive agent in toothpastes and face washes and also as a whitener and neutralizer in cosmetics. It has no known toxicity.

Candida albicans A yeast that causes thrush and, in more severe cases, symptoms affecting the whole body. Recent studies have shown that tea tree oil can be very effective at treating this infection locally.

Capric acid A fatty acid that is used as an emollient in creams. It occurs as glycerides in the milk of goats and cows, and in coconut and palm oil.

Caramel A concentrated solution of heated sugar that can be used as a natural colouring agent.

Carbomer-934 A polymer of acrylic acid that is used as a thickener. It is considered to be of essentially low toxicity.

Carboxymethyl hydroxycellulose A derivative of cellulose that has been chemically modified for use as a thickener and stabilizer in creams, lotions and ice cream. It is considered non-toxic externally.

Carmine A red substance used as a dye and colourant, obtained from the female cochineal insect.

Carotene One of the most important colouring matters of green leaves. It is found in all plants and in many animal tissues. Beta-carotene (provitamin A) is the yellow colouring matter of carrots and egg yolk. It is used as a natural colourant in cosmetics.

Casein A protein found in the mammals' milk. It is used as a hair thickener and conditioner and as an emulsifier. It has no known toxicity.

Cationic surfactant see Surfactant.

Caustic soda (sodium hydroxide) A common reagent that is widely used in the manufacture of soap.

Cellulose gum A synthetic gum, of which the starting material is cellulose, used as a thickener in cosmetics and foods, and stabilizer.

Ceteareth-5 Cetearyl alcohol, which has been rendered soluble in water by condensing it with ethylene oxide. Used as a thickener and emulsifier in creams and lotions; it has no known toxicity.

Cetearyl alcohol Also known as cetyl stearyl alcohol or emulsifying wax, this is a mixture of cetyl and stearyl alcohols, which may be animal, vegetable or petrochemical derived. It is used as an emulsifier, emollient and thickener and is excellent for use in homemade creams and conditioners. It has no known toxicity.

Cetrimonium chloride A cationic surfactant, which is a quaternary ammonium salt. It is used in conditioners and also as an antiseptic and preservative. Concentrated solutions can irritate the skin, and it is toxic internally.

Cetyl alcohol An alcohol consisting of mainly n-hexadecanol. It is used as a thickener and emulsifier. See also Cetearyl alcohol.

Chelatory agent A substance that binds minerals to itself. In cosmetic manufacture it refers to chemicals that mop up free ions, such as metals, in formulae and inhibit them from causing deterioration of the product.

Chloromethyl isothiarzolinone One of the components of Kathon GG, which is the trade name for a commonly used preservative. Its popularity is due to its effectiveness at very low concentrations. Skin sensitization is possible.

Chlorophyll The green pigment of plants that is essential for photosynthesis. It is used as a natural colourant.

Chloroxylenol An antimicrobial agent used in treatment shampoos and antiseptic lotions. It is apparently non-irritant at low dilutions of less than 5 per cent.

Citric acid A component of citrus fruits used as a pH modifier in cosmetics and foods. It has no known toxicity.

Clay A natural aluminosilicate – that is, a compound based on aluminium, silicon and oxygen. It is used in face masks because of its absorbing, cleansing ability and also as a thickener in some shampoo ingredients.

Coal tar Tar obtained during the distillation of coal. It is used as an anti-dandruff ingredient. It can cause dermatitis on the skin.

Cocamide DEA An unchanged (non-ionic) surfactant, derived from chemically modified coconut oil and used in shampoos and cleansers.

Cocamidopropyl betaine Properly called cocamidopropyl dimethyl glycine, it is used as a mild foaming and cleansing agent to reduce the irritancy of harsher surfactants in shampoos.

Cocobetaine An amphoteric surfactant, which is based on chemical modifications to coconut oil. It is included in shampoos and cleansing rinses and, used correctly, will help render certain other surfactants more mild.

Cocotrimonium chloride An antionic surfactant used as a hair conditioner. It can be an irritant to the eyes.

Co-emulsifiers Secondary emulsifiers that improve the stability of emulsion systems when making creams and lotions.

Collagen The most abundant protein in the body, containing mainly glycerine, hydroxyproline and prioline. It is found in all connective tissues, such as skin. When the collagen in the skin deteriorates, due to ageing or overexposure to the sun, the appearance of the skin is affected by wrinkles. It is sometimes used in cosmetics and toiletries, although there is no evidence that external application is effective.

Concrète The by-product obtained from solvent extraction of an aromatic material. The solvent is generally evaporated off to leave behind the absolute and the concrète – for example, rose absolute and rose concrète.

Contact dermatitis A condition in which the skin has become damaged through topical contact with chemicals. Two types exist: primary irritation, which occurs at the time of contact and can cause itchy swelling and redness, and allergic sensitization, in which symptoms arise after several exposures to the chemical.

Coupling agent A material used to increase the solubility of one ingredient in another.

Cream The source of highly concentrated proteins, which are readily absorbed by the skin.

DEA lauryl sulphate Diethanolamine salt of lauryl sulphate, used as a foaming and cleansing agent. It may be irritant in concentration.

Decyl alcohol An anti-foaming agent, fixative, lubricant and emollient. It occurs naturally in some plant oils but is commercially extracted from coconut oil or paraffin. It has no known toxicity.

Dimethicone Dimethicone copolyol, a polymer based on silicone, which is used as a conditioner in hair-care products and as a skin protectant. It has a tendency to build up on the hair shaft, eventually making the hair appear dull and is not, therefore, currently favoured. It is not considered toxic.

Deodorant Any product that masks the odour produced by the action of bacteria or sweat. Unlike an antiperspirant, a deodorant does not interfere with the production of sweat.

Depilatory A preparation designed to aid hair removal. This may be chemical, as in hair-dissolving creams, or mechanical, as in wax.

Detergent A chemical used as a cleansing agent and unlike soap does not derive directly from fats and oils. Detergents modify the interface between two surfaces (see Surfactant). They may derive from petroleum (most household detergents) or vegetable oil.

Dimethyl stearamine see Surfactant.

Dioctyl sodium sulfosuccinate Used as a dispersing agent and solubilizer – usually to disperse essential oils in a cosmetic product. It is non-irritant in dilution.

Dipentene Another name for limonene – see also Limonene.

Dipropylene glycol see Propylene glycol.

Disodium EDTA A compound used as an antioxidant, preservative and chelating agent to form complexes with elements and stop any catalytic reactions from occurring. It is not generally considered to be toxic externally, although sensitization is possible.

Disodium monococamido sulfosuccinate see Dioctyl sodium sulfosuccinate.

Disodium phosphate see Sodium phosphate.

DMDM hydantoin A water-soluble preservative. It can be toxic at a high level, but used within the guidelines is essentially safe. See also Disodium EDTA.

EDTA Ethylene diamine tetra acetic acid, used as a chelating agent in shampoos and also as an antioxidant. It is chemically synthesized. See also Disodium EDTA.

Elastin A protein of elastic tissue of the skin, ligaments and arterial wall. It is structurally related to collagen.

Electrolyte A substance that undergoes partial or complete dissociation into ions in solution. Electrolytes are important in cosmetics and toiletries because they can affect viscosity and other properties of the product. Salt, for example, is a common electrolyte used to thicken some shampoos.

Emollient Any substance that prevents water loss from the skin. Most natural oils perform this function.

Emulsifier A substance that holds oil in water or water in oil. Examples include borax, beeswax and cetearyl alcohol. Emulsifiers are necessary in the manufacture of creams and lotions.

Emulsifying wax A wax used to prepare stable emulsions such as creams and lotions. See also Cetearyl alcohol.

Emulsion A mixture of two incompatible substances. Most creams on the cosmetic market are emulsions consisting of oil-soluble ingredients mixed with water-soluble ingredients by the use of emulsifiers.

Enzyme A biological catalyst that acts to speed up chemical reactions. Digestive enzymes are necessary for the breakdown of protein, carbohydrates and fats – for example, pancreatin and pepsin.

Epsom salts Magnesium sulphate used as a purgative and in bath salts used for detoxifying and relaxation.

Essential fatty acid A fatty acid that must be supplied in the diet as the body cannot produce it itself. They include linoleic, linolenic and arachidonic acids. The first two are found in evening primrose oil and the latter in beeswax.

Essential oil The odorous, volatile product of a known botanical origin. Most essential oils are produced by steam distillation, although some are mechanically expressed; they are used therapeutically in aromatherapy. When using essential oils at home, it is important to know the plant species, origin, chemotype and the method of extraction of the oil if you are looking for a therapeutic benefit. See also Absolute.

Ester A derivative of an acid. Many esters have fruity smells and are used in artificial fruit essences.

Ethanol Alcohol is manufactured by the fermentation of sugar, starch and other carbohydrates. Ethanol, or ethyl alcohol, used in cosmetic formulation such as perfumes and aftershaves is usually denatured by the addition of an unpleasant-tasting chemical to stop consumption.

Ethanolamine A component manufactured by heating ethylene oxide under pressure with concentrated aqueous ammonia. They form soaps with fatty acids. They are used for pH control or, when linked to fatty acids, as solubilizers and thickeners. The di- and tri-ethanolamines are able to form highly toxic nitrosamines under certain conditions and so their manufacture must be carefully monitored. Can be irritant in high concentrations.

Ethoxylate A substance – often a detergent – that has had ethylene oxide added to render it more water soluble. There is some concern about the impact of the ethoxylation process on the environment because of the presence of 1,4 Dioxane, a by-product of the process and a suspected carcinogen.

Ethyl parabens see Parabens.

Eucalyptol Also known as 1,8 Cineole. The chief component of the essential oil derived from *Eucalyptus globulus*.

Eugenol The chief constituent of clove oil but also found in cinnamon oil and bay oil. It has excellent antiseptic properties.

Exfoliate To remove surface layers of the skin, especially dead skin cells, generally by the use of an abrasive agent.

Expression Describes the technique used for extracting essential oils from citrus products. See also Essential oil.

Fat A greasy solid that is an ester of fatty acids and glycerol. Fats can be used in the soap-making process, and glycerol is generally a by-product.

Fatty acid A monobasic acid containing only the chemicals carbon, hydrogen and oxygen. Found in vegetable and animal fats, they are important for maintaining a healthy skin and are excellent emollients.

Fatty acid alkanolamides see Ethanolamine.

F D & C colours Refers to colours that are permitted in the USA in food, drugs and cosmetics.

Fixative A material that helps to slow the rate of evaporation of components of perfume formulations, thereby making the fragrance last longer. Certain essential oils, for example sandalwood, have fixative properties.

Filtration The process of separating a solid from a liquid or gas by the use of a membrane that will allow only the liquid or gas to pass through.

Fixed oil It is chemically the same as a fat, but is generally liquid. Examples include almond oil, apricot kernel oil and grapeseed oil.

Flashpoint Refers to the lowest temperature at which the vapour above a flammable liquid will ignite on application of a flame. Alcohol has a low flashpoint.

Flavoprotein One of a group of proteins containing riboflavin. They act as oxygen carriers in biological systems.

Fluoride This inorganic substance and some of its compounds are used in toothpastes to slow tooth decay. In some countries it is added to the water supply prior to reaching the consumer. High doses can cause dental fluorosis, nausea, vomiting and even death.

Foam A coarse dispersion of a gas in a liquid, observed as bubbles. Many modern shaving gels contain low boiling point gases, which boil off and cause foaming when applied to the face. Foam does not actually enhance either cleansing ability or mildness.

Follicle A small cavity in the skin containing the hair root.

Formaldehyde An antimicrobial used in many household products and toiletries. It is irritating to the mucous membranes and can be toxic. Its use is banned or restricted in many countries these days.

Free radicals Molecules or ions with impaired electrons that are extremely reactive. They cause many of the rancidity reactions that occur in natural oils and antioxidants are added to products to prevent this.

Freeze drying The removal of water from a frozen solid.

Fuller's earth An absorptive clay consisting of fine siliceous material, used in face masks to draw out impurities from the skin. It may be used instead of talc.

Fungicide A substance that is able to kill at least some types of fungi.

Fungistatic A material inhibiting the growth and multiplication of some types of fungi.

Gas chromatography (also gas liquid chromatography, GLC) A method of analysis often used to help determine the components of essential oils and other liquids.

Gel A suspension of solid and liquid particles that exists as a solid or semi-solid mass. It usually refers to a water-based product that has been thickened by the addition of a gelling agent.

Gelatin Gelatin is manufactured from the bones and hides of animals by purifying the protein collagen. It is used as a thickener, to form gels and in the manufacture of capsule shells.

Geraniol A fresh-smelling alcohol that exists naturally in many essential oils such as geranium and palmarosa.

Glucose glutamate A reaction product formed from glucose and glutanic acid which is used as a conditioning/moisturising agent. It is essentially non-toxic.

Glycereth The product resulting from the condensation of glycerol with ethylene oxide. It is a humectant to provide moisturising. See also Glycerin.

Glyceryl stearate A white, waxy solid that is prepared by combining glycerol and stearic acid chemically. It is used as an emulsifier and a moisturizing ingredient. It is considered non-toxic.

Glycerin A colourless, odourless, viscous liquid with a very sweet taste. Known technically as glycerol, it is a form of alcohol that is used as a solvent, sweetener and humectant in cosmetics and can be manufactured from animal or plant material. It is non-toxic.

Glycerol see Glycerin

Glycol stearate Also known as glycol distearate, this is a reaction product of glycol and stearic acid commonly used as an emulsifier in creams. It has no known toxicity.

Glycolic acid An acid used for pH control. It can be extremely irritating to the skin.

Glycols The materials containing the alcohol groups. They tend to be very thick, humectant liquids which are often used as solubilizers and to impart a moisturizing effect.

Glycyrrhizic acid An acid derived from liquorice root. It has antibacterial properties, which make it particularly suitable for use in deodorants.

Guar hydroxypropyltrimonium chloride A cationic surfactant derived from chemically modified guar gum. It is used in some detergent products, such as shampoos.

Hardness of water Refers to water containing alkaline earth salts, which prevent formation of a lather with soaps. Detergents can help remove the hardness of water.

Hectorite A mineral found in bentonite clay used as a thickening agent and for its absorption and conditioning properties.

Histamine A chemical released via the body's immune system in response to allergens.

Humectant A substance that reduces water loss from the skin and aids moisturization.

Hydrocarbon A molecule consisting of just hydrogen and carbon. They are generally petrochemical derived and are used as propellants in aerosols and as emollients in cosmetics.

Hydrochloric acid A strong acid used for pH adjustment in some toiletries. It is highly irritant in concentration.

Hydrogenated oil An oil that has hydrogen added to solidify it.

Hydrogen peroxide A chemical used in cosmetics for bleaching and perming hair. It also has antiseptic properties. It is very potent and in concentration can cause damage to the hair shaft and burning on the skin.

Hydrolysed animal protein An animal protein that has been broken down chemically to remove hydrogen and used in toiletries to improve the feel of skin and hair. Some reactions can occur with milk protein.

Hydroscopic Capable of absorbing moisture from the atmosphere.

Hypoallergenic In the strictest sense means without fragrance, but more broadly refers to products that are unlikely to cause skin irritation.

Hydrolysis A decomposition reaction that involves the splitting of water into its ions at the formation of a weak acid or base, or both.

Hydromethylcellulose A chemically modified form of cellulose that is used as a thickening agent in products such as eye gels.

IFRA The International Fragrance Association, which provides information, recommendations and guidelines on the legislative, toxicological and dermatological aspects of perfumery.

Imidazolidinyl urea An antimicrobial agent, commonly used as a preservative in toiletries. It can release formaldehyde into formulations if not used correctly. It can cause sensitization but is generally considered to be of low toxicity.

IMS Industrial Methylated Spirits, generally of ethanol, which has a chemical added to make it unsuitable for internal consumption.

Infusion The liquid resulting from boiling plant material with water in order to extract water-soluble plant components.

Insecticide A material used to control insects. Citronella essential oil provides an excellent natural insecticide.

Insoluble Material that does not dissolve in a solvent.

Iron oxide A pigment used to colour cosmetics.

Irritant Any compound that causes a negative skin reaction on application or sometimes after application.

Isoluitane A propellant used in aerosol products.

Isoprene The smallest building block of terpenes and found in certain essential oils.

Isopropyl myristate A chemically modified fatty acid that has emollient properties and used in certain skin creams. It is generally considered to be non-toxic, although there is concern that its use increases the ability of the skin to absorb other more toxic compounds – nitrosamines, for example.

Kaolin A white powdery clay, also known as china clay, which arises following decomposition of feldspars in granites. It is used in face powder and clay masks for its absorption properties.

Kathon CG The trade name for the preservative octhilinone, which is used as a fungicide and preservative in shampoos and cosmetics. Sensitization is possible.

Keratin A fibrous protein found in hair and nails.

Keralolytic An agent that causes skin shedding and removes surface layers of skin.

Laneth-16 A mixture of ethoxylates produced from lanolin alcohol used for emulsifying and solubilizing. It can be a mild irritant.

Lanolin A preparation of cholesterol and its esters obtained from wool fat. The lanolin is washed off the wool of living sheep. In the past many people thought they were allergic to lanolin; they were actually allergic to the detergent that was used to extract the lanolin from the wool. In recent years only mild detergent is used. Anhydrous lanolin refers to lanolin that does not contain water. Lanolin is an excellent emollient and thickener and is used in creams, conditioners and so on. It is protective to the skin and well tolerated by people with sensitive skin.

Lanolin alcohol A mixture of alcohols obtained by hydrolysis of lanolin, used for its moisturizing properties.

Lauramide MIPA A non-ionic surfactant used for emulsifying properties. See also Lauric acid.

Laureth 1 to 23 Products of the combination of ethylene oxide with lauryl alcohol to enhance emulsifying properties.

Lauric acid A fatty acid occurring in milk, laurel oil, coconut oil, palm oil and other vegetable oils. It is used to make soaps, detergents and lauryl alcohol.

Lauryl alcohol A fatty alcohol often obtained from coconut oil, used to make anionic surfactants such as sodium laureth sulphate. It has good foaming qualities, hence it is used in products such as shampoos. It is mildly irritant in concentration but it is non-sensitizing.

Lauryl betaine A synthetic detergent based on vegetable-derived raw materials which is used to create milder formulations when combined with detergents such as sodium lauryl sulphate. It is commonly used in shampoos. See also Lauric alcohol.

Lauryl sulphate Derived from lauryl alcohol, this is used to make detergents as in ammonium lauryl sulphate, sodium lauryl sulphate.

Lecithin An excellent natural emulsifier present in all living organisms but usually commercially derived from the processing of soya oil. It contains a mixture of stearic, palmitic and oleic acid compounds and has antioxidant and emollient properties. It is used in skin and hair care products.

Lethal dose (LD/50) The lethal dose of a substance that, when administered to a group of experimental animals over a period given, causes the death of 50 per cent of them.

Lignin A naturally occurring polymer found with cellulose in lignified plant tissues. Kelp seaweed is a rich source of lignin, which is thought to help detoxify the body as it passes through the system.

Lime soap An insoluble calcium and magnesium fatty acid soap formed when soluble soaps are added to hard water.

Limonene A component of many essential oils. Also manufactured synthetically for use in household cleaners. Irritant in concentration.

Linalool An alcohol that is a component in many essential oils, such as lavender and coriander.

Linoleic acid An unsaturated fatty acid that occurs in some vegetable oils, especially linseed oil.

Lipids Natural substances of a fat-like nature.

Liposomes Artificial microscopic sacs used for the introduction of various agents into cells in vitro. They can be manufactured from a variety of substances, including phospholipids. Some manufacturers incorporate them into skin creams and claim they can be used to deliver certain substances to the underlying layers of the skin.

Litmus A natural colouring matter obtained from lichens used as an indicator of the presence of certain chemicals.

Lake An insoluble pigment obtained by the combination of an

organic colouring matter with an inorganic compound. Lakes are used primarily in colour cosmetics.

Lye Potassium or sodium hydroxide, a strong alkaline base found in hair straighteners.

Magnesium aluminium silicate A component of natural clays that is used as a thickener and suspending agent.

Magnesium sulphate see Epsom salts.

Malic acid An acid found in certain herbs and fruits. It has antioxidant and astringent properties.

Medicated products Products that contain active ingredients to produce a specific physiological action.

Melanin The dark pigment of hair, skin and eyes. It arises by oxidation of tyrosine by the action of tyrosinase, especially during exposure to the sun.

Methyl parabens see Parabens.

Mica Silicate compounds used in eye colour cosmetics to create a glittery effect.

Milk A cleanser, emollient, moisturizer and softener, readily absorbed by the skin. Milk is high in protein, calcium and vitamins. Sensitization is possible.

Mineral oil An oil obtained as a by-product of petroleum refinement, frequently used in cosmetics and toiletries such as lipsticks and baby oil for its emollient and lubricant properties. Mineral oil is not readily absorbed by the skin and tends to block the pores. It can be useful in producing barrier creams. It is not considered toxic.

Mucous membranes Thin layers of tissue that line the respiratory, intestinal and genito-urinary tracts. They produce mucus as a protective film. They tend to be more sensitive and permeable to all types of preparations than other areas of skin.

Mud Draws impurities through the skin and removes excess surface oil, dirt and grime. It can also be used to cleanse the hair. Mud packs have long been used for cleansing and therapeutic purposes.

Musk The dried secretion from the sexual glands of the male musk deer. In the past it was much valued for its use in perfumes as a fragrance and fixative. Its use has declined in recent years as it has been replaced with the synthetic musk ambrette.

Myristalkonium chloride A quaternary ammonium compound used as a cationic surfactant in conditioning rinses. It can be irritant to eyes and skin in concentration.

Myristic acid A solid organic acid occurring naturally in many animal and vegetable fats, notably coconut oil. It is combined with potassium to produce a soap with a copious lather. It has no known toxicity.

Myristyl alcohol An emollient prepared from fatty acids and used in creams and lotions. It is non-toxic.

Nail polish A varnish used to colour the nails that is a cocktail of many chemicals, including nitro-cellulose, butyl acetate, toluene, alkyl esters, glycol derivatives, gums, hydrocarbons, lakes and ketones. Nail polish is one of the most toxic and irritant of all cosmetics.

Nail polish remover The main active ingredient in most nail polish removers is acetone, but many commercial formulae also contain conditioning agents. Acetone is a synthetic ingredient that is highly dangerous if taken internally – be sure to wash nails thoroughly after using remover to avoid any being ingested. In fact, acetone is already banned or restricted in many countries.

Natural No official definition exists, but this term generally refers to products that exist in nature and are not further processed.

Natural colouring Food and cosmetic dyes which are unprocessed. The range of colours is limited and they are more prone to fading than synthetic dyes. The accepted natural colourings are less likely to be toxic than synthetic dyes. See also Carmine, Carotene.

Nerol An alcohol found in many essential oils including neroli, lemongrass, orange and rose.

Niacin Vitamin B3.

Nitrosamines Compounds formed by the combination of a secondary amine with an oxide of nitrogen. They are highly carcinogenic in even minute quantities (parts per million).

They are found in food products such as cured bacon, beer and also in cosmetics. In formulating products, care must be taken to prevent the formation of nitrosamines by monitoring pH and using antioxidant compounds. Some raw materials by their nature have the potential to cause nitrosamine formation and these must be especially closely monitored when used in formulae.

Non-ionic surfactant A surface active agent that has no electrical charge on it. Examples include polysorbate 20, cetyl stearyl alcohol. They can render formulations much milder.

Nonoxynol-10 A non-ionic emulsifier that is a derivative of phenol. It is irritant in concentration.

Occlusive agent A substance that prevents compounds from leaving a surface. On the skin, oils can act as occlusive agents by preventing the evaporation of water.

Octyl dimethyl paba see PABA.

Oil Describes a naturally occurring hydrocarbon that can be plant, animal or mineral derived.

Ointment base A base to which you can add your own tinctures or essential oils – available from Neal's Yard Remedies stores. It contains de-ionized water, glycerine, polysorbate-20, cetyl stearyl alcohol, beeswax, jojoba oil, methyl parabens and propyl parabens.

Oleakonium chloride A quaternary ammonium compound that is a cationic surfactant with conditioning and antistatic properties.

Oleic acid An emollient with good skin-penetrating properties. Obtained from animal or vegetable fats, it oxidizes rapidly on exposure to the air. It is mildly irritant.

Oleoresin A plant extract consisting of essential oil and resin extracted using a solvent. Oleoresins may then be further diluted using a base oil – for example, benzoin extract, carrot extract.

Oleth 2-20 Oily products derived from fatty alcohols and used as surfactants. They have no known toxicity.

Oleyl alcohol An oily product that is obtained from tallow, fish oil and vegetable oils, such as palm oil. It is used in the manufacture of detergents as an antifoam agent and for its emollient properties. It has no known toxicity.

Opacifying agent A substance used to make cosmetics and toiletries appear opaque and improve their aesthetic appeal.

Organic Describes products that have been certified as grown without the use of artificial pesticides and fertilizers by the Soil Association or other certifying authority.

Oxidation A chemical reaction involving oxygen and causing rancidity to many natural oils. Antioxidants are often added to prevent this happening.

Ozokerite A naturally occurring mineral wax that is used as a thickener. It has no known toxicity.

PABA A water-soluble acid (para-aminobenzoic acid) found in B vitamins and used as a sunscreen agent. Natural PABA is a skin sensitizer; synthetically produced octyl dimethyl PABA is not.

Pantothenic acid (B5) A B-complex water-soluble vitamin, used in hair and skin-care products for its moisturizing actions. It has no known toxicity.

Parabens Parahydroxybenzoic acid esters used as preservatives in foods, cosmetics and toiletries. They have a broad spectrum antimicrobial action. They are found in nature, but for commercial purposes are synthetically produced. They have a long history of relatively safe use, but like all synthetic preservatives they do have some potential for irritation. Commonly used parabens include methyl parabens, propyl parabens, ethyl parabens and butyl parabens. Effective levels are 0.1–0.3 per cent concentration in the overall product. See also Propyl parabens.

Paraffin wax Wax derived from petrochemicals, used as a moisturizer and thickener.

Patch test Describes the technique of applying a small amount of a product prior to full use to see if any allergic reaction occurs. The best places to try a patch test are on the inside of the elbow or, if that is not appropriate, the inside of the wrist. Leave at least two hours for each test. Doing a patch test is strongly advisable prior to buying or trying a new product for anyone with sensitive skin.

Pearlizing agent see Opacifying agent.

Pectin The dried extract of various fruit rinds or vegetables, used as a natural thickener.

PEG derivatives Derivatives of polyethylene glycol, which is prepared from ethylene oxide and water, dihydroxyethane or diethylene glycol plus a base. The amount of ethylene oxide present will dictate the water solubility. These are used as humectants, solubilizers and moisturizing agents. PEG products can be combined with oils such as castor oil (for example, PEG 20 Castor Oil) and lanolin to produce a range of non-ionic surfactants which can be used as emulsifiers and conditioners. PEG is usually written with a number after it, for example PEG 24, the number referring to the viscosity; the lower the number the more liquid the product. PEG derivatives are not considered toxic; those with a higher number (lower molecular level), for example, PEG 200-400, may be sensitisers.

Perfume A product used for fragrancing the body, generally based on a combination of fragrant oils with alcohol. Throughout history essential oils and flower waters have been used as perfume materials, though since the 1920s most famous perfumes have also included synthetic fragrances. Perfume or fragrance is often the most likely ingredient in a product to cause sensitization; hence hypoallergenic products are without fragrance. Eau de parfum is highly concentrated, eau de toilette less so.

Petroleum jelly (petrolatum, vaseline) A salve-like material derived from petroleum which is used as a lubricant and emollient in many cosmetics and toiletries. It is not considered toxic; however, sensitization is possible.

Phenoxyethanol An antimicrobial agent (preservative) often used in combination with parabens. It is manufactured by combining phenol (coal tar derived) with ethylene oxide. It is irritant at high concentrations and sensitization is possible. See also Parabens.

Phosphoric acid Used for pH adjustments of products. Irritant in concentration, but not considered toxic in cosmetic use.

Phytosterols Fatty alcohols that are derived from plants.

Phytotherapy Using plants and herbs for their therapeutic value.

Polyacrylamide A polymer produced by a combination of acrylamide and sodium acrylate that is used as a thickener and additive in tanning products and nail polish. It is toxic and irritant.

Polymer Whenever many small molecules are combined the result is called a polymer. Examples include plastics and animal tissue. In cosmetics it generally refers to a group of non-ionic surfactants based on fatty acid esters of Sorbiton that are used as foaming, cleansing and dispersing agents.

Polyquaternium companiol A synthetic polymer that is combined with ammonium to produce a positively charged nitrogen, rendering it a cationic surfactant. They are used in hair-care products because of their substantivity to hair. See also Quaternary ammonium compound.

Polysorbates 1-85 Products of the combination of lauric acid with sorbitol, which is condensed with ethylene oxide to render it water-soluble. They are generally considered mild and non-toxic. Their main functions are as solubilizers and emulsifiers.

Preservative A substance added to products to prevent their deterioration. Bacteria and fungi will grow in any product with a significant water content. Preservatives are added to inhibit (bacteriostatic) or kill (antibiotic) those microbes that would otherwise cause spoilage. To have a realistic shelf life, most commercially manufactured products contain preservatives; otherwise products must be kept in the refrigerator and replaced every few days.

Propane A propellant used in aerosols.

Propolis A substance produced by bees to protect their hive from viral or bacterial attack. Propolis has a preservative and antibiotic action. It is available as a tincture and may be combined into cosmetic formulations.

Propylene glycol A colourless, almost odourless liquid, synthetically produced. It is used in perfumes and flavourings and as a solvent, humectant and moisturizing ingredient in a wide range of cosmetics and toiletries. Sensitization is possible.

Propyl parabens A commonly used broad-spectrum preservative. Recent evidence suggests that people with certain types of cancer produce an excess of propyl parabens and due to this link the popularity of this substance is declining. There is no evidence to date that propyl parabens causes cancer. See also Parabens.

Protein Building blocks of the human body, which are composed of a combination of amino acids. Keratin, which makes up the hair, is an example.

Quaternary ammonium compound A compound based on ammonium salts where the hydrogen atoms have been replaced by other chemical groups. These compounds are cationic and can be combined with other materials to provide a range of chemical functions, mainly preservatives and surfactants. Examples are Quaternarium 1-30 and Benzalkonium chloride. Many are irritant in concentration. Sensitization is possible.

Resorcinol A synthetically derived alcohol that is used in dandruff shampoos to prevent itching; it also acts as a preservative and reduces skin greasiness. It is a known sensitizer and is irritant in concentration.

Retinoids Derivatives of vitamin A, used in anti-ageing creams and acne treatments. They are toxic in concentration.

Rosin The residue left after distilling off the volatile oil from the oleoresin obtained from *Pinus palustris* and other species of pine trees. It is used in cosmetics and toiletries in soaps, lacquers and depilatory waxes. Sensitization is possible.

Rum Alcohol produced from the distillation of fermented molasses or sugar-cane. Rum reduces the production of oil by the sweat glands and is a traditional hair tonic, especially for greasy hair.

Salicylic acid This occurs naturally as methyl salicylate – for example, in oil of wintergreen, from which it can be obtained by treatment with alcoholic potassium hydroxide. The synthetic version, which is more often used commercially, is used in cosmetics as an antiseptic and preservative and for treating acne. Sensitization is possible.

Salt see Sodium chloride.

Saponification The process used in soap-making whereby an oil or fat is reacted with a strong base, for example caustic soda, to produce a soap.

Saponins A group of sugar-based substances forming solutions that foam on shaking. Saponins occur naturally, for example in soapwort herb and quillaja bark, and are also produced synthetically. They are used in cosmetics and drinks for their foaming properties.

SD alcohol An alcohol that has been denatured by the addition of a compound that renders it undrinkable.

Sensitizer A product that causes an allergic reaction. Initial exposure to the product may not cause a noticeable reaction, but subsequent or repeated exposure may cause a severe inflammatory response.

Shellac A resinous substance excreted by various insects on to trees, used as a lacquer and binder. Sensitization is possible.

Silicone A widely used group of oils and compounds derived from the mineral silica. Silicones are water repellent and very stable. There is no known toxicity when used externally.

Silicone derivatives These products, based on silicone, are used in hair-care and skin-care products. Their use in hair care is becoming less popular because they have a tendency to cause build-up. They have no known toxicity.

Simethicone A mixture of dimethicone and silica, used as a conditioning agent. It has no known toxicity.

Sodium ascorbate Salt form of vitamin C used as an antioxidant and preservative in cosmetics.

Sodium benzoate An antiseptic and preservative used in food and cosmetics. It is non-toxic externally.

Sodium bicarbonate An alkaline substance used in deodorants and toothpastes for its absorption properties and as a pH neutralizer.

Sodium borate see Borax.

Sodium carbonate Known as washing soda when hydrated. It is used in glass, soap and chemical detergents. Sensitization is possible.

Sodium chloride Common salt, used as an astringent and antiseptic. It also appears in some cosmetic formulations, such as shampoos, as a thickener. It is considered non-toxic and non-irritant externally in dilution.

Sodium citrate Salt of citric acid, used medicinally as a blood anticoagulant and in cosmetics as a buffering agent and sequestrant. It is non-toxic externally.

Sodium hydroxide see Caustic soda.

Sodium lactate A thick colourless liquid that is a natural component of the skin's upper layers, used for its moisturizing properties.

Sodium lauryl sulphate A synthetic detergent of which the origins may be plant (coconut and palm kernel oil) or animal. It is one of the most common ingredients used in shampoos and toothpastes for its foaming and detergent properties. It can be irritant in concentration, but correct formulation renders it functional with low irritancy.

Sodium laureth sulphate Similar to sodium lauryl sulphate except that it contains ethylene oxide to render it more water-soluble and consequently milder. See also Ethoxylate.

Sodium monofluorophosphate Used in toothpastes to provide fluoride to prevent tooth decay. See also Fluoride.

Sodium silicate A mineral-derived component often found in clays such as kaolin and bentonite.

Sodium tetraborate see Borax.

Soft detergents Detergents that are biodegradable.

Solvent A substance used to dissolve solute or extract components from solid material.

Solvent extraction The removal of soluble material from a solid mixture by means of a solvent or the removal of components from a liquid mixture by use of a solvent with which the liquid is unmixable, or nearly so.

Sorbic acid Obtained from the berries of the rowan tree (*Sorbus aucuparia*) or synthetically manufactured, sorbic acid is used as a preservative, binder and humectant in cosmetics. It is non-toxic and non-irritant in dilution. Sensitization is possible.

Sorbitan fatty acid esters Mixtures of fatty acids with esters of sorbitol, for example sorbitan oleate and sorbitan stearate. They have wide-ranging use in cosmetics as emulsifying, stabilizing, surfactant and thickening agents. They are generally considered to be non-toxic and non-irritant, although they may cause blackheads in susceptible individuals.

Sorbitan oleate A reaction product of oleic acid and sorbitol, used as a thickener and emollient. It has been reported to cause blackheads.

Sorbitol Alcohol derivative of glucose used as a humectant, binder and sweetener in cosmetics. It occurs naturally in certain fruits. It is non-toxic externally.

SPF Sun protection factor, an indicator of the degree of sun protection that a sunscreen offers. As a rule, for each SPF number 20 minutes of sun protection is offered by correct use of the product. Low SPF products tend to be in the SPF range of 1–6; medium SPF 7–11; and high 12 to 30+. There is some debate as to whether an SPF over 20 does in fact offer greater protection. The SPF rating applies to UVB protection only. See also Sunscreens.

Squalene A component of various animal and vegetable oils, commercially extracted from shark-liver oil, which has lubricant and fixative properties. It has no known toxicity.

Starch A sugar polymer derived from plant sources, used in cosmetics for its absorbent and soothing properties. Sensitization to various forms of starch is possible.

Stearalkonium chloride see Quaternary ammonium compound.

Steareth compounds Compounds produced by ethoxylation of stearyl alcohol, which are used as solubilizers and co-emulsifiers.

Stearic acid A waxy, fatty acid that can be derived from tallow and other animal fats, but also from cocoa butter and other vegetable fats. It is used as an emulsifier and emollient in soaps, creams and lotions. It is non-toxic. Sensitization is unusual but possible.

Stratum corneum The outer hardened layer of the skin.

Sunscreens Substances used to block out the sun's burning rays. Sunscreens may act in two main ways: chemical sunscreens, for example PABA, which refract the sun's rays; and physical sunscreens, for example titanium dioxide, which block the sun's rays from reaching the skin. Sunscreens are also divided into those that

protect against UVB light, which causes immediate burning (and this is what the SPF system is based on); and those that protect against UVA light, which is thought to cause longer term but less immediately obvious damage and premature ageing. See also SPF.

Surfactant A substance with the ability to reduce the surface tension at the interface between two unlike surfaces. Soap is an example, as are all detergents. Amphoteric surfactants have both a positive (cationic) group and a negative (anionic) group. The final pH of a product will dictate which group is more dominant. At an intermediate pH, both forms are present. At a pH of less than 7 the cationic group is more prevalent, and at a pH of over 7 the anionic group is more prevalent. They tend to be very mild and are often found in baby products. Anionic surfactants are negatively charged surface active agents used widely in shampoo and foaming baths as the primary cleansing agent. These are chemically produced, although the raw materials used to produce them can be vegetable, animal or mineral derived. Examples include ammonium lauryl sulphate and sodium laureth sulphate. Cationic surfactants are detergents of which the ions are positively charged. They are used mainly in conditioners. See also Detergent.

Talc Magnesium silicate, obtained by mining, also known as talcum powder or French chalk. It has soothing, absorbtive and anti-chafing properties and is used in body powders and as a base for many colour cosmetics. It is irritant if inhaled. There is some evidence of toxicity if it is absorbed through the skin.

Tallow Fat obtained from the fatty tissue of animals (usually cows and sheep), used to make some soaps, emulsifiers and glycerol.

Tannins A large group of substances found in plants. They are used for their astringency.

Terpinol One of the active components of tea tree oil, also found in other oils.

Tincture An extract that has been prepared using alcohol and water to extract plant components.

Titanium dioxide A mineral salt that is used as a white pigment in makeup and as a physical sunblock in high SPF sunscreen lotions. It has no known external toxicity.

Tocopherol A form of vitamin E, usually extracted from soya oil. It is used as an antioxidant in a wide range of cosmetics and toiletries. It is non-toxic and non-sensitizing. Also known as vitamin E acetate.

Tragacanth A gum which is used as a thickener. Sensitization is possible.

Triclosan A white powder which is used as an antimicrobial and deodorant. It is a known sensitizer.

Triethanolamine A frequently used dispersing agent and emulsifier. It is irritant in concentration and sensitization is possible.

Urea A product of protein metabolism present in urine. It is used in cosmetics and toiletries as an antiseptic and preservative. It has no known toxicity externally.

Vegetable oil An oil extracted from a plant as opposed to an animal or mineral.

Vinegar Dilute acetic acid, used in cosmetics as an astringent and pH adjuster.

Viscosity Degree of pourability or stickiness. A highly viscous product is thick and sticky, for example treacle, while a product with low viscosity is readily pourable and 'thin' – water, for example.

Wax Fatty acid esters that are water-repellent and have plasticity.

Wetting agent A substance that increases the spreading of a liquid by reducing the tension between two surfaces.

Wool wax see Lanolin.

Xanthan gum Also known as corn sugar gum, this is a polysaccharide produced from bacteria (*Xanthomonas campestris*) fermented with a carbohydrate. It is used in food and cosmetics as a thickener, emulsifier and stabiliser. It has no known toxicity.

Zinc oxide A soft white powder used as a white pigment. It has antimicrobial, preservative and water-repellent properties. It is frequently used in baby creams to prevent nappy rash and is also effective as a sunscreen. It is not considered toxic in cosmetic use.

Zinc pyrithione A synthetic anti-dandruff active ingredient. It is a sensitizer and possible irritant.

glossary of therapies

As awareness of the inextricable link between mind and body grows, and as we take more responsibility for our own health, so different alternative therapies offer different healing paths to rediscovering ourselves through the places where we have become diseased. Alternative therapies offer a renewal of the relationship between our bodies, our minds and our lives.

Acupuncture A traditional form of Chinese medicine based on the understanding that the body is linked by energy pathways called meridians. Illness is seen as an imbalance of energy or a blockage of energy flow (qi). Practitioners use fine, sterile needles, which they insert into specific points on the meridians. This rebalances the person's energy, thus treating the underlying cause of the symptom.

Alexander technique An educational therapy which improves overall mental and physical well-being through changes in the physical use of your own body. Practitioners teach you how to use your body properly and how to develop balance and poise with minimum tension and energy and so avoid pain and strain.

Anthroposophical medicine A system of medicine using mainly plant and low potency homoeopathic remedies. Medicinal baths, massage, art therapy, eurythmics and counselling are also employed. It is based on the teachings of Rudolph Steiner, the founder of anthroposophy.

Aromatherapy The use of essential oils of flowers and plants in holistic treatments to improve health and prevent disease. Essential oils may be administered by massage, friction, inhalation, compresses and baths. Knowledge of the medicinal effects of individual essential oils has been acquired by use through the ages.

Ayurveda An ancient Indian system of healing based on the three main elements (doshas) in the body – in order to stay healthy the natural balance of these doshas must be maintained. Pulse diagnosis is used to help establish the body's imbalances. Herbal medicine, massage, diet and meditation may all be part of the overall treatment.

Autogenic training A technique of relaxation whereby you are taught to give yourself a series of suggestions and then taught to observe the result in your body of each suggestion. Leads to a heightened state of both relaxation and awareness.

Bach flower remedies see Flower therapies.

Bates method Through the repetition of simple processes a person can make themselves aware of how they are using their eyes, particularly if that person is suffering from eyestrain. By learning to use our eyes properly we can experience dramatic improvements in our sight.

Biomagnetic therapy A system of treatment based on the principles of acupuncture, using magnets instead of needles. Practitioners put small magnets on the meridians to rebalance the body's structure and energy flow.

Chinese medicine Chinese herbs (and often acupuncture) are used to bring the body back to its natural balance. Aimed at restoring the flow of qi (vital energy) between the yin and yang forces within the body. See also Acupuncture.

Chiropractic A system of physical manipulation based on the theory that diseases are mainly caused by impingements on spinal nerves and can be corrected through spinal and other adjustments. However, most people tend only to visit chiropracters for bad backs.

Colonic irrigation Using enema-type equipment and water, all toxic waste is washed out from the colon – cleaning the bowels is an excellent way to revitalize them. Colonic irrigation is very effective as part of a detoxifying programme and it is also a very good way to begin a fast.

Colour therapy The impact of colour on mood is widely recognised and colour can be used in coloured oils, as light, in crystals, in drawing, and so on, to treat mental, emotional and spiritual problems.

Counselling The client is given an empathetic space to talk about the things that are worrying him or her. A good counsellor will not offer solutions but help his client to find his or her own. Counselling is a branch of psychotherapy. See also Psychotherapy.

Cranial osteopathy Using subtle manipulation of the joints of the skull and attuning to and regulating the deep pulsing energy, as perceived by the cranial osteopath through the skull, deep changes in the rest of our bodies can be effected.

Crystal therapy Crystals focus healing energies. Crystal therapy is a preventative and curative form of treatment using crystals that focus healing vibrations and which act on the body's energy field. Crystals can be placed on specific parts of the body that need treatment.

Feldenkrais method Named after its originator, the therapist uses gentle touch to help the patient find alternative and more efficient patterns of movement and body organization. The patient learns to recognize unnecessary and destructive patterns in movement and behaviour, and to integrate more intelligent and constructive ones. The inner wisdom of the body is gently re-awakened; life can then be lived more easily with less pain or disturbance.

Feng shui The ancient Chinese art of creating and maintaining harmony and balance in your environment through the placement of objects, such as furniture and plants. Good feng shui can enhance energy and feelings of well-being.

Flower therapy A healing system to treat physical and other symptoms via presenting emotional symptoms. The remedies are made from the flowers of wild plants, bushes and trees and work to restore balance, a positive outlook and good health. The first collection of flower remedies was discovered in England by Edward Bach, hence Bach's flower remedies. Since then collections of healing flower remedies, such as the Australian bush remedies or the North American flower essences, have been gathered the world over.

Healing therapy (also known as Spiritual healing therapy) This therapy uses touch and the transfer of energy: the healer becomes the medium through whom healing energies are channelled to the patient.

Herbalism The practice of using plants to treat and prevent disease. These may be given in the form of teas, extracts, tinctures and tablets. Knowledge of the medicinal effects of different plants has been acquired since time immemorial.

Homoeopathy The word 'homoeopathy' comes from the Greek, meaning 'similar suffering'. Homoeopathy is based on the law of similars: 'like cures like.' This means that a remedy, given frequently to a healthy person, will produce the symptoms which that remedy can heal in a sick person. The correct homoeopathic remedy will stimulate the sick person's vitality to send healing energy where it is needed. Homoeopathic remedies do not work directly on the physical body, but rather by correcting imbalances – mental, emotional or psychic. Once rebalanced, the natural forces of the body then work to further restore physical health and harmony.

Hydrotherapy Waist compresses, body compresses, water jets, and so on, are all used to stimulate the circulation and the flow of energy through the body. Hydrotherapy is often used in conjunction with Naturopathy. See also Naturopathy.

Hypnotherapy By placing the client in a trance – making the conscious part of the brain temporarily less active – the hypnotherapist has the chance to unearth very deep hidden past experiences, which may be negatively affecting the client's present life. Powerful suggestions can be given while under hypnosis, which can effect conscious or unconscious behavioural changes.

Iridology A method of diagnosis rather than a treatment, based on the principle that different parts of the body are reflected in different parts of the eyes. Using a magnifier and a torch the practitioner examines the eyes to pin-point physical weaknesses or potential areas of trouble.

Kinesiology Using a series of simple muscle tests a practitioner can detect energy blockages and imbalances which cause illness. These may be the result of what has happened to the patient in the past, or from subtle allergies to different foods or substances. Dietary corrections and some direct physical rebalancing by the practitioner can lead to better health.

Massage The different parts of the body are systematically kneaded and rubbed, usually with oil, which results in an increased circulation of the blood and lymph flow. Essential oils which are added to massage oils are usually used for their therapeutic properties. Massage is usually very relaxing. The direct physical touch of the masseur can be healing too.

Meditation The technique of centering and gaining control of one's mind through exercises in self-observation, such as watching one's breath. Meditation brings about a state of increased awareness, inner harmony and profound relaxation.

Metamorphic technique A very light working of just a few areas on the feet, hands and head can effect profound healing changes by freeing one's own life force for healing. The technique is easily learned and self-treatment is also encouraged.

Naturopathy Our bodies function best when we avoid refined or toxic foods and eat only those foods which are completely natural. Naturopaths suggest different natural diets for different conditions to restore the body's ability to heal itself. Naturopathy is often used in conjunction with hydrotherapy and osteopathy. See also Hydrotherapy and Osteopathy.

Nutritional therapy Prevention and treatment of illness can be effected through the use of food and dietary supplements – for example, vitamins and minerals. Identified allergens are avoided and nutrient deficiencies are supplemented with tablets and/or a healthy diet.

Osteopathy The structure of the body, including bones, joints, ligaments, tendons, muscles and general connective tissue, are worked on in osteopathy. Practitioners will use manipulation, massage and stretching techniques. If the musculo-skeletal system is correctly aligned then other body systems, including healing, will function properly, too.

Pilates Through an instructor, pilates addresses the needs of individual clients with stretching exercises specially designed and carefully structured to strengthen the body. The stretches are slow and controlled, focusing on individual muscles or groups of muscles.

Polarity therapy By placing his or her hands on different parts of a patient's body, a therapist completes the vital energy (qi) circuit through his or her own body, thereby rebalancing the energy between different parts of the patient's body. Rebalanced energy leads to renewed health.

Psychotherapy Present day problems find their origins in early childhood experiences and problems. These are unearthed during psychotherapy. Through seeing the habitual patterns he or she is stuck in the client has a chance to change these for the better. A good psychotherapist will not offer solutions but help the client to find his or her own. See also Counselling.

Radionics Using a lock of your hair or a blood sample, for example, the practitioner employs dowsing techniques and/or uses radionic equipment to assess your condition to determine what treatment to give. It may not even be necessary to visit the radionic practitioner because once the practitioner has your 'witness' (that is, hair or blood sample, for example) he can 'broadcast' any remedy you may need to you over any distance using his radionic equipment.

Reflexology A system of treatment that works on the principle that specific areas of the feet – reflex points – correspond to different body organs. Pressure massage of the reflex points brings about healthy changes in the corresponding organs. Excellent results can be obtained in many acute first-aid situations, as well as ongoing chronic ones.

Reiki Illness tends to block our life-force energy. Practitioners of reiki channel universal energy to the recipient. This encourages the body to heal itself physically and emotionally.

Rolfing Deep, and often painful, manipulation of muscles and connective tissue helps to unknot the body and release trapped emotions, rebalancing the body. Posture is improved and injuries are relieved, and clients often report positive changes in their outlook.

Shamanism Drumming, chanting, spirit journeys and communing with non-ordinary states of reality are employed on this path towards self-development and healing.

Shiatsu Like acupuncture, this is a treatment which works on pressure points and energy pathways (meridians). Instead of needles, as in acupuncture, the practitioner uses his or her fingers and thumbs – and sometimes elbows, knees, hands and feet – to massage or apply firm pressure to the meridians to release and rebalance the flow of energy (qi).

Tomates Through a course of individually-tailored high frequency audio tapes one can improve not only one's hearing, but also release many negative experiences which have become trapped in one's body.

Traditional Chinese medicine see Chinese medicine

Yoga By adopting ancient stretching postures and breathing techniques, a person can maintain an excellent level of general health and flexibility.

useful addresses

The addresses below are arranged by therapy. As well as UK-based organizations, there are addresses for Australia and North America, and a complete list of Neal's Yard Remedies' outlets.

UK

COMPLEMENTARY MEDICINE

British Complementary Medicine Association (BCMA)
Kensington House, 33 Imperial Square
Cheltenham, Gloucestershire GL50 1QZ
tel: 01242 519911
web: www.bcma.co.uk

Complementary Medical Association
The Meridian, 142a Greenwich High Road
London SE10 8NN
tel: 020 8305 9571
web: www.phe-cma.org.uk

Council for Complementary & Alternative Medicine (CCAM)
63 Jeddo Road, London W12 9HQ
tel: 020 8735 0632

Institute for Complementary Medicine
PO Box 194, London SE16 7QZ
tel: 020 7237 5165
web: www.icmedicine.co.uk

British Register of Complementary Practitioners administered by **Institute for Complementary Medicine** (see above)

Natural Medicines Society
PO Box 232
East Molesey, Surrey KT8 1YF
tel: 020 8974 1166

ACUPUNCTURE

British Acupuncture Council
63 Jeddo Road, London W12 6HQ
tel: 020 8735 0400
web: www.acupuncture.org.uk

Society of Auricular Acupuncture
Nurstead Lodge, Nurstead
Meopham, Kent DA13 9AD
tel: 01474 813902
e-mail: paulineronson@
    nurstead49.fsbusiness.co.uk

ALEXANDER TECHNIQUE

Society of Teachers of the Alexander Technique
129 Camden Mews, London NW1 9AH
tel: 020 7284 3338
web: www.stat.org.uk

ANTHROPOSOPHICAL MEDICINE

Anthroposophical Medical Association
c/o Park Attwood Clinic, Trimpley
Bewdley, Worcestershire DY12 1RE
tel: 01299 861561
e-mail: movementoffice@btinternet.com

AROMATHERAPY

Aromatherapy Organizations Council
PO Box 19834, London SE25 6WF
tel: 020 8251 7912
web: www.aromatherapy-uk.org

The International Society of Professional Aromatherapists
82 Ashby Road, Hinckley
Leicester, Leicestershire LE10 1SN
tel: 01455 637987
web: www.the-ispa.org.uk

The Tisserand Institute
65 Church Road
Hove, East Sussex BN3 2BD
tel: 01273 206640
web: www.tisserand.com

International Federation of Aromatherapists
182 Chiswick High Road, London W4 1PP
tel: 020 8742 2605
web: www.int-fed-aromatherapy.co.uk

AUTOGENIC TRAINING

British Autogenic Society
c/o The Royal London Homoeopathic Hospital
60 Great Ormond Street
London WC1N 3HR
tel: 020 7713 6336
web: www.autogenic-therapy.org.uk

AYURVEDA

Ayurveda Medical Association
The Hale Clinic, 7 Park Crescent
London W1N 3HE
tel: 020 7631 0156
web: www.ayurveda.co.uk

Maharishi Ayurveda Health Centre
The Golden Dome, Woodley Park
Skelmersdale, Lancashire WN8 6UP
tel: 01695 51008
web: www.maharishi.co.uk

BACH FLOWER REMEDIES
see *FLOWER REMEDIES*

BATES METHOD
The Bates Association
PO Box 25, Shoreham by Sea
East Sussex BN43 6ZF
tel: 01273 422090
web: www.seeing.org

BIOMAGNETIC THERAPY
The British Biomagnetic Association
The Williams Clinic, 31 St Marychurch Road
Torquay, Devon TQ1 3JF
For more information please send an SAE

BIRTH
Active Birth Centre
25 Bickerton Road, London N19 5JT
tel: 020 7482 5554
web: www.activebirthcentre.com

CHINESE MEDICINE
Register of Chinese Herbal Medicine
PO Box 400, Middlesex HA9 9NZ
tel: 07000 790332
web: www.rchm.co.uk

The Chinese Heritage
15 Dawson Place, London W2 4TH
tel: 020 7229 7187
web: www.dao-hua-qigong.com

CHIROPRACTIC
General Chiropractic Council
344–354 Gray's Inn Road
London WC1X 8BP
tel: 020 7713 5155
web: www.gcc-uk.org

COLONIC IRRIGATION
Colonic International Association
16 Drummond Ride
Tring, Hertfordshire HP23 5DE
tel: 01442 827687
web: www.colonic-association.com

COLOUR THERAPY
**Aura Soma International Academy of
Colour Therapeutics (A.S.I.A.C.T.)**
South Road, Tetford, Lincolnshire LN9 6QB
tel: 01507 533581
web: www.aura-soma.co.uk

The International Association of Colour
46 Cottenham Road, Histon
Cambridge, Cambridgeshire CB4 9ES
tel: 01223 563403
e-mail: iac@kgrevis.freeserve.co.uk

COUNSELLING
British Association for Counselling
1 Regent Place
Rugby, Warwickshire CV21 2PJ
tel: 01788 550899
web: www.bac.co.uk

National Council of Psychotherapists
PO Box 6072, Nottingham NG6 9BW
tel: 0115 913 1382
web: www.natcouncilofpsychotherapists.org.uk

UK Council for Psychotherapy
167–169 Great Portland Street
London W1N 5FB
tel: 020 7436 3002
web: www.psychotherapy.org.uk

**The British Association of
Psychotherapists**
37 Mapesbury Road, London NW2 4HJ
tel: 020 8452 9823
web: www.bap-pscyhotherapy.org

CRANIOSACRAL OSTEOPATHY
Craniosacral Therapy Association
27 Old Gloucester Street
London WC1N 3XX
tel: 020 8450 7627

The Upledger Institute UK
2 Marshall Place, Perth PH2 8AH
tel: 01738 444404
web: www.upledger.co.uk

CRYSTAL THERAPY
**Affiliation of Crystal Healing
Organizations**
PO Box 344, Manchester M60 2EZ
tel: 01479 841450

International College of Crystal Healing
PO Box 738, Canterbury, Kent KT2 9GA
tel: 01227 472435
web: www.crystaltherapy.co.uk

FELDENKRAIS
Feldenkrais Guild UK
PO Box 370, London N10 3XA
tel: 07000 785506
web: www.feldenkrais.co.uk

FENG SHUI
Feng Shui Network International
PO Box 2133, London W1A 1RL
tel: 07000 336474
web: www.fengshuinet.com

Feng Shui Association
31 Woburn Place
Brighton, East Sussex BN1 9GA
tel: 01273 693844
web: www.fengshuiassociation.co.uk

FLOWER REMEDIES

Bach Flower Remedies

Bach Centre, Mount Vernon

Baker's Lane, Brightwell-cum-Sotwell

Wallingford, Oxfordshire OX10 0PZ

tel: 01491 834678

web: www.bachcentre.com

Julian Barnard Healing Herbs

PO Box 65, Herefordshire HR2 0UW

tel: 01873 890218

web: www.healing-herbs.co.uk

HEALING

The Confederation of Healing Organizations

The Red & White House, 113 High Street

Berkhamsted, Hertfordshire HP4 2DJ

tel: 01442 870660

web: drive.2/cho

College of Healing

Runnings Park, Croft Bank

West Malvern, Worcestershire WR14 4DU

tel: 01684 566450

National Federation of Spiritual Healers

Old Manor Farm Studio, Church Street

Sunbury-on-Thames, Middlesex TW16 6RG

tel: 0891 616080

web: www.nfsh.org.uk

HERBALISM

National Institute of Medical Herbalists

56 Longbrook Street

Exeter, Devon EX4 6AH

tel: 01392 426022

web: www.btinternet.com/~nimh/

International Register of Consultant Herbalists & Homoeopaths

32 King Edwards Road, Swansea SA1 4LL

tel: 01792 655886

web: www.irch.org

HOMOEOPATHY

The Society of Homoeopaths

4a Artizan Road, Northampton

Northamptonshire NN1 4HU

tel: 01604 621400

web: www.homeopathy-soh.org

The British Homoeopathic Association

27a Devonshire Street

London WC1N 3HZ

tel: 020 7935 2163

web: www.nhsconfed/bha

Homoeopathic Trust

15 Clerkenwell Close, London EC1R 0AA

tel: 020 7566 7800

web: www.trusthomeopathy.org

British Homoeopathic Dental Association

15 Clerkenwell Close, London EC1R 0AA

tel: 020 7566 7827

British Association of Homoeopathic Veterinary Surgeons

The Honorary Secretary

Alternative Veterinary Medicine Centre

Chinham House, Stanford-in-the-Vale

Faringdon, Oxfordshire SN7 8NQ

tel: 01367 718115

web: www.bhbs.com

HYPNOTHERAPY

Association for Professional Therapists

Katepwa House, Ashfield Park Avenue

Ross-on-Wye, Herefordshire HR9 5AX

tel: 01989 566676

web: www.hypnotherapists.org

British Hypnotherapy Association

67 Upper Berkeley Street

London W1H 7QX

tel: 020 7723 4443

British Society of Clinical Hypnosis

15 Connaught Square, London W2 2HG

tel: 020 7402 9037

web: www.bsch.org.uk

British Society of Medical & Dental Hypnosis (national office)

17 Keppel View Road, Kimberworth

Rotherham, South Yorkshire S61 2AR

tel: 07000 560309

web: www.bsmdh.org

The National Council for Hypnotherapy

PO Box 5779, Burton-on-the-Wold

Loughborough, Leicestershire LE12 5ZF

tel: 0800 952 0545

web: www.hypnotherapists.org.uk

The National Register of Hypnotherapists and Psychotherapists

12 Cross Street, Nelson

Lancashire BB9 7EN

tel: 01282 716839

web: www.nrhp.co.uk

IRIDOLOGY

Guild of Naturopathic Iridologists

94 Grosvenor Road, London SW1V 3LF

tel: 020 7821 0255

web: www.gni-international.org

KINESIOLOGY

Association for Systematic Kinesiology

39 Browns Road, Surbiton, Surrey KT5 8ST

tel: 020 8399 3215

web: www.kinesiology.co.uk

MASSAGE

British Federation of Massage Practitioners

78 Meadow Street

Preston, Lancashire PR1 1TS

tel: 01772 881063

web: www.jolanta.co.uk

The Academy of On-Site Massage
Avon Road, Charfield, Wotton-under-Edge
Gloucestershire GL12 8TT
tel: 01454 261900
web: www.aosm.co.uk

MEDITATION
Transcendental Meditation Association
Freepost, London SW1P 4YY
tel: 08705 143733
web: www.t-m.org.uk

NATUROPATHY
General Council & Register of Naturopaths
Goswell House, 2 Goswell Road
Street, Somerset BA16 0JG
tel: 01458 840072
web: www.naturopathy.org.uk

NUTRITIONAL THERAPY
British Association of Nutritional Therapists
PO Box 17436, London SE13 7WT
tel: 0870 606 1284

Institute for Optimal Nutrition
Blades Court, Deodar Road
London SW15 2NU
tel: 020 8877 9993
web: www.ion.ac.uk

**The British Society for Allergy,
    Environmental and Nutritional Medicine**
PO Box 7, Knighton LD7 1WT
tel: 09063 020010
web: www.bsaenm.org.uk

OSTEOPATHY
Osteopathic Information Service
Premier House, 10 Greycoat Place
London SW1P 1SB
tel: 020 7357 6655
web: www.osteopathy.org.uk

College of Osteopaths
13 Furzehill Road, Borehamwood
Hertfordshire WD6 2DG
tel: 020 8905 1937

PILATES
The Body Control Pilates Centre
17 Queensbury Mews West
London SW7 2DY
tel: 020 7581 7041

The Body Control Pilates Information Line:
0870 169 0000

POLARITY THERAPY
UK Polarity Therapy Association
Monomark House, 27 Old Gloucester St,
London WC1N 3XX
tel: 0700 705 2748

RADIONICS
The Radionic Association
Baerlein House, Goose Green
Deddington, Oxon OX15 0SZ
tel: 01869 338852
web: www.radionic.co.uk

REFLEXOLOGY
Association of Reflexologists
27 Old Gloucester Street
London WC1N 3XX
tel: 0990 673320
web: www.reflexology.org/aor

Holistic Association of Reflexology
92 Sheering Road
Old Harlow, Essex CM17 0JW
tel: 01279 429060
web: www.footreflexology.com

International Institute of Reflexology
255 Turleigh
Bradford on Avon, Wiltshire BA15 2HG
tel: 01275 373359
web: www.reflexology-uk.co.uk

REIKI
Reiki Association
Cornbrook Bridge House, Clee Hill
Ludlow, Shropshire SY8 3QQ
tel: 01981 550829
web: www.reikiassociation.org

ROLFING
The Rolfing Institute
PO Box 14793, London SW1V 2WB
tel: 020 7834 1493
web: www.rolf.org

To find a local practitioner:
0117 946 6374

SHAMANISM
The Sacred Trust
PO Box 603, Bath, BANES BA1 2ZU
tel: 01225 852615
web: www.sacredtrust.org

SHIATSU
The Shiatsu Society
Eastlands Court, St Peter's Road
Rugby, Warwickshire CV21 3QP
tel: 01788 555051
web: www.shiatsu.org

YOGA
Yoga Therapy Centre
c/o The Royal London Homoeopathic
    Hospital
60 Great Ormond Street
London WC1N 3HR
tel: 020 7419 7195
web: www.yogatherapy.org

GENERAL INFORMATION
Internet Health Library
Suite 1–10, Ground Floor Offices
Orchard Villa, Porters Park Drive
Shenley, Hertfordshire WD7 9DS
tel: 01923 856222
web: www.internethealthlibrary.com

The Hale Clinic

7 Park Crescent, London W1N 3HE

tel: 020 7631 0156

web: www.haleclinic.com

AUSTRALIA

ALEXANDER TECHNIQUE

Australian Society for Teachers of the Alexander Technique

PO Box 716, Darlinghurst, NSW 2010

tel: (+613) 952 92372

web: www.alexandertechnique.org.aus

AROMATHERAPY

Australasian College of Natural Therapies

620 Harris Street, Ultimo, NSW 2007

tel: (+617) 221 26699

COUNSELLING

Australian Institute of Professional Counsellors

PO Box 260, Lutwyche, Queensland 4030

tel: (+617) 385 72277

Australian Psychological Society

PO Box 126, Carlton South, Victoria 3053

tel: (+613) 966 36166

web: www.aps.psychsociety.com.au

FELDENKRAIS

Australian Feldenkrais Guild

PO Box 285, Ashfield, NSW 1800

tel: (+612) 955 51374

HERBALISM

National Herbalists' Association

PO Box 65, Kingsgrove, NSW 2208

tel: (+617) 278 74523

HOMOEOPATHY

Australian Association of Professional Homoeopaths

80 Essenden Road

Anstead, Queensland 4070

tel: (+617) 320 26517

e-mail: ann_tacey@telstra.easymail.com.au

Australian Homoeopathic Association

Federal Body, C/- 65 Brosely Road

Toowong, Queensland 4068

tel: (+617) 337 17245

NORTH AMERICA

ALEXANDER TECHNIQUE

The American Society for the Alexander Technique

30 North Maple, PO Box 60008

Florence, MA 01062, USA

tel: (+1) 413 584 2359

web: www.alexander.org

CHIROPRACTIC

American Chiropractic Association

1701 Clarendon Boulevard, Arlington

Virginia, VA 24203, USA

tel: (+1) 703 276 8800

COUNSELLING

Canadian Guidance & Counselling Association

220 Laurier Avenue West, Ottawa

Ontario K1P 5Z9, Canada

tel: (+1) 613 237 1099

Council for Accreditation of Counselling

University of Florida

1215 Norman Hall, Gainsville

Florida, FL 32605, USA

tel: (+1) 904 392 0733

CRANIOSACRAL OSTEOPATHY

Upledger Institute Inc.

1121 Prosperity Farms Road

Palm Beach Gardens

Florida FL 33410-3487, USA

tel: (+1) 561 622 4706

web: www.upledger.com

FELDENKRAIS

Feldenkrais Guild Canada

1012 Rue Mont Royalest, Bureau 107

Montréal, Quebec H2J 1X6, Canada

tel: (+1) 514 522 8027

Feldenkrais Guild North America

3611 SW Hood Avenue, Suite 100

Portland OR 97201, USA

tel: (+1) 800 775 2118

web: www.feldenkrais.com

HOMOEOPATHY

Ontario Homeopathic Association

PO Box 258, Station P

Toronto, Ontario M5S 2S7, Canada

tel: (+416) 488 9685

web: www.ontariohomeopath.com

Syndicat Professionel des Homéopaths du Quebec

1600 de Lorimier, Suite 382

Montréal, Quebec H2K 3W5, Canada

tel: (+514) 525 2037

e-mail: sphq@total.net

National Center for Homeopathy

801 North Fairfax Street

Alexandria, VA 22314, USA

tel: (+1) 703 548 7790

NEAL'S YARD REMEDIES

Neal's Yard Remedies' products can be obtained in many parts of the world. Contact the UK head office for details of your nearest outlet:

Head office
26–34 Ingate Place
London SW8 3NS
tel: 020 7498 1686
web: www.nealsyardremedies.com

Mail order
29 Dalton Street
Manchester M2 6DS
tel: 0161 831 7875
fax: 0161 835 9322

Customer services
tel: 020 7627 1949
e-mail: cservices@nealsyardremedies.com

Neal's Yard Remedies' outlets worldwide:

UK

15 Neal's Yard
Covent Garden
London WC2H 9DP
tel: 020 7379 7222

Chelsea Farmers Market
Sydney Street
London SW3 6NR
tel: 020 7351 6380

9 Elgin Crescent
London W11 2JA
tel: 020 7727 3998

68 Chalk Farm Road
Camden
London NW1 8AN
tel: 020 7284 2039

2a Kensington Gardens
Brighton
East Sussex BN1 4AL
tel: 01273 601464

126 Whiteladies Road
Clifton
Bristol BS8 2RP
tel: 0117 946 6034

The Glades Shopping Centre
Bromley
Kent BR1 1DD
tel: 020 8313 9898

23–25 Morgan Arcade
Cardiff CF1 2AF
tel: 029 2023 5721

9 Rotunda Terrace
Montpellier Street
Cheltenham
Gloucestershire GL50 1SX
tel: 01242 522136

46a George Street
Edinburgh EH2 2LE
tel: 0131 226 3223

2 Market Street
Guildford GU1 4LB
tel: 01483 450434

29 John Dalton Street
Manchester M2 6DS
tel: 0161 831 7875

19 Central Arcade
Newcastle-upon-Tyne NE1 5BQ
tel: 0191 232 2525

26 Lower Goat Lane
Norwich NR2 1EL
tel: 01603 766681

5 Golden Cross
Oxford
Oxfordshire OX1 3EU
tel: 01865 245436

ASIA

4-9-3 Jingumae
Shibuya-ku
Tokyo 150-0001
Japan
tel: (+81) 35 771 2455

KNK Building 3F
3-5-17 Kita Aoyama
Minato-ku
Tokyo 107-0061
Japan
tel: (+81) 33 405 7207

NORTH AMERICA

79 East Putnam Avenue
Greenwich
Connecticut
CT 06830-5644
USA
tel: (+1) 203 629 0885

SOUTH AMERICA

Rua Melo Alves 383
Jardins
Sao Paulo
CEP 01417 010
Brazil
tel: (+5511) 3064 1662

further reading

GENERAL INTEREST

Campbell, J., *An Open Life: Joseph Campbell in Conversation with Michael Toms* (Harper Perennial, 1990)

Capra, F., *The Turning Point* (Flamingo, 1983)

Heindel, M., *The Vital Body* (Fowler, 1950)

Howe, Dr E. Graham, *The Mind of the Druid* (Skoob Books, 1989)

Tompkins, P., *The Secret Life of Nature* (Thorsons, 1997)

Whitefield, P., *Permaculture in a Nutshell* (Permanent Publications, 1993)

Yeoman, J., *Self-reliance: A Recipe for the New Millennium* (Hyden House, 1999)

Zukav, G., *The Dancing Wu Li Masters* (Rider, 1991)

HEALTH – GENERAL

Bottomley, R., *You Don't Have to Feel Unwell* (Gill & Macmillan Newleaf, 2000)

Castro, M., *Homoeopathic Guide to Stress* (St Martin's Press, 1997)

Dethlefson, T. & Dahlke, R., *The Healing Power of Illness* (Element Books, 1990)

Hill, S., *Reclaiming the Wisdom of the Body* (Constable, 1997)

Kenton, L., *Quick Fix to Beat Stress* (Vermilion, 1996)

Kenton, L., *Ten Day Anti-fatigue Plan* (Ebury Press, 1999)

Litchfield, C., *The Organic Directory 2000/2001* (Green Books, 2000)

McKenna, J., *Alternatives to Tranquilisers* (Gill & Macmillan Newleaf, 1999)

AROMATHERAPY

Curtis, S., *Neal's Yard Remedies: Essential Oils* (Aurum, 1996)

Davis, P., *Aromatherapy: An A–Z* (CW Daniel, 1988)

Lawless, J., *The Encyclopedia of Essential Oils* (Element Books, 1995)

Maury, M., *Marguerite Maury's Guide to Aromatherapy* (CW Daniel, 1989)

Price, S., *Practical Aromatherapy* (Thorsons, 1983)

Tisserand, R., *The Art of Aromatherapy* (CW Daniel 1977)

Tisserand, R. & Balacs, T., *Essential Oil Safety* (Churchill Livingstone, 1995)

Worwood, V., *The Fragrant Pharmacy* (Bantam, 1991)

Valnet, Dr J., *The Practice of Aromatherapy* (CW Daniel, 1982)

BODYWORK AND MASSAGE

Liechti, E., *The Complete Illustrated Guide to Shiatsu* (Element Books, 1999)

Lundberg, P., *The Book of Shiatsu* (Gaia Books, 1999)

Mitchell, S., *The Complete Illustrated Guide to Massage* (Element Books, 1999)

Shivapremananda, S., *Yoga for Stress Relief* (Gaia Books, 2000)

Sivananda Yoga Centre, The, *The New Book of Yoga* (Ebury Press, 2000)

Thomas, S., *Massage for Common Ailments* (Gaia Books, 1992)

DIET AND NUTRITION

Alexander, J., *The Detox Plan* (Gaia Books, 1998)

Carper, J., *Food: Your Miracle Medicine* (Simon & Schuster, 1995)

Cochrane, A., *Safe Natural Remdies for Babies and Children* (Thorsons, 1997)

Holford, P., *The Optimum Nutrition Bible* (Piatkus Books, 1998)

Meek, J. & Holford, P., *Boost Your Immune System* (Piatkus Books, 1998)

Mervyn, L., *Thorsons' Complete Guide to Vitamins and Minerals* (Thorsons, 2000)

Mindell, E., *The Vitamin Bible* (Arlington Books, 1985)

Murray, M., *Encyclopedia of Nutritional Supplements: The Essential Guide For Improving Your Health Naturally* (Prima Publications, 1996)

FLOWER REMEDIES

Bach, E., *Heal Thyself* (CW Daniel, 1996)

Bach, E., *The Twelve Healers* (CW Daniel, 1952)

Barnard, J., *A Guide to the Bach Flower Remedies* (CW Daniel, 1979)

Chancellor, P., *Handbook of the Bach Flower Remedies* (CW Daniel, 1980)

White, I., *Australian Bush Flower Remedies* (Findhorn Press, 1993)

HERBS

Bartram, T., *The Encyclopaedia of Herbal Medicine* (Constable Robinson, 1998)

Brooke, E., *A Woman's Book of Herbs* (The Women's Press, 1992)

Green, J., *The Male Herbal* (Crossing Press, 1991)

Grieve, M., *A Modern Herbal* (in two volumes) (Dover Publications, 1972)

Hoffman, D., *The New Holistic Herbal* (Element Books, 1990)

McIntyre, A., *The Complete Woman's Herbal* (Gaia Books, 1999)

Ody, P., *The Herb Society's Home Herbal* (Dorling Kindersley, 1995)

Tierra, M., *The Way of Chinese Herbs* (Pocket Books, 1999)

Tierra, M., *The Way of Herbs* (Pocket Books, 1999)

HOMOEOPATHY

Castro, M., *The Complete Homoeopathy Handbook*
(Papermac, 1991)

Curtis, S., *A Handbook of Homoeopathic Alternatives to Immunisation*
(Winter Press, 1994)

Goodwin, J., *The Biochemic Handbook* (Thorsons, 1980)

Lockie, A., *The Family Guide to Homoeopathy* (Hamish Hamilton,
1989)

MacEoin, B., *Homoeopathy and the Menopause* (Thorson, 1996)

Miles, M., *Homoeopathy for Human Evolution* (Winter Press, 1988)

Phatak, Dr S., *The Materia Medica of Homoeopathic Medicine*
(IBPS, 1982)

Shepherd, D., *Homoeopathy for the First Aider*
(CW Daniel, 1953)

Speight, P., *Before Calling the Doctor* (CW Daniel, 1976)

Vithoulkas, G., *Medicine of the New Man* (Thorsons, 1979)

Watson, I., *A Guide to the Methodologies of Homoeopathy*
(Cutting Edge Publications, 1991)

Wells, R., *Neal's Yard Remedies: Homoeopathy* (Aurum, 2000)

LIFE AND DEATH

Kubler-Ross, E., *On Death and Dying* (Routledge, 1990)

Lagrand, L., *After-death Communication: Final Farewells*
(Llewellyn Publishing, 1997)

Singh, K., *The Grace in Dying* (Gill & Macmillan, 1999)

NATURAL COSMETICS AND BEAUTY

Carvo, J., *Natural Facelift* (Century Publishing Co., 1991)

Cousin, P-J., *Facelift at Your Fingertips* (Quadrille Publishing, 1999)

Neal's Yard Remedies, *Neal's Yard Remedies: Make Your Own
Cosmetics* (Aurum, 1997)

PARENT AND BABY

Burgess, A., *Fatherhood Reclaimed* (Vermilion, 1998)

Castro, M., *Homoeopathy for Pregnancy, Birth and Your Baby's First Year*
(St Martin's Press, 1993)

England, A., *Aromatherapy and Massage for Mother and Baby*
(Vermilion, 1999)

Maxted-Frost, T., *The Organic Baby Book* (Green Books, 1999)

Walker, P., *Baby Massage* (Piatkus Books, 1995)

PREGNANCY AND CHILDBIRTH

Balaskas, J. & Petersen, G., *New Natural Pregnancy: Practical Well-being
from Conception to Birth* (Interlink Publishing Group, 1999)

Gaskin, I., *Spiritual Midwifery* (The Book Publishing Company, 1990)

Kitzinger, S., *The New Pregnancy and Childbirth* (Penguin, 1997)

Kitzinger, S., *The Year After Childbirth* (Oxford Paperbacks, 1994)

Thomas, P. (ed.) & Kitzinger, S., *Every Birth is Different* (Headline, 1998)

REFLEXOLOGY

Crane, B., *Reflexology: An Illustrated Guide* (Element Books, 1998)

Kunz, K. & Kunz, B., *A Complete Guide to Foot Reflexology*
(Thorsons, 1999)

WOMEN'S HEALTH

Blum, J., *Woman Heal Thyself* (Element Books, 1996)

Campion, K., *Holistic Woman's Herbal* (Bloomsbury, 1995)

Campion, K., *Menopause Naturally* (Gill & Macmillan Newleaf, 1998)

Curtis, S. & Fraser, R., *Natural Healing for Women* (Thorsons, 1992)

Drake, K. & J., *Natural Birth Control* (Thorsons, 1984)

Kenton, L., *Passage to Power* (Vermilion, 1996)

Nissim, R., *Natural Healing in Gynaecology* (Thorsons, 1986)

Phillips, A. & Rakusen, J., *The New Our Bodies, Ourselves* (Penguin, 1996)

Index